Concepts and Activities

Pediatric Nursing

Concepts and Activities

Pediatric Nursing

Maureen L. Thompson, RN, PhD
Assistant Professor
College of Nursing
Syracuse University
Syracuse, New York

Springhouse Corporation
Springhouse, Pennsylvania

Staff

Executive Director, Editorial
Stanley Loeb

Senior Publisher, Trade and Textbooks
Minnie B. Rose, RN, BSN, MEd

Art Director
John Hubbard

Editors
Diane Labus, David Moreau, Helen Hamilton, Kathy Goldberg

Copy Editors
Diane M. Armento, Pamela Wingrod

Clinical Consultants
Maryann Foley, RN, BSN; Patricia Kardish Fischer, RN, BSN

Designers
Stephanie Peters (associate art director), Mary Stangl (book designer), Donald G. Knauss, Laurie Mirijanian, Anita Curry (cover design)

Typography
Diane Paluba (manager), Elizabeth Bergman, Joyce Rossi Biletz, Phyllis Marron, Robin Mayer, Valerie L. Rosenberger

Manufacturing
Deborah Meiris (director), Anna Brindisi, Kate Davis, T.A. Landis

Editorial Assistants
Caroline Lemoine, Louise Quinn, Betsy K. Snyder

Printed in the United States of America.

CAPN-021297

℞ A member of the Reed Elsevier plc group

Library of Congress Cataloging-in-Publication Data

Thompson, Maureen L.
  Pediatric nursing / Maureen L. Thompson.
    p. cm. — (Concepts and activities)
  Includes bibliographical references and index.
  1. Pediatric nursing I. Title. II. Series
  [DNLM: 1. Pediatric Nursing—methods. 2. Acute Disease—in infancy & childhood. 3. Child Development—nurses' instruction. WY 159 T474p 1994]
RJ245.T49 1994
610.73'62—dc20
 DNLM/DLC
ISBN 0-87434-577-4   94-15346
                   CIP

Contents

Reviewers

Andrea T. Chonin, RN,C, MSN
Pediatric Nursing Instructor
Jackson Memorial Hospital
School of Nursing
Miami

Susan Galea, RN, MSN, CCRN
Clinical Nurse Specialist, Surgical ICU
University of Pennsylvania
Philadelphia

Ginger Peterson Kee, RN, MSN, EDd
Associate Professor, Clinical Nursing
University of Texas
Health Science Center
Houston

Linda Owen Rimer, RN, MSE
Associate Professor
University of Arkansas
Little Rock

Acknowledgments

This book would not have been possible without the encouragement and assistance of many people. I would like to thank Barbara MacDermott, RN, MS, for convincing me to accept this challenge and for her continued encouragement and support in completing this project. I also would like to express my gratitude to my colleagues and my family, who supported me during the many months of writing and editing. Special thanks goes to Beth Ann Lipke, RN, MS, who helped with the development of the chapters related to respiratory and gastrointestinal disorders.

Preface

As one of the first books in a new series, *Concepts and Activities: Pediatric Nursing* delivers a unique way for nursing students to study an important core subject. Each chapter provides a combination of key concepts that crystallize essential, need-to-know information, followed by various study activities designed to challenge the student and boost information retention.

This new series gives students basic information about core nursing subjects as well as a forum for testing and applying that knowledge. Each volume covers a separate nursing subject and provides sufficient information and clear graphics (numerous illustrations, charts, and diagrams) to be used as a free-standing reference. Although not as comprehensive as a textbook, each book provides sufficient detail for students to understand the subject's essential concepts and complete all of the book's study activities.

Concepts and Activities: Pediatric Nursing is written for nursing students in BSN, AD, and diploma programs who need to master the basics of assessing, diagnosing, planning, implementing, and evaluating the nursing care of pediatric patients. It is especially useful in curricula that do not require a large core text. In other curricula, it can serve as a supplement to a major text or as a study guide.

This book provides extensive information about children's health, pediatric growth and development, and other related issues as well as a comprehensive review of major disorders and surgical procedures encountered by the pediatric nurse. Almost every chapter includes pertinent information on patient assessment, laboratory findings, nursing diagnoses, care planning and implementation, medical findings, and evaluation—a functional framework for providing holistic nursing care.

All chapters are formatted for easy access and use. Each begins with a list of objectives to focus the reader's attention, followed by an overview of concepts that clearly presents core information and establishes the data base from which the reader can complete the study activities. Activities may include multiple-choice questions, true-or-false statements, carefully selected fill-in-the blank statements, matching exercises, and short-answer questions. Each chapter concludes with a list of study activities answers, including rationales whenever the answer is not immediately apparent.

To provide the most current, accurate, and clinically appropriate information, *Concepts and Activities: Pediatric Nursing* was reviewed extensively by nurses from appropriate specialty areas. Their combined efforts have produced a valuable information source and a ready-reference for years to come.

CHAPTER 1

Evolution of child health care and pediatric nursing

OBJECTIVES
After studying this chapter, the reader should be able to:
1. Describe changes in child health care practices from 1700 to 1993.
2. Identify primary child health care issues in the United States.
3. Describe the role of the pediatric nurse.

OVERVIEW OF CONCEPTS
This chapter discusses the evolution of child health care, detailing child health care practices from the 17th century to the present time. It explores critical issues relating to child health care in the United States, then discusses the role of the pediatric nurse as provider of health care for children.

Evolution of child health care

Throughout most of history, the health care of children received no special attention. In recent centuries, however, changing societal influences and evolving scientific understanding of child development have shaped policies related to child health.

17th and 18th centuries

Before and throughout the 18th century, society viewed children as miniature, incomplete adults who grew into maturity through parental care and guidance. Because physicians were few and only the wealthy had access to medical care, sick children, like most sick adults, were cared for at home by family members. Children received the same remedies as adults.

Unsanitary conditions contributed greatly to the high incidence of illness and death in children. Childhood illness was so common that fewer than 50% of children lived beyond age 5. In fact, illness and death during early childhood seemed almost inevitable.

At the same time, overwhelming poverty caused widespread abandonment of infants and children. This led to the establishment of foundling homes. By the mid-18th century, the rate of abandonment was so great that foundling homes were severely overtaxed; children in these homes had a staggering death rate.

Eventually, high mortality among children led some physicians to look more closely at prevailing child-care practices. They noted that infants were swaddled tightly in three or four layers of clothing. Few infants were breast-fed. Instead, infants received boiled bread and sugar or thin gruels within hours after birth, and up to 10 times a day. Various spices and wine or ale commonly were added for flavoring.

In 1748, William Cadogan's "Essay on Nursing" called attention to unhealthy child-care practices and identified overdressing, overfeeding, and poor diet as factors contributing to childhood illness. Cadogan encouraged breast-feeding and urged parents to dress infants in loose, lightweight gowns. For infants who could not be breast-fed, he recommended feeding with milk alone for the first 3 months and cautioned against waking infants for feeding. To introduce solid feedings, he recommended light broths boiled with bread or rice. However, despite the early efforts of Cadogan and others, child-care practices were slow to change.

19th century

During the early 19th century, infirmaries were established to care for the sick. However, adults and children received care in the same wards. Because many of these children had communicable diseases, the spread of infection was rampant. To help control contagion, infirmaries began to separate children from adult patients. Both children and adults, however, continued to receive the same types of treatment.

Nevertheless, the burgeoning recognition that childhood diseases differ from adult diseases led to the establishment of hospitals devoted solely to caring for children. Such facilities, opened in the mid-19th century, provided a homelike atmosphere in which parents were encouraged to help care for their children, nurses and physicians wore street clothing, and children were allowed to wear their usual clothing and play with their own toys.

During the late 19th century, the care of sick children again changed dramatically as scientists proved that many diseases were caused by bacteria. In an effort to prevent infection, hospital wards were closed to visitors. Moreover, parental visits were noted to cause distress, especially when the parents had to leave. Thus, parental visitation was considered emotionally stressful to hospitalized children. To prevent both infection and emotional distress, parents were prohibited from visiting hospitalized children.

Concern about contagion led to other changes as well. Hospitals began to require personnel to wear uniforms, restricted toys, and commonly limited social contact between children in the wards. These new policies, instituted to reduce the spread of infection, persisted well into the early 20th century. While hospital care focused on curing physical diseases and preventing their spread to others, the emotional health of hospitalized children received little consideration.

20th century

During the 1940s and 1950s, the pioneering work of R. Spitz and J. Bowlby stimulated research on the emotional well-being of hospitalized children. Spitz (1945) observed the behavior of children in a foundling home where the staff provided competent physical care but rarely talked to or handled the children. He reported that these children began to show emotional reactions to separation from their mothers at approximately age 6 months. Their first reaction was loud, persistent crying that lasted for the first month of separation. During the second month, the children became wary of people. During the third month, their activity level decreased. During the fourth month, they became withdrawn and apathetic; their facial expressions were flat and they no longer screamed. By the sixth month, the children were silent and unresponsive emotionally.

However, Spitz reported that the emotional effects of separation could be reversed if children were reunited with their mothers before the third month of separation. If separation lasted longer than 6 months, behavioral changes seemed irreversible.

In a classic earlier study (which was published in 1953), Bowlby observed the effects of separation on children who were removed from their homes in London during World War II and relocated to the countryside to escape air raids. These children, who were expected to be psychologically healthier than those who had stayed in London, developed severe behavioral changes similar to those described by Spitz.

Influenced by the work of Bowlby and Spitz, J. Robertson (1970) studied the effects of hospitalization on young children. He reported similar behavioral patterns after even relatively short hospitalizations. Robertson organized these patterns into three stages: protest, despair, and denial.

During the *protest* stage, children cried loudly; some rejected comforting measures. This stage persisted for several hours to several days. Next came *despair,* in which the children became less active, their crying became mournful, and some turned away from a parent's approach; others lost weight or developed insomnia. During *denial,* the final stage, children became quiet and regained superficial interest in their surroundings, but repressed feelings for their mothers.

Current practice

In response to growing knowledge about the emotional effects of illness and hospitalization, hospital policies related to pediatric care have changed slowly during the late 20th century. In the United States, for example, the Association for the Care of Children's Health (ACCH) emerged as a major force in promoting humanized pediatric care. As a result of these efforts, parental visitation was encouraged and hospital stays were shortened.

Despite these changes, nurses and researchers noted that hospitalization of children continued to cause emotional distress; clearly, separation from parents was not its only cause. Growing contributions of developmental theorists identified other issues and sources of anxiety related to pediatric hospitalization. This information helped shape current practices regarding the care of sick children.

Now, children routinely are prepared emotionally for medical procedures. Along with their parents, they are fully informed about scheduled procedures, offered choices when appropriate, and encouraged to participate actively in their care. To help nurses assume a more emotionally supportive role, nursing systems are designed to assign one primary nurse to a child's care. In many hospitals, Child Life Programs help children and their families cope with the stress of illness and hospitalization, which affects the entire family. Recent trends, such as pediatric ambulatory care, home care, and day surgery, also help to minimize the stress of illness and hospitalization on children and their families.

Primary issues: 1990 to 2000

Despite better understanding of the importance of well-child care, adequate nutrition, immunization, and prompt medical attention for illness and injury, American children have significantly higher mortality and morbidity rates than those in other developed countries. For example, the United States has a higher infant mortality rate than many other developed countries and a higher childhood mortality rate and lower immunization rate for preschool-age children than European countries. High rates of pregnancy, abortion, and childbirth among adolescents also contribute to the development of health problems in both the childbearing adolescent and her child.

Factors contributing to morbidity and mortality

Barriers to preventive health care are major factors contributing to morbidity and mortality in American children. The most common barriers are poverty, lack of health insurance, and inadequate provider systems. In view of this, R. Williams and C. Miller (1991) urged the U.S. government to work toward the goal of making preventive health services available for all women of childbearing age and their children. To reach this goal, they recommended the following actions:

• Ensure health insurance coverage for all infants, children, and childbearing women.
• Establish national health care standards for children. Identify areas of deficient performance for intensified preventive effort.
• Establish methods to identify and track high-risk children.
• Increase the numbers of mid-level professional health workers, including nurse practitioners, outreach workers, and health care coordinators.

Roles of pediatric nurses

Pediatric nurses are involved in all aspects of child health care. They assume various roles in monitoring child growth and development, promoting health, preventing illness, and providing care during illness. These roles, which primarily include caregiver advocate, counselor, health teacher, and researcher, may be carried out either in ambulatory care settings that focus on promoting health and preventing illness or in acute care settings that focus on health restoration and rehabilitation.

STUDY ACTIVITIES

Short answer

1. Identify child-care practices that contributed to the high incidence of childhood illness during the 18th century.

_____

_____

2. Describe how research has influenced pediatric hospitalization policies in the United States.

_____

_____

_____

_____

_____

3. List at least four problems associated with childhood morbidity and mortality in the United States.

_____

_____

True or false

4. Cadogan's "Essay on Nursing" called attention to 19th-century child-care methods.
☐ True   ☐ False

5. During the 19th century, children were separated from adults in infirmaries to prevent emotional distress.
☐ True   ☐ False

6. The earliest recognition of the need for separate medical care for children and adults grew out of concern over children's communicable diseases.
☐ True   ☐ False

7. During the 19th century, the recognition that bacteria cause disease led to the decline of infirmaries for sick children.
☐ True   ☐ False

8. Foundling homes were relatively unimportant in the evolution of children's health care.
☐ True   ☐ False

9. Numerous factors — not just separation anxiety — can cause emotional distress in hospitalized children.
☐ True   ☐ False

10. Cadogan, Spitz, and Bowlby studied the effects of hospitalization on children.
☐ True   ☐ False

11. Bowlby found that British children who were relocated to escape wartime air raids avoided the behavioral effects of separation anxiety.
☐ True   ☐ False

12. In the mid-20th century, researchers reported that children's behavioral changes reflecting separation anxiety could not be reversed if separation lasted longer than 6 months.
☐ True   ☐ False

13. During the second stage of separation anxiety, children cry loudly for several hours or days.
☐ True   ☐ False

Fill in the blank

14. Robertson's three stages of separation anxiety are _____, _____, and _____.

15. Three pioneering researchers of separation anxiety in hospitalized children were _____, _____, and _____.

16. The primary roles of the pediatric nurse are _____, _____, _____, _____, and _____.

ANSWERS   **Short answer**

1. Deleterious child care practices during the 18th century included tight swaddling and overdressing, inappropriate diet (overfeeding, wine or ale use for flavoring, minimal breast-feeding, and too early feeding of solid foods), and overcrowding in foundling homes.

2. Spitz, Bowlby, and Robertson studied the effects on children of separation from parents. Their research influenced hospital policies regarding parent visitation and length of hospital stays. As a result of such efforts, parental visitation was encouraged and hospital stays were shortened. Despite these changes, however, nurses and researchers noted that hospitalization of children continued to cause emotional distress; clearly, separation from parents was not its only cause. Growing contributions of developmental theorists identified other issues and sources of anxiety related to pediatric hospitalization; this information helped shape current practices regarding the care of sick children. For example, children now routinely are prepared emotionally for medical procedures. Along with their parents, they are fully informed about scheduled procedures, offered choices when appropriate, and encouraged to participate actively in their care. Nursing systems are designed to assign one primary nurse to a child's care. In many hospitals, Child Life Programs help children and their families cope with the stress of illness and hospitalization, which affects the entire family.

3. Childhood morbidity and mortality problems in the United States include high infant mortality; low immunization rates; poverty; high rates of pregnancy, abortion, and childbirth among adolescents; high childhood mortality; and lack of health insurance.

True or false

4. False. Cadogan studied 18th-century child-care methods.

5. False. Children were separated from adults to prevent contagion.

6. True.

7. True.

8. False. The high mortality in foundling homes provoked pioneering studies of child-care practices.

9. True.

10. False. Spitz, Bowlby, and Robertson studied the effects of hospitalization on children.

11. False. Bowlby found that relocated British children developed typical patterns of separation anxiety.

12. True.

13. False. Children cry loudly during the first stage of separation anxiety.

Fill in the blank

14. Protest, despair, denial

15. Spitz, Bowlby, Robertson

16. Advocate, caregiver, counselor, health teacher, researcher

CHAPTER 2

Pediatric nursing concepts

OBJECTIVES
After studying this chapter, the reader should be able to:
1. Discuss major concepts of growth and development.
2. Describe family developmental tasks.
3. Relate family developmental tasks to child health.
4. Describe patterns of genetic inheritance.
5. Identify major disorders related to various patterns of genetic inheritance.

OVERVIEW OF CONCEPTS
Child health is influenced by patterns of growth and development, family achievement of developmental tasks, and genetic factors. To plan nursing care effectively, the pediatric nurse must understand these concepts and how they influence a child's health.

This chapter discusses major concepts of growth and development, describes the family's role in promoting child health, and details genetic influences on child health.

Growth and development

Growth refers to an increase in size, notably height and weight. *Development* refers to maturation of body structures and acquisition of physical, psychosocial, cognitive, and language skills.

Human growth and development progress cephalocaudally, from head to toe; proximodistally, from the trunk to the tips of the extremities; and from the general to the specific (for example, from reaching to grasping). Growth follows a predictable pattern during the developmental periods of infancy, toddler stage, preschool age, school age, and adolescence. (See *Physical growth patterns during childhood*.)

Developmental theories provide direction for assessing child development and for planning care aimed at promoting the child's socioemotional health. For basic information on three commonly used developmental theories — Sigmund Freud's psychosexual theory, Erik Erikson's psychosocial theory, and Jean Piaget's cognitive theory — see *Theories of child development,* page 10. For additional information on child development during specific childhood stages and implications for pediatric nurses, see chapters 6 through 10.

Physical growth patterns during childhood

This chart outlines human growth patterns from infancy through adolescence.

AGE	WEIGHT	HEIGHT
Infancy: Birth to 6 months	• Monthly gain: $1\frac{1}{2}$ lb • Birth weight doubles by age 6 months	• Monthly gain: 1″
6 to 12 months	• Monthly gain: $\frac{3}{4}$ lb (12 oz) • Birth weight triples by age 12 months	• Monthly gain: $\frac{1}{2}$″
Toddler: 1 to 3 years	• Yearly gain: 4 to 6 lb • Birth weight quadruples by age $2\frac{1}{2}$	• Yearly gain: 3″ to 4″
Preschool age: 3 to 6 years	• Yearly gain: 4 to 6 lb	• Yearly gain: 2″ to 3″
School age: 6 to 13 years	• Yearly gain: 4 to 6 lb	• Yearly gain: 2″
Adolescence: 13 to 21 years	*Females:* • Highly variable; gain of 15 to 50 lb over span of $2\frac{1}{2}$ to 3 years • Growth spurt begins at average age of 11 *Males:* • Highly variable; gain of 15 to 60 lb over span of 3 to 4 years • Growth spurt begins at average age of 13	*Females:* • Highly variable; gain of 2″ to 8″ over span of $2\frac{1}{2}$ to 3 years *Males:* • Highly variable; gain of 4″ to 12″ over span of 3 to 4 years

Family influences The quality of family life influences the health of family members, which in turn plays an essential role in promoting health and preventing illness. Family developmental theory postulates successive stages of family development, during which the family unit must accomplish specific tasks. By assessing the family's developmental stage and its achievement of the corresponding tasks, the nurse obtains information that aids in planning for the family's health needs as it progresses through certain transition points — including parenthood, adjustment to children's development stages (such as entering school or becoming adolescents), and adjustment to middle life and retirement.

According to Evelyn Duvall (1977), the family life cycle progresses through eight stages, each associated with specific developmental tasks. In families with more than one child, the family's primary stage corresponds to the age of the oldest child. (However, stages overlap somewhat.) To move to the next stage smoothly, the family must

Theories of child development

The child development theories discussed in this chart should not be compared directly, because they measure different aspects of development. Erik Erikson's psychosocial-based theory is the most commonly accepted model for child development, although it cannot be empirically tested. Jean Piaget's cognitive theory does not translate well into psychomotor skills. Sigmund Freud's psychosexual approach, a precursor of more recent theories, no longer serves as the primary model.

AGE-GROUP	PSYCHOSOCIAL THEORY	COGNITIVE THEORY	PSYCHOSEXUAL THEORY
Infancy	Age 0 to 18 months	Age 0 to 2	Age 0 to 6 months
	Trust vs. mistrust (consistency of needs being met allows infant to predict responses)	Sensorimotor (can't learn without doing; reflexive behavior)	Oral passive (id develops; biological pleasure principle)
			Age 7 to 18 months
			Oral aggressive (teething begins; everything is put into mouth; oral satisfaction decreases anxiety)
Toddlerhood	Age 18 months to 3 years	Not applicable	Age 18 months to 3 years
	Autonomy vs. shame and doubt (desire to do things independently)		Anal (bowel and bladder training occur; child projects feelings onto others; elimination and retention are used to control and inhibit)
Preschool age	Age 3 to 6	Age 2 to 4	Age 4 to 5
	Initiative vs. sense of guilt (mimics; more purposeful and active in goal setting)	Preoperational-preconceptual (egocentric, animistic, magical thinking; no cause-effect reasoning; uses symbols)	Phallic (ego develops [objective conscious reality]; Oedipal complex — love of opposite-sex parent)
School age	Age 6 to 13	Age 4 to 7	Age 6 to 12
	Industry vs. inferiority (using hands to make things; being helpful; mastering tasks)	Intuitive-preoperational (begins to use cause-effect reasoning)	Latent (superego develops morality; repressed sexual drive)
		Age 7 to 11 Concrete operations (collecting; mastering facts)	
Adolescence	Age 13 to 18	Age 11 to 15	Not applicable
	Identity vs. confusion (defining self in relation to others)	Formal operations (abstract ideas; reality-based)	

Source: Selekman, J. Springhouse Notes: *Pediatric Nursing*, 2nd ed. Springhouse, Pa.: Springhouse Corp., 1993.

achieve the developmental tasks within each stage. Achieving these tasks accomplishes the family's six basic functions:
- affective function — meeting family members' socio-emotional needs
- socialization function — assisting family members to behave in appropriate sex- and age-related roles, including child-rearing practices
- provision of physical necessities, such as food, clothing, shelter, and health care
- reproductive function — family planning behaviors and birth of new family members
- economic function — providing and allocating financial and material resources
- coping function — promoting such behaviors as problem solving during times of family stress and crisis.

For more information on Duvall's family stages and the developmental tasks within each stage, see *Family development: Stages and tasks,* pages 12 and 13.

Genetic influences

Genetic factors probably play a role in virtually every disease and disorder. Certain diseases, such as muscular dystrophy and cystic fibrosis, result from a specific genetic defect. In others, such as cancer, a genetic defect is suspected but has not been identified.

Disorders known to result from genetic factors are classified as cytogenetic, monogenetic, or multifactorial.

Cytogenetic disorders

Cytogenetic disorders result from a deviation in the structure or number of chromosomes. The normal number of chromosomes is 46, or 23 pairs. Structural abnormalities include losses, additions, rearrangements, or exchanges among the genes on a chromosome, and weak or fragile chromosome sites. Abnormalities of number include the loss or addition of entire chromosomes. Losses and additions involving autosomes (chromosomes 1 to 22) typically cause more severe problems than those involving sex chromosomes X and Y (pair 23). Common cytogenetic disorders include cri du chat, fragile X syndrome, Kleinfelter's syndrome, trisomy 13, trisomy 18, trisomy 21 (Down syndrome), Turner's syndrome, and XYY syndrome.

Monogenetic disorders

Monogenetic (single-gene) disorders result from a defect in a single gene located on a specific chromosome, or from a defective gene on the X chromosome. Defective genes may be either recessive or dominant; they are inherited according to Mendelian principles.

A disorder caused by a recessive gene is expressed only in the presence of two recessive genes — one from each parent. In a person who inherits just one recessive gene, the normal gene on the paired chromosome overcomes the effect of the recessive gene; thus, this person is a carrier for the attributed disorder but does not manifest the disorder. In

Family development: Stages and tasks

This chart presents the eight stages of the family life cycle proposed by Duvall and describes the developmental tasks and nursing responsibilities associated with each stage.

DEVELOPMENTAL STAGE	DEVELOPMENTAL TASKS	NURSING RESPONSIBILITIES
Stage 1: Beginning family (no children)	• Establishment of couple identity • Realignment of relationships with extended families • Decision-making about parenthood	• Assist couple with sexual and marital role adjustment. • Teach couple about family planning. • Provide prenatal education.
Stage 2: Early childbearing family (oldest child is under age 30 months)	• Integration of infant into family unit • Accommodation of new parenting and grandparenting roles • Maintenance of marital bond	• Assist couple in adjusting to parenting role. • Monitor developing parent-child relationship. • Teach well-infant care. • Provide child development counseling. • Encourage couple to attend to individual physical, sexual, and social needs.
Stage 3: Family with pre-school-age child (oldest child is age $2\frac{1}{2}$ to 5)	• Accommodation to child's need for exploration • Socialization of child • Integration of new family members • Adjustment to separation • Taking on of outside interests by child	• Provide parents with anticipatory guidance on child environmental safety, discipline, sibling rivalry, growth and development, and school entry. • Encourage parents to attend to their own needs.
Stage 4: Family with school-age child (oldest child is age 6 to 13)	• Development of peer relationships by child • Adaptation by parents to peer and school influences on child's development • Maintenance of marital relationship, which may diminish during escalating external demands (such as work, school, and community responsibilities)	• Encourage parents to support child's increased independence. • Support child's endeavors to join school- or community-related organizations. • Support parental unit.
Stage 5: Family with adolescent (oldest child is age 13 to 20)	• Development of adolescent autonomy • Focusing on midlife marital and career issues • Maintenance of family ethical and moral standards	• Provide drug and sex education. • Support parental unit. • Encourage parents to allow adolescent's increasing responsibility and independence. • Support family problem-solving processes during parent-adolescent conflict.
Stage 6: Launching center family (period during which first through last child leave home)	• Establishment of independent identities for parents and young adult child • Renegotiation of marital relationship • Expansion of family circle	• Support continuing communication between young adult children and their parents. • Assist parents in role transition.
Stage 7: Family of middle years (from departure of last child to parents' retirement)	• Reinvestment in couple identity, concurrent development of independent interests • Realignment of relationships to include grandparenting role • Assisting of aging and ill members of extended family	• Assist couple to participate in leisure activities and pursue personal interests. • Assist couple in transition to grandparenting role. • Assist couple in assuming responsibility for aging family members.

Family development: Stages and tasks *(continued)*

DEVELOPMENTAL STAGE	DEVELOPMENTAL TASKS	NURSING RESPONSIBILITIES
Stage 8: Family in retirement and old age (from retirement to death of both partners)	• Maintenance of satisfying living relationships • Adjustment to reduced income • Adjustment to full or partial retirement • Adjustment to declining health • Adjustment to loss of spouse	• Refer couple to support services if one or both partners need assistance to maintain independent lifestyle. • Refer couple to community organizations that provide recreational and social activities. • Encourage couple to participate in volunteer activities. • Refer couple to financial planning services, as appropriate. • Provide physical and emotional support during aging. • Provide emotional support during grieving.

contrast, a dominant gene produces its effect even in someone with one normal gene for a given trait. Autosomal dominant disorders include achondroplasia, Marfan's syndrome, neurofibromatosis, osteogenesis imperfecta, progeria, retinoblastoma, tuberosis sclerosis, and von Willebrand's disease. Autosomal recessive disorders include albinism, congenital adrenal hyperplasia, cystic fibrosis, galactosemia, phenylketonuria, sickle cell anemia, Tay-Sachs disease, thalassemia major, and Werdnig-Hoffman disease.

Monogenetic disorders also may result from spontaneous mutation of a gene, as from exposure to an environmental mutagen (such as high temperatures, chemicals, or radiation).

Disorders caused by X-linked inheritance patterns are transmitted through a defect in a gene on the X chromosome. Because males have only one X chromosome, a defective gene on that chromosome always leads to expression of the disease. X-linked disorders may follow either a dominant or recessive inheritance pattern.

Disorders of X-linked dominant inheritance may occur in both males and females. Disorders of X-linked recessive inheritance occur only in males; they are transmitted through carrier females who pass on the disorder to their sons. X-linked dominant disorders are rare. Common X-linked recessive disorders include color blindness, Duchenne muscular dystrophy, hemophilia A, hemophilia B, and Wescott-Aldrich syndrome.

Multifactorial disorders

Multifactorial disorders have no clear inheritance pattern but are believed to be genetic because certain families show an increased susceptibility. Presumably, these disorders result from interaction among many genes and environmental influences. They include congenital defects and a wide range of common diseases and disorders, such as bipolar affective disorder, cleft lip and palate, clubfoot, congenital heart defects, diabetes mellitus, neural tube defects, psoriasis, pyloric stenosis, schizophrenia, and tuberculosis.

Diagnosis of genetic disorders

Defective genes can be detected from genetic screening tests. Besides detecting a disease or the potential for transmitting one, such tests are performed to provide reproductive information and genetic counseling and to gain information about the incidence of certain diseases in the population.

Prenatal diagnosis

Prenatal diagnosis of genetic disorders involves ultrasonography, amniocentesis, chorionic villi sampling, and fetal blood sampling. Ultrasonography may reveal physical manifestations of neural tube defects, Down syndrome, and hydrocephaly. Amniocentesis and chorionic villi sampling may detect abnormalities in chromosome number as well as Tay-Sachs disease, sickle cell anemia, Duchenne muscular dystrophy, and cystic fibrosis. Elevated alpha-fetoprotein levels in the amniotic fluid may indicate neural tube defects. Fetal blood sampling may reveal a deficiency in coagulation factors VIII and IX, as in hemophilia. If a congenital disorder is detected prenatally, the family may decide to terminate the pregnancy.

Postnatal diagnosis is accomplished through a comprehensive history and physical examination for typical manifestations of certain disorders. Chromosome analysis, enzyme assays, and serologic studies also may be performed.

Genetic counseling

Genetic counseling aims to provide the family with complete and accurate information about genetic disorders. The goals of genetic counseling include:
- promoting informed decisions by involved family members
- clarifying the family's options, available treatments, and prognosis
- examining alternatives to reduce the risk of genetic disorders
- decreasing the incidence of the genetic disorder
- reducing the impact of the disorder.

To achieve these goals, genetic counseling must include an accurate diagnosis and nondirective counseling, which provides information in a nonthreatening, unbiased manner and reserves related decisions for the family. Such counseling also must be confidential and completely truthful, upholding the family's right to know what to expect (including the prognosis of the fetus or child). Also, it must be timed appropriately — preferably, before pregnancy (or, less ideally, just after prenatal or postnatal diagnosis).

A team approach that involves the physician, nurse, and social worker is essential. The nurse plays an important role in follow-up, clarifying information, providing continuous support to the family, and assisting the family with the grieving process as appropriate.

To decrease the risk of transmitting a genetic disorder or to reduce the impact of the disorder, a genetic counselor may discuss with the couple who wishes to have a family such alternatives as adoption, artificial insemination, surrogate pregnancy, prenatal diagnosis with selective abortion or prenatal treatment, curative treatment with gene splicing, and fetal surgery.

STUDY ACTIVITIES **Short answer**

1. Differentiate cephalocaudal growth and development from proximodistal growth and development.

_____

2. Compare and contrast cytogenetic, monogenetic, and multifactorial disorders.

_____

_____

3. List the five goals of genetic counseling.

_____

_____

_____

Multiple choice

4. An infant's birth weight triples by what age?
   A. 6 months
   B. 12 months
   C. 18 months
   D. 24 months

5. When does adolescent growth begin in females?
   A. Age 9
   B. Age 11
   C. Age 13
   D. Age 17

6. Jimmy, age 4, comes to the clinic for a well-child visit. The nurse notes that he grew 1½″ during the last year. Which statement about Jimmy's height gain is true?
   A. It is slightly less than expected.
   B. It is average.
   C. It is slightly more than expected.
   D. It is typical for a 4-year-old boy.

7. The best time for genetic counseling is:

A. When a couple is planning to start a family.

B. During the pregnancy.

C. Just after the birth of a child with a genetic disorder.

D. Before a second pregnancy, if the woman has had a child with a genetic disorder.

8. Susan, age 3, comes to the physician's office with her mother for a well-child visit. Which question would be the most appropriate one for the nurse to ask Susan's mother?

A. "What birth control measures do you practice?"

B. "Do you plan to have more children?"

C. "Have you considered nursery school for Susan?"

D. "Have you taught Susan how to cross the street safely?"

ANSWERS

Short answer

1. Cephalocaudal growth and development progresses from head to toe; proximodistal growth and development progresses from the trunk to the tips of the extremities.

2. Cytogenetic disorders are caused by an abnormality of the structure or number of chromosomes. Monogenetic disorders result from a defect in a single gene located on a specific chromosome, or from a defective gene on the X chromosome; these disorders also may occur when a gene spontaneously undergoes mutation. Multifactorial disorders presumably result from an interaction among many genes and environmental influences.

3. The goals of genetic counseling include promoting informed decision-making by involved family members; clarifying the family's options, available treatments, and prognosis; examining alternatives to reduce the risk of genetic disorders; decreasing the incidence of the disorder; and reducing the impact of the disorder.

Multiple choice

4. B. Birth weight triples by about age 12 months.

5. B. In females, adolescent growth begins at approximately age 11.

6. A. The preschool-age child grows approximately 2″ to 3″ per year.

7. A. Ideally, genetic counseling should take place before pregnancy.

8. C. Parents with a preschool-age child may consider nursery school placement. The nurse can provide anticipatory guidance to help parents evaluate and select a nursery school and handle separation issues.

CHAPTER 3

The nurse–child–family relationship

OBJECTIVES

After studying this chapter, the reader should be able to:
1. Describe the characteristics of the nurse–child–family relationship.
2. Discuss the four phases of the nurse-patient relationship.
3. Describe the characteristics of therapeutic communication.
4. Identify effective techniques for communicating with children and parents who have trouble expressing themselves.

OVERVIEW OF CONCEPTS

The nurse–child–family relationship establishes a positive environment for health care and helps the nurse meet the child's and family's health needs. Effective communication forms the basis for this relationship; it is especially important during assessment. Effective communication also can stimulate positive changes and professional growth in the nurse.

This chapter describes the characteristics of the nurse–child–family relationship, emphasizing the importance of empathy, mutuality, and caring. It identifies the phases of the nurse-patient relationship, including the tasks that must be accomplished during each phase. Then the chapter discusses therapeutic communication and describes special communication techniques the nurse can use when interacting with children and parents.

The nurse–child–family relationship: A helping bond

The nurse–child–family relationship focuses on meeting the child's and family's health care needs. Ideally, it promotes a climate that brings about positive change and growth in both the child and family.

Characteristics

Optimally, the nurse–child–family relationship leads the child and family to trust that their health care needs will be met. This relationship is based on respect, honesty, consistency, and hope. To establish such a relationship, the nurse can use various strategies. (See *Establishing trust within the nurse–child–family relationship,* page 18.)

Establishing trust within the nurse–child–family relationship

The nurse can use the following strategies to help establish a trusting relationship with the child and family.
- Recognize that each child is an individual.
- Convey warmth and caring, such as by maintaining a warm, friendly tone of voice.
- Establish eye contact with the child and family.
- Use active listening techniques.
- Use postures that signal attention to the child and family, such as keeping the arms, legs, and body relaxed and leaning slightly toward the child or family member.
- Provide adequate information.
- Allow time for questions.
- Remain honest and open.
- Provide complete information about the child's health and health care.
- Follow through with commitments.
- Maintain confidentiality.

As in any effective nurse-patient relationship, the nurse caring for a pediatric patient must express empathy, mutuality, and caring. *Empathy* is the capacity to perceive another's emotions and state of mind and to understand the meaning and significance of that person's behavior. (*Sympathy,* in contrast, is the capacity to share another person's feelings.) The nurse can express empathy by:
- accepting the patient, as shown by using the patient's correct name, maintaining eye contact, and responding to nonverbal cues
- listening attentively, as shown by nodding and smiling while the patient speaks, offering encouraging responses, and using therapeutic silence at appropriate times
- clarifying, such as by asking open-ended questions, restating the problem, and validating the patient's perceptions.

To convey *mutuality,* include the child and family in collaborative health care planning to meet health goals. Other nursing actions that promote mutuality include discussing health goals with the family, expressing personal feelings about the nurse–child–family relationship, encouraging the child and family to express their thoughts and feelings, and collaborating to develop mutually agreed-upon health goals.

To convey a sense of *caring,* the nurse must show a commitment to the family through willingness to be involved in the child's care and to be available to the family. Other ways to convey caring include showing mutual respect and positive regard for the child and family and recognizing the child as an individual.

Phases of the nurse-patient relationship

The nurse-patient relationship has four phases: preinteraction (preparatory phase), orientation, working, and termination.

During *preinteraction,* the nurse reviews the child's record, identifies initial problems, and evaluates the potential impact of the child's and family's values or personal characteristics on the nurse-patient relationship. Such issues must be acknowledged and managed before the relationship begins.

During *orientation*, the nurse initiates the nurse-patient relationship by establishing contact, defining roles, identifying the child's and family's needs, and establishing a therapeutic contract.

To establish initial contact, the nurse identifies herself or himself and describes the nursing role to be undertaken, including its purpose and how long it will continue. For example, a nurse caring for a child might say, "Good morning, Susan and Mrs. Davis. I'm Jean Graft, a staff nurse on the pediatric unit. I'll be taking care of Susan until 3 o'clock this afternoon." After a brief social conversation to show interest in the patient, the nurse continues the orientation, explaining the nurse's role (which is to help the child and parents understand the child's health status and treatment plan) and the child's and family's responsibility (which is to take an active part in health care and to carry out mutually agreed-upon therapeutic activities).

Continuing the orientation phase, the nurse identifies the child's health problems, helps the child and family become aware of these problems, focuses on the problems, and explores potential solutions. To promote orientation, the nurse may use such techniques as attentive listening, asking open-ended questions, paraphrasing, and clarifying (discussed later in this chapter).

At completion of the orientation phase, the nurse, child (as appropriate), and family establish a nurse-patient contract — an agreement that specifies the location and frequency of contact, duration of the relationship, and expected behaviors of the nurse, child, and family. At the end of this meeting, the child and family should understand clearly the relevant health care issues and the nurse's interest in the child's care.

During the *working phase* (active intervention), the nurse promotes a climate of mutuality, defines the child's health problem, explores solutions, and formulates a realistic plan of care. To aid this process, the nurse may use open-ended questions and explore cause-and-effect relationships. After identifying the child's health care problem, the nurse formulates nursing diagnoses and establishes collaborative health goals with the child and family. To help achieve these goals, the nurse writes patient outcomes and implements appropriate nursing interventions.

The *termination phase* begins once the child's health goals have been achieved. During this phase, the child, family, and nurse reflect on the therapeutic experience and review both positive and negative aspects. The nurse should allow adequate time to share feelings. After verifying that health goals have been attained, the nurse, child, and family say their good-byes.

Promoting effective communication

Communication — the reciprocal exchange of messages by two or more people — involves a complex interplay in which the participants send, receive, decode, and return verbal messages (words and voice tones) and nonverbal messages (facial expressions, body movements, gestures, and touch).

Just as mutual understanding is the basis for all relationships, effective communication is essential in establishing the nurse–child–family relationship. Poor communication inevitably leads to disordered thoughts, emotions, and behavior — problems that can jeopardize the nurse–child–family relationship.

Factors that influence the effectiveness of communication include the participants' developmental and cognitive levels, values, emotions, and sociocultural factors. For example, when talking to a young child, the nurse must assess the child's cognitive level and modify word choice and sentence length to match the child's ability to comprehend.

When communicating with a child, the nurse may aim to influence as well as inform. By using confirming responses — those that validate the child's and family's worth, convey respect and acceptance, and support their right to have and express feelings — the nurse can exert a positive therapeutic influence.

In contrast, a nurse who uses disconfirming responses shows disregard for the validity of the patient's feelings and exerts a negative therapeutic influence. Such responses include ignoring the patient's feelings, imposing value judgments on the patient, inappropriately changing the topic, offering unrealistic reassurance, or presuming to know what the patient means without seeking validation.

Therapeutic communication

Therapeutic communication encompasses patient-focused exchanges that aim to achieve clear, mutually established therapeutic goals. Such communication is limited to the scope of the patient's problem, is problem oriented, and supports the patient's needs.

To promote therapeutic communication, provide a quiet environment and allow a comfortable position for both the nurse and patient. Make sure to allow adequate interpersonal space; at least 2′ to 4′ should separate nurse and patient.

Goals of therapeutic communication

Therapeutic communication serves these purposes:
• elicits additional information when the patient's message is unclear
• ensures that the nurse has understood the patient's message correctly
• informs the patient of the nurse's feelings or focuses on patient behavior that must be changed
• allows for recovery during emotionally laden situations.

Eliciting information

The nurse can use the *clarifying* technique to gain additional information and thus enhance understanding of the patient's message. Nurse: "I'm not sure I understand what you mean. Could you tell me again?"

By *restating,* in which the nurse repeats the important part of the patient's message, the nurse can focus on a specific part of the message. Patient: "I don't want to go to physical therapy today." Nurse: "You don't want to go to physical therapy *today?*"

Using minimal cues or leads encourages the patient to continue with the message. Nurse: "Uh-huh" (while nodding the head).

Asking open-ended questions also helps elicit information. Patient: "I don't want to go to physical therapy today." Nurse: "Tell me about your physical therapy."

Ensuring that the nurse understands the message

When *paraphrasing,* the nurse states the patient's message, conveying the meaning in another form. Paraphrasing helps the patient elaborate on the content of the message and confirms that the nurse understands the message. Paraphrased responses should be more concise than the patient's message. Patient: "I have pain here" (points to his arm). Nurse: "Your arm hurts?"

Reflecting addresses the emotional content of the message, calling attention to and clarifying the patient's feelings. Patient: "I don't want to go to physical therapy today." Nurse: "You sound angry."

When *summarizing,* the nurse paraphrases or reflects on the patient's statements at the end of the interaction to confirm that the nurse understands the patient's message.

Validating involves turning the patient's statement into a question, reflecting the nurse's understanding of the patient's message. Validation confirms the accuracy of the message received. Patient: "I don't feel so good today." Nurse: "You feel worse than you felt yesterday?"

Conveying the nurse's feelings or focusing on needed change in patient behavior

To tell the patient about the nurse's feelings or to help change unacceptable patient behavior, the nurse may use "I" statements. For example, if a patient refuses to go to physical therapy for the fourth day in a row, the nurse might say, "I'm getting frustrated by your refusal to adhere to the treatment plan we both agreed to follow."

Defusing emotionally laden situations

Silence, in which the nurse briefly refrains from speaking in response to a patient's message, helps the patient regain composure while the nurse's continued presence offers support. The nurse can use *humor,* as in jokes or light, humorous comments, to provide momentary relief from a difficult issue at hand. Through *touch,* such as holding hands, hugging, or stroking, the nurse conveys acceptance and support.

Encouraging the child and parents to express themselves

If the child and parents have trouble expressing themselves, the nurse may use several techniques. *Third-person statements,* which describe a related situation, can help determine if the child or parents feel the same way. For example, if a hospitalized child seems upset, the nurse might say, "Some children in the hospital feel angry when their parents can't stay with them all the time. Are you feeling angry now?"

Encouraging *storytelling* can help a child express feelings or fears. Nurse: "Tell me a story about a little boy who's waiting to have his tonsils taken out."

Keeping a diary of thoughts and feelings can encourage expression of feelings by parents as well as children over age 8. (However, young children may need reminders and direction to help focus their thoughts.) For example, the nurse may ask a child to describe feelings experienced when a cast was removed; afterward, the nurse may ask permission to read what the child wrote or may ask the child to discuss it.

In *bibliotherapy,* the nurse reads to the child, or has the child read, a story portraying another child experiencing similar events. Afterward, the nurse asks the child to talk about what happened in the story. Bibliotherapy also may be effective for parents. For example, the nurse may ask them to read a book or brochure about families experiencing similar events.

Drawing also promotes expression of feelings, and can be effective with parents and children. For example, the nurse might say to a child, "Draw me a picture about Mom and Dad bringing home your new baby brother." After the child draws the picture, the nurse can ask the child to talk about the picture. With training in art therapy, the nurse also may interpret a child's spontaneous drawings to gain insight into the child's feelings and experiences. This technique commonly is used to elicit information about child abuse.

In *sentence completion,* the nurse asks the child to respond to an open-ended, incomplete statement, such as "The worst thing about having diabetes is . . ."

In *therapeutic play,* used exclusively with children, the nurse sets up a play situation and asks the child to act it out. Doing this helps the child express thoughts and feelings indirectly. For example, the nurse may ask a hospitalized child in traction to play with a doll in traction, with mother and father dolls, or with a nurse or doctor doll. The nurse then observes the child playing with the dolls to gain insight into the child's thoughts and feelings about hospitalization and confinement in traction.

STUDY ACTIVITIES

Short answer

1. Describe at least five nursing actions that promote trust within the nurse–child–family relationship.

_____

_____

_____

2. Identify at least three actions the nurse can take to convey mutuality within the nurse–child–family relationship.

_____

_____

_____

3. List the tasks to be accomplished during the orientation phase of the nurse-patient relationship.

_____

_____

4. What type of environment should the nurse provide to promote therapeutic communication?

_____

_____

5. What are some factors that influence the effectiveness of communication?

_____

_____

Multiple choice

6. The nurse formulates the patient's plan of care during which phase of the nurse-patient relationship?
  A. Preinteraction
  B. Orientation
  C. Working phase
  D. Termination

7. Which communication technique helps to elicit more information from a patient?
  A. Validating
  B. Paraphrasing
  C. Using "I" statements
  D. Restating

8. By using reflecting as a communication technique, the nurse can:
  A. Focus on the emotional content of the patient's message.
  B. Encourage the patient to elaborate on the message.
  C. Ensure that the patient's message was heard correctly.
  D. Allow the patient to reconsider the message.

9. Therapeutic play provides an opportunity for the child to:
  A. Improve fine motor development.
  B. Express thoughts and feelings indirectly.
  C. Socialize with other children.
  D. Become distracted from problems.

ANSWERS **Short answer**

  1. Actions that promote trust within the nurse–child–family relationship include recognizing that each child is an individual, conveying warmth and caring, establishing eye contact, using active listening techniques, using postures that signal attention to the child and family, allowing time for questions, remaining honest and open, following through with commitments, providing complete information, and maintaining confidentiality.

  2. To convey mutuality, the nurse can include the child and family in collaborative health care planning, discuss health goals with the family, encourage the child and family to share their thoughts and feelings, express personal feelings about the nurse–child–family relationship, and collaborate to develop mutually agreed-upon health goals.

  3. Tasks to be accomplished during this phase include establishing contact, defining roles, identifying the patient's needs, and establishing a therapeutic contract.

  4. To promote therapeutic communication, the nurse should provide a quiet environment and allow adequate interpersonal space, with 2′ to 4′ separating nurse and patient.

  5. Factors that influence the effectiveness of communication include the participants' developmental and cognitive levels, values, emotions, and sociocultural factors.

Multiple choice

  6. C. The nurse formulates the plan of care during the working phase.
  7. D. Restating allows the nurse to focus on a specific part of the message and thus elicit more information.
  8. A. Reflecting helps to focus on the emotional content of the patient's message.
  9. B. Therapeutic play allows the child to express thoughts and feelings indirectly.

CHAPTER 4

Health promotion

OBJECTIVES After studying this chapter, the reader should be able to:
1. Describe principles related to health promotion.
2. Discuss guidelines for supervision of child health.
3. Discuss immunization principles and the nurse's role in pediatric immunization.

OVERVIEW OF CONCEPTS This chapter presents a summary of concepts related to health promotion. It describes three levels of illness prevention and discusses the nursing role in health promotion. The chapter provides guidelines for supervision of child health, then discusses childhood immunizations and outlines the related nursing role.

Health promotion The concept of health promotion, which encompasses both health maintenance and illness prevention, includes activities that help the child and family achieve their optimal function. Health maintenance involves activities that support the child's and family's present state of health. Illness prevention, in contrast, involves activities that prevent development and transmission of illness and disease.

Levels of illness prevention

The model of illness prevention proposed by Leavell and Clark (1965) includes three levels of prevention: primary, secondary, and tertiary. *Primary prevention* includes health promotion and specific activities aimed at protecting against disease, such as immunization. It also addresses illness prevention and health maintenance.

Secondary prevention includes early diagnosis and prompt treatment of illness and disease, with the goal of restoring the patient's previous state of health as quickly as possible. Secondary prevention also includes screening for disease.

Tertiary prevention encompasses activities undertaken when disease leads to permanent disability. Such activities aim to prevent further complications and disability and to help the patient achieve optimal functioning within the constraints of the disability.

Nursing roles

Nursing roles that aid child health promotion include teacher, child and family advocate, counselor, and consultant.

Teacher

As a teacher of health promotion activities, the nurse provides the child and family with information they need to maintain or improve health and to prevent illness. The nurse also helps them to use this information to incorporate health-promoting behaviors into their daily lives. In a special form of teaching, the nurse provides anticipatory guidance to inform the family and prepare them to deal with anticipated events in the child's life or environment. For instance, the nurse may provide information about parental or child concerns, routine child care, child growth and development, child behavior, care-giving schedules, family stressors, family supports, and safety issues.

Child and family advocate

The nurse may serve as a child and family advocate by supporting passive or active health promotion strategies. Passive health promotion strategies require no direct action by the child or family. For example, the nurse acts as a child and family advocate when supporting local water fluoridation systems to reduce dental caries in children.

Active health promotion strategies require the child's and family's personal involvement in adopting and carrying out behaviors designed to promote health, such as encouraging the family to keep well-child visits and providing immunization. To support these activities, the nurse helps the child and family become responsible for their own health care, such as by informing them about the child's health status, health care options, and health care rights; by helping the child and family make health care decisions; and by supporting them in their choices.

Counselor

The nurse uses the nurse-patient relationship to help the child and family solve problems. Using warmth, empathy, and active listening techniques, the nurse can help them move toward independent problem solving.

Consultant

The nurse acts as a consultant to community agencies, legislative bodies, and others to provide information about health promotion and illness prevention related to specific child health issues.

Supervision of child health

Supervision of child health encompasses both primary and secondary prevention. During routine health supervision visits, the physician and nurse provide guidance on issues related to child growth, development, and health. Routine health supervision also provides an opportunity for the physician and nurse to screen for specific diseases and to detect changes in the child's growth, development, and health status. Once identified, the health care team can address such changes promptly and plan appropriate interventions.

The American Academy of Pediatrics recommends a specific schedule and activities for routine child health supervision. (See *Routine child health supervision: Schedule and activities,* page 28.) For details on how to obtain the child's health history and perform the physical examination, see Chapter 5, Child health assessment.

Immunizations

A major component of child health supervision, immunizations protect against disease and thus are considered a primary prevention strategy. Immunizations confer artificial active immunity, thus providing potentially lifelong protection against a given disease by exposing the patient to the causative agent and stimulating formation of antibodies.

Immunizing agents include live vaccines, killed vaccines, genetically engineered vaccines, and toxoids. *Live vaccines* use an attenuated form of the pathogen to achieve immunity. Examples include measles, mumps, and rubella virus vaccine (MMR) and the Sabin polio vaccine. *Killed vaccines* use dead forms of the pathogen to achieve immunity. Examples include the pertussis and Salk polio vaccines. *Genetically engineered vaccines*, such as recombinant DNA hepatitis B vaccine, use an artificially produced pathogen. *Toxoids* are bacterial toxins that have been treated to destroy toxic properties while stimulating antitoxin formation. Examples include tetanus toxoid and diphtheria toxoid.

The nurse's role in immunization includes:
- assessing the child's immunization status
- administering required immunizations
- informing parents about the immunization and potential adverse effects
- accurately documenting the immunization administered.

Schedule

Whenever possible, children should receive routine immunizations at specific ages. (See *Pediatric immunization schedule,* page 29.) A child can receive immunizations safely even during a minor afebrile illness, such as a cold, allergy, mild diarrhea, or otitis media. Deferring immunizations in such children commonly results in missed doses.

Contraindications

Routine immunizations are contraindicated in some circumstances. For instance, live vaccines should not be administered to children with congenital disorders of immune function. (However, such children can receive killed vaccines safely.) The oral live poliovirus vaccine (OPV) is contraindicated in children with human immunodeficiency virus; these children can safely receive the inactivated poliovirus vaccine (IPV). OPV also should not be administered to family members of an immunocompromised child because this virus may be transmitted through respiratory secretions. Children with leukemia who are in re-

Routine child health supervision: Schedule and activities

The American Academy of Pediatrics (1987) recommends that children undergo routine health supervision activities at the ages specified below. For immunization information, see the chart on the next page.

DEVELOPMENTAL PERIOD: Infancy
Age: Birth
Health supervision activities:
- History (pre- and postnatal, including labor, delivery)
- Routine examination, including length, weight, and head circumference
- Gestational age assessment
- Metabolic screening for phenylketonuria (PKU), thyroxine (T_4)

Age: 2 weeks to 12 months
Health supervision activities:
- History at 2 weeks and at 2, 4, 6, 9, and 12 months
- Routine examination, including length, weight, and head circumference at 2 weeks and at 2, 4, 6, 9, and 12 months
- Sensory screening (subjective data taken from history) at 2 weeks and at 2, 4, 6, 9, and 12 months
- Developmental assessment at 2 weeks and at 2, 4, 6, 9, and 12 months
- Anticipatory guidance at 2 weeks and at 2, 4, 6, 9, and 12 months
- Laboratory screening: urinalysis at 6 months; hemoglobin, hematocrit, and tuberculin test at 9 months

DEVELOPMENTAL PERIOD: Toddler stage
Age: 15 to 36 months
Health supervision activities:
- History at 15, 18, 24, and 30 months
- Routine examination, including height and weight at 15, 18, 24, and 30 months; head circumference at 15 and 18 months
- Sensory screening (subjective data taken from history) at 15, 18, 24, and 30 months
- Developmental assessment at 15, 18, 24, and 30 months
- Anticipatory guidance at 15, 18, 24, and 30 months
- Laboratory screening: hemoglobin and hematocrit at 18 months; serum lead levels at 18, 24, and 30 months

DEVELOPMENTAL PERIOD: Preschool age
Age: 3 to 5 years
Health supervision activities:
- History at ages 3, 4, and 5
- Routine examination, including height, weight, and blood pressure at ages 3, 4, and 5
- Sensory screening: subjective data taken from history at age 3; objective vision and hearing screening using standardized instruments at ages 4 and 5
- Developmental assessment at ages 3, 4, and 5
- Anticipatory guidance at ages 3, 4, and 5
- Laboratory screening: serum lead levels at 3 years; urinalysis and tuberculin test at age 4
- Referral for routine dental supervision at age 3

DEVELOPMENTAL PERIOD: School age
Age: 6 to 13 years
Health supervision activities:
- History at ages 6, 8, 10, and 12
- Routine examination, including height, weight, and blood pressure, at ages 6, 8, 10, and 12
- Sensory screening: objective vision and hearing screening, using standardized instruments at ages 6 and 12, using subjective data from history at ages 8 and 10
- Developmental assessment at ages 6, 8, 10, and 12
- Anticipatory guidance at ages 6, 8, 10, and 12
- Laboratory screening: hemoglobin, hematocrit, urinalysis, and tuberculin test at age 10

DEVELOPMENTAL PERIOD: Adolescence
Age: 13 to 19 years
Health supervision activities:
- History at ages 14, 16, and 18
- Routine examination, including height, weight, and blood pressure at ages 14, 16, and 18
- Sensory screening: objective vision screening using standardized instruments at ages 14, 16, and 18
- Developmental assessment at ages 14, 16, and 18
- Anticipatory guidance at ages 14, 16, and 18
- Laboratory screening: hemoglobin, hematocrit, urinalysis, and tuberculin test at age 16

Source: Committee on Psychosocial Aspects of Child and Family Life. *Guidelines for Health Supervision, II.* Elk Grove Village, Ill.: American Academy of Pediatrics, 1987.

Pediatric immunization schedule

Immunizations are preventive health measures that involve a primary dose followed by a booster dose. This chart shows recommended ages for childhood immunizations. (Note: These ages are not absolute.)

	DTP[1]	Polio[2]	MMR	Hepatitis B[3]	Haemophilus[1]	Tetanus-Diphtheria
Birth				√		
1 to 2 months				√		
2 months	√	√			♦	
4 months	√	√			♦	
6 months	√				♦	
6 to 18 months				√		
15 months			√		♦	
15 to 18 months	●	√				
4 to 6 years	●	√				
11 to 12 years			★	#		
14 to 16 years				#		√

[1] The HbOC-DTP combination vaccine may be substituted for separate vaccinations for Haemophilus and DTP.

[2] Children in close contact with immunosuppressed individuals should receive inactivated polio vaccine.

[3] Infants of mothers who tested seropositive for hepatitis B surface antigen (HBsAg+) should receive hepatitis B immune globulin (HBIG) at or shortly after the first dose. These infants also will require a second hepatitis B vaccine dose at age 1 month and a third hepatitis B vaccine injection at age 6 months.

♦ Depends on which *Haemophilus influenzae* type b vaccine was given previously.

● For the fourth and fifth dose, the acellular (DTaP) pertussis vaccine may be substituted for the DTP vaccine.

★ Except where public health authorities require otherwise.

Where resources permit, the hepatitis B vaccine series of three immunizations should be given to previously unimmunized preadolescents or adolescents.

Used with permission of the American Academy of Pediatrics, ©1993.

mission should not receive live vaccines unless they received their last dose of chemotherapy at least 3 months previously.

Premature infants should receive routine immunizations at the specified age. The exception is OPV, which is administered only after the infant has been discharged from the hospital.

MMR is contraindicated in children with severe allergies to eggs, chickens, ducks, or feathers because it may cause a systemic anaphylactic reaction.

Diphtheria and tetanus toxoids and pertussis vaccine (DTP) is contraindicated in children with neurologic disorders (such as encephalopathy or seizures). DTP also is contraindicated in children who have had the following reactions to the pertussis component: seizures, persistent crying lasting 3 or more hours, temperature of 104.9° F (40.5° C), or anaphylactic reaction.

In children with febrile illness, immunizations should be deferred until the fever subsides.

Indications for tetanus toxoid

Children who have sustained a wound should receive tetanus toxoid according to the following recommendations:

• A child with a clean, minor wound who has received fewer than three DTP immunizations or who received the last DTP or Td (adult tetanus toxoid and diphtheria toxoid) more than 10 years ago can receive Td immunization. A child with a clean, minor wound who has received three DTP immunizations and received the last DTP or Td immunization within the past 10 years needs no further immunization.

• A child with a more serious, contaminated wound who has received fewer than three DTP immunizations or who had the last DTP or Td immunization within the past 5 years should receive Td immunization and tetanus immune globulin. A child who has received three DTP immunizations and received the last DTP or Td immunization within the past 5 years needs no further immunization.

STUDY ACTIVITIES

Matching related terms

Match the nursing activity on the left with the level of illness prevention—primary, secondary, or tertiary— listed on the right.

1. ___ Obtain a urine sample from a 4-year-old child.

A. Primary illness prevention

2. ___ Administer MMR to a 15-month-old child.

B. Secondary illness prevention

3. ___ Administer antibiotics to a 6-year-old child with streptococcal pharyngitis.

C. Tertiary illness prevention

4. ___ Instruct parents how to provide a balanced diet for a 2-year-old child.

5. ___ Teach a child with neurologic deficits resulting from a head injury how to get from the bed to a chair.

Multiple choice

6. At what age should routine blood pressure monitoring begin?
   A. Birth
   B. Age 1
   C. Age 3
   D. Age 4

7. At what age can routine measurement of head circumference be discontinued?
   A. 12 months
   B. 15 months
   C. 18 months
   D. 24 months

8. At what age are infants routinely screened for tuberculosis?
   A. 4 months
   B. 6 months
   C. 9 months
   D. 12 months

9. Which immunization can a 2-month-old hospitalized, premature infant safely receive?
   A. OPV
   B. DTP
   C. Td
   D. MMR

10. Which circumstance contraindicates administration of DTP?
   A. The mother reports that the child had a fever of 103° F (39.4° C) after the last DTP injection.
   B. The mother reports that the child had a seizure shortly after birth.
   C. The mother reports that the child developed a rash after the last DTP injection.
   D. The mother reports that the child's brother is being treated for cancer.

11. What is the most important action the nurse should take before administering MMR vaccine?
   A. Ask the mother if the child has a history of food allergies.
   B. Ask the mother how the child reacted to other immunizations.
   C. Ask the mother if the child has ever had a high fever.
   D. Ask the mother if the child cried excessively after previous immunizations.

ANSWERS **Matching related terms**

    1. A
    2. A
    3. B
    4. A
    5. C

Multiple choice

    6. C. Routine blood pressure monitoring should begin at age 3.

    7. C. Routine measurement of head circumference may be discontinued at age 18 months, by which time the fontanels generally have closed.

    8. C. Routine tuberculosis screening takes place at age 9 months.

    9. B. A hospitalized, premature infant can safely receive DTP.

10. B. DTP is contraindicated in children with a history of seizures.

11. A. A child with an allergy to eggs may have a severe reaction to the MMR vaccine.

CHAPTER 5

Child health assessment

OBJECTIVES   After studying this chapter, the reader should be able to:
1. Discuss the components of child health assessment.
2. Describe general guidelines for the health history interview.
3. Identify the normal ranges for heart rate, respiratory rate, and blood pressure in children.
4. Describe developmental and home pediatric assessment instruments.

OVERVIEW OF CONCEPTS   Child health assessment is an important component of primary prevention nursing practice. Based on principles of the nurse–child–family relationship and effective communication (described in Chapter 3, The nurse–child–family relationship), child health assessment starts with a comprehensive health history, followed by a physical examination. It may include a complete developmental assessment and, for some children, a home assessment. Additional relevant information may be obtained from other sources, such as medical records and laboratory test results.

   This chapter presents concepts related to assessing a child's health. It describes the components of and procedures used in child health assessment, including instruments for developmental and home assessments. The chapter describes vision and hearing screening tests and presents normal ranges of selected vital signs for pediatric patients.

Health history   Obtained by interview, the health history provides an opportunity for the nurse to establish a therapeutic relationship with the child and family. The history serves as a source of information about the child's past and present health status and health practices.

   The format of the health history depends partly on the reason for the health care contact. Typically, the nurse obtains a complete history during the initial health care visit, then updates it on subsequent patient contacts. For a sick child, the history focuses on the current illness.

General guidelines

Obtain the child's history in a quiet, well-lit room. Make sure chairs are available for the nurse, child, and parent. If appropriate, provide toys to distract an active child so the parent and nurse can talk with minimal interruption.

Whenever possible, include the child in the health history interview. Most children over age 2 can provide some helpful information. In some circumstances — for example, if the patient is an adolescent — separate interviews with the child and parent may be warranted.

Begin by explaining the purpose of the health history to the child and parent. Then proceed to broad, open-ended questions to encourage them to provide additional information. To make sure the nurse understands the child's and parent's statements clearly, use the clarifying and summarizing techniques discussed in Chapter 3, The nurse–child–family relationship. To maintain their interest and participation in the interview, keep writing to a minimum while recording important details.

Required content

Obtain a comprehensive health history including immunizations, allergies, and medication use (both prescription and nonprescription). Be sure to obtain the information outlined below. For examples of specific interview questions that elicit such information, consult a textbook on pediatric nursing care.

Identification. Ask for the patient's name, nickname (if any), name and relationship of the person interviewed (if other than the patient), patient's date of birth, age (in years and months), sex, race, languages spoken, languages understood, home telephone number, emergency telephone number, and address.

Reason for contact. Find out the reason for the visit from the parent or child.

Present illness (if illness is the reason for the visit). Gather information about the patient's chief complaint, including its onset, duration, and description; whether it is a new or recurrent complaint; if it is a recurrent complaint, how it was managed in the past and the patient's response to treatment; and whether the patient currently is receiving treatment and, if so, its effect.

Family history. Record the names and ages of the child's parents and siblings. Note any health problems experienced by parents, siblings, grandparents, aunts, and uncles, particularly those listed below:
• *Skin:* eczema
• *Head:* headaches
• *Eyes:* vision problems
• *Ears:* hearing problems, ear infections
• *Nose:* allergies, sinus problems, frequent colds
• *Throat:* frequent infections
• *Lungs:* asthma, chronic bronchitis, frequent coughing

- *Heart:* heart disease, hypertension
- *Blood:* anemia, hemophilia, sickle cell anemia
- *Gastrointestinal:* ulcers, constipation, diarrhea, rectal bleeding, hemorrhoids
- *Kidneys:* bed-wetting, bladder infections, painful urination
- *Endocrine:* diabetes, thyroid problems
- *Skeletal:* scoliosis, arthritis, congenital hip dislocation
- *Neurologic:* seizures, mental retardation, mental illness, learning disabilities
- *Other:* cancer, obesity, hereditary diseases.

Consider using a pedigree to show the interrelationships, ages, and health status of family members.

Prenatal and childbirth history. Find out when the mother began prenatal care, how much weight she gained during pregnancy; if she experienced pregnancy complications (such as bleeding, edema, headaches, high blood pressure, high blood glucose level, infections, or exposure to rubella); if she used drugs, tobacco, or alcohol during pregnancy; where labor and delivery took place; if labor was spontaneous or induced; length of labor and any medications used; delivery presentation; delivery method; and the child's gestational age at birth.

Neonatal history. Obtain the child's birth weight and Apgar score. Note whether the child had congenital anomalies, respiratory problems, jaundice, feeding difficulty, vomiting, or infections. Record the length of the neonate's hospital stay.

Social history. Find out the parents' occupations and marital status. Obtain information about the home environment, including the type of housing (whether rented or owned, its age, and its general condition).

Determine the extent of the parents' schooling (for example, if they are high school or college graduates). Also, ask if they participate in sports or club activities, and note their hobbies and personal interests.

Find out the age at which the child began toilet training, achieved daytime bladder and bowel control, and achieved nighttime bladder and bowel control. Ask about such habits as pacifier use, thumb-sucking, and nail-biting; sleep habits and requirements; and bedtime fears.

Obtain a description of the child's personality (for example, aggressive, shy, or quiet). Ask about the child's relationships with parents, siblings, and peers and the child's degree of self-control. Determine what discipline strategies the parents use and how the child responds.

Depending on the child's age, ask if the child uses alcohol, drugs, or tobacco. Find out if the child is sexually active, and, if so, ask if the child takes measures to prevent sexually transmitted diseases and pregnancy.

Nutritional history. Find out which infant feeding method the patient used. If the patient was breast-fed, note the duration of breast-feeding; if formula-fed, determine the type of formula used and the duration of formula-feeding. Find out if the child had feeding problems (such as vomiting, diarrhea, or colic).

Ask if the child received vitamins or fluoride as an infant. Note the patient's age when solids were introduced to the diet and when the infant first slept through the night.

Find out about the child's present diet, including appetite, food likes and dislikes, vitamin supplementation, fluoride intake, number of daily meals, where meals are eaten (such as at home, school, or fast-food restaurants), daily milk consumption, and snack habits. Obtain a 24-hour dietary recall, and ask if the child has lost or gained weight recently.

Developmental history. Obtain information about the child's past and current development.

Past development. Find out at what age the child first rolled over, sat unassisted, crawled, walked, spoke the first words, and dressed without help.

Current development. Administer the Revised Prescreening Developmental Questionnaire (R-PDQ). On this test, the parent's responses to questions provide information about the child's achievement of age-appropriate developmental behaviors. (For more information on this test, see the section on developmental assessment later in this chapter.)

Previous illnesses. Ask if the child has ever been hospitalized, had surgery, or been injured; obtain a description of the event and record the date. Also find out if the child has had communicable diseases.

Next, conduct a review of all body systems. This review should include the following:

- *Skin* (including the scalp). Ask about eczema, rashes, flaking, and hair loss.
- *Head.* Ask about a history of headaches.
- *Eyes.* Ask if the child has had vision problems or strabismus. Find out if the child wears eyeglasses or contact lenses or uses visual aids.
- *Ears.* Determine if the child has had hearing problems, earwax, drainage, or ear infections.
- *Nose.* Ask about any difficulty breathing, nasal drainage, frequent colds, allergies, nosebleeds, and snoring.
- *Mouth.* Ask whether the child has seen a dentist. Find out about the child's oral hygiene practices. Ask about chancres or cold sores.
- *Throat.* Ask if the child has frequent sore throats, hoarseness, or difficulty swallowing.
- *Lungs.* Note any history of bronchitis, pneumonia, asthma, croup, or cough.
- *Heart.* Ask if the child has a history of heart murmurs or edema, and determine the child's energy level.
- *Gastrointestinal system.* Ask if the child experiences diarrhea, constipation, or stomach pain. Ask for a description of the color, consistency, and frequency of stools.

- *Genitourinary system.* Ask about bladder infections, vaginal discharge, bed-wetting, painful urination, and anal itching.
- *Musculoskeletal system.* Ask about joint or bone pain, swelling, and injuries.
- *Neurologic system.* Ask if the child has ever fainted, felt dizzy, or had seizures.
- *Metabolic system.* Note any history of jaundice or excessive thirst.

Developmental assessment

After completing the health history, proceed with a developmental assessment, if indicated. For best results, perform the developmental assessment *before* the physical examination because the child is more likely to be cooperative.

A complete developmental assessment includes a developmental history, developmental screening, and, if warranted, a diagnostic developmental test. Diagnostic developmental tests commonly are administered by psychologists, developmental clinical nurse specialists, and nurse practitioners with training in developmental testing and evaluation.

Developmental screening tests

Developmental screening tests are designed to rapidly identify children whose developmental levels fall below their age norms; they are *not* intelligence tests. These tests are administered by nurses with special training; however, they are relatively easy to administer and interpret and can be completed quickly. Children who receive atypical scores are referred to a specialist for further evaluation.

Developmental screening tests include the R-PDQ, Denver Developmental Screening Test-Revised (DDST-R), Goodenough Draw-A-Person Test, Minnesota Infant Development Inventory/Minnesota Child Development Inventory, Denver Articulation Screening Examination (DASE), Emergent Language Milestone Scale (ELM), and Preschool Readiness Experimental Screening Scale (PRESS).

R-PDQ

When obtaining the child's developmental history, the nurse may use the R-PDQ. If test results reveal that the child is functioning below the expected age level, further assessment is warranted, using additional tests that rely on observation as well as parental report. (Parental report may yield inaccurate data due to parental error or denial.)

Denver Developmental Screening Test-Revised

This test provides information about four categories of a child's development: personal-social, language, fine motor-adaptive, and gross motor development. It relies both on observation and parental report. The child is asked to demonstrate certain behaviors; other behaviors are ascertained through parental report.

DDST-R is appropriate for children from birth to age 6. It was developed using Caucasian middle-class children. When administered to children from other races and socioeconomic groups, it may yield biased results.

Goodenough Draw-A-Person Test

This test provides information about the child's intellectual development based on observation. The examiner asks the child to draw the best possible picture of a person, then evaluates it according to the number of body parts drawn. This test is appropriate for children ages 3 to 10.

Minnesota Infant Development Inventory/Minnesota Child Development Inventory

This test provides information about the child's gross motor, fine motor, language, comprehension, and personal-social development. It obtains information through both observation and parental report. Although observation of the child's behavior and skills is preferred, the inventory may be completed by parental report alone. Data evaluation yields a profile of the child's strengths and weaknesses. The infant development inventory is appropriate for use in children from birth to age 15 months; the child development inventory, from ages 1 to 6.

Denver Articulation Screening Examination

This language screening test provides information about the child's speech articulation (pronunciation) and intelligibility. The examiner asks the child to repeat selected words, then totals the number of correct pronunciations and evaluates intelligibility (whether the child is easy to understand, understandable half the time, or not understandable). DASE may be used to test children ages 2½ to 6.

Emergent Language Milestone Scale

This test uses both observation and parental report to obtain information about the auditory expressive, auditory receptive, and visual components of the child's language. ELM is appropriate for children from birth to age 36 months.

Preschool Readiness Experimental Screening Scale

This test provides information through observation of five areas of school readiness: knowledge of numbers, general numbers, drawing coordination, overall performance, and maturity. The child receives a score of high, above average, average, borderline, or insufficient. PRESS is appropriate for children ages 4 to 6.

Physical examination

After completing the developmental assessment, perform a physical examination of the child.

Techniques

Physical examination techniques include inspection, palpation, percussion, and auscultation.

To *inspect,* use sight, hearing, and smell. Make sure lighting is adequate. Check body areas for shape, color, symmetry, odor, and abnormalities.

To *palpate,* use the hands to assess temperature, hydration, texture, shape, size, tender areas, and pulses. Use the palms to gauge movement and vibration. Be sure to warm the hands before palpating, and keep fingernails clipped short to avoid accidental scratching. If appropriate, use distraction techniques, including conversation, to help the child relax.

To *percuss,* use tapping motions with the fingertips to produce sound waves, then evaluate the intensity, pitch, duration, and quality of the elicited sounds. Percussion sounds include:
• tympany — an intense, high-pitched, drumlike sound of moderate duration, normally heard over the stomach and gas-filled intestinal areas
• resonance — a low-pitched, hollow sound of moderate to high intensity and long duration, normally heard over the lungs
• hyperresonance — an intense, low-pitched booming sound of long duration heard over the lung fields of a young child or a patient with air trapped in the lungs
• dullness — a high-pitched sound of soft to moderate intensity and moderate duration, normally heard over the liver
• flatness — a high-pitched sound of low intensity and short duration, normally heard over muscles.

To *auscultate,* use a stethoscope to hear body sounds. Use the bell of the stethoscope to listen for low-pitched sounds, such as heart sounds; use the diaphragm (the flat part of the stethoscope) to listen for higher-pitched sounds, such as breath sounds and bowel sounds.

Examination sequence
Before proceeding with the physical examination, warm the hands and equipment, and make sure the room is comfortably warm. As appropriate, tailor the examination to the child's age. (See *Modifying the pediatric physical examination,* page 40.)

During the physical examination, gather the data described below. (For detailed procedures to follow during the physical assessment, consult a standard pediatric nursing text.)
General appearance and behavior. Determine the child's body build, size, alertness, and activity level.
Vital signs, height, weight, and head circumference. Measure the patient's temperature, heart and respiratory rates, and blood pressure (in children age 3 and over). (For normal ranges, see *Pediatric heart rate, respiratory rate, and blood pressure ranges,* page 41.)

Measure the patient's height and weight, and plot the results on a growth curve. In children from birth to age 18 months, measure head circumference and plot the result on a growth curve.
Skin. Inspect for odor, color, pigmentation, scaling, and lesions. Palpate for moistness, temperature, texture, and turgor.

Modifying the pediatric physical examination

During the physical examination, the nurse should tailor the approach, sequence, or technique to the child's age. Follow the guidelines below.

Infant

Ask the parent to remove all the infant's clothing except the diaper. Have the parent hold the infant for as much of the examination as possible. A young infant may be placed supine or prone on the parent's lap; an older infant may sit on the parent's lap.

Approach the infant quietly. If needed, use distraction, such as conversation, "peek-a-boo," or mobiles suspended over the examination area. If the infant cries, offer a bottle or pacifier, if appropriate.

Perform less disruptive examination procedures first, while the infant is cooperative. For instance, check heart and respiratory rates and auscultate the lungs, heart, and abdomen first. Examine the throat, mouth, nose, and ears last because this examination is likely to make the infant cry. During the ear examination, have the parent hold the infant firmly.

Toddler

Ask the parent to remove all the child's clothing except underpants; suggest that the toddler help with this.

Before starting the examination, show the child the equipment and allow the child to handle it.

Let the child remain close to or held by the parent. Allow the child to hold comfort objects, such as toys or a blanket. Approach the toddler quietly. Use distraction as needed, and praise cooperative behavior.

While the child is quiet and cooperative, check the heart and respiratory rates and auscultate the lungs, heart, and abdomen. Just before genital and anal examination, have the parent remove the child's underpants. Examine the throat, mouth, nose, and ears last because the toddler may protest inspection of these areas.

Preschool-age child

Ask the child to remove all clothing except underpants, and offer the child a gown. Allow the child to remain close to the parent.

Show the child the examination equipment and allow the child to handle it. Demonstrate how to listen with the stethoscope. Use games to encourage cooperation. For example, say, "Show me how you can wiggle your toes."

Proceed from head to toe; examine the genitalia last.

School-age child

Let the child decide whether the parent should be present during the examination. Ask the child to remove all clothing except underpants. Offer a gown, and allow the child to undress in privacy. Explain the purpose of the equipment and allow the child to handle it.

Proceed from head to toe, exposing only the area to be examined. Examine the genitalia last.

Adolescent

Let the adolescent decide if the parent should be present. Ask the patient to remove all clothing except underpants. Offer a gown, and allow the patient to undress in privacy. Explain the purpose of the equipment, and let the patient handle it.

Proceed from head to toe, explaining the purpose of each assessment technique. Examine the genitalia last.

Explain assessment findings. Emphasize that the adolescent is developing normally (if appropriate).

Head. Inspect the patient's head for size and shape. In an infant, assess the degree of head control and palpate fontanels and suture lines.
Scalp and hair. Inspect hair color and distribution, and check for flaking, hair loss, and scalp lesions. Assess hair texture.
Face. Inspect for symmetry of features. Percuss the sinus areas if infection or congestion is suspected.
Eyes. Inspect for size and shape, and check for epicanthal folds, wide-set eyes (hypertelorism), or close-set eyes (hypotelorism). Inspect pupils for size, shape, equality, and reactivity to light. Check the iris for color, shape, notches, spots, and irregular coloring. Inspect eyelids for ptosis (when the eyelid partially covers the pupil or lower part of the

Pediatric heart rate, respiratory rate, and blood pressure ranges

This chart shows average normal ranges for heart rate, respiratory rate, and blood pressure in pediatric patients, measured when the child is awake and quiet. Ranges may vary slightly by sex.

AGE	HEART RATE (beats/minute)	RESPIRATORY RATE (breaths/minute)	BLOOD PRESSURE (mm Hg)
Newborn (birth to 1 week)	100 to 180	35 to 60	45 to 84 systolic 40 to 70 diastolic
1 week to 3 months	100 to 200	30 to 45	65 to 110 systolic 35 to 70 diastolic
3 to 12 months	80 to 150	25 to 35	70 to 110 systolic 38 to 70 diastolic
1 to 2 years	80 to 140	25 to 30	70 to 110 systolic 38 to 70 diastolic
2 to 4 years	70 to 120	24 to 30	72 to 112 systolic 40 to 72 diastolic
4 to 6 years	70 to 110	22 to 30	75 to 115 systolic 40 to 74 diastolic
6 to 8 years	70 to 110	20 to 26	78 to 117 systolic 41 to 75 diastolic
8 to 10 years	70 to 110	20 to 26	81 to 120 systolic 45 to 78 diastolic
10 to 12 years	70 to 110	20 to 26	86 to 122 systolic 47 to 80 diastolic
12 to 14 years	70 to 105	18 to 22	90 to 128 systolic 46 to 82 diastolic
14 to 18 years	60 to 90	16 to 20	92 to 130 systolic 48 to 84 diastolic

iris), irritation, crusting, drainage, and excessive blinking. Inspect conjunctivae for color and excessive tearing.

Assess eye muscle function by having the child's eyes follow the examiner's finger. Assess visual acuity using the Denver Eye Screening Test or Snellen E test, and check for strabismus. With special training, the nurse may perform an ophthalmoscopic examination to elicit the red reflex and assess the fundus.

Ears. Inspect for size, shape, symmetry, and position. Palpate the auricle and mastoid areas and the postauricular lymph nodes.

Perform an otoscopic examination, inspecting the external canal for inflammation, color, earwax, and discharge and the tympanic mem brane for color, light reflex, bony landmarks, mobility, bulging, flatness, and retraction. Also assess the patient's auditory acuity using the sound localization, whisper, Rinne, and Weber tests.

Nose. Inspect for size, shape, mucosal color, discharge, and septum position.

Mouth. Inspect the lips for symmetry, lesions, and color; the gums for color and lesions; the tongue for color, position, shape, and movement; the teeth for number, position, and caries; and the palate for shape, color, cleft, and arch. Assess for mouth odor.

Throat. Inspect the uvula for symmetry and shape. Check the tonsils for symmetry, shape, size, color, exudate, and ulcerations.

Neck. Inspect for size, shape, masses, neck veins, and range of motion. Palpate the anterior and posterior cervical lymph nodes. Palpate the trachea for position and the thyroid for size.

Lungs and chest. Inspect the chest for shape, size, symmetry, and mobility. Check respiratory depth and rate, and auscultate breath sounds for stridor, grunting, wheezing, snoring, cough, and vocal resonance.

Palpate the supraclavicular and axillary lymph nodes. Also palpate for tactile fremitus, and check the breasts for masses, lumps, nipple discharge, and secondary sex characteristics. (For more information on adolescent sexual development, see Chapter 10, The adolescent and family.) Percuss the entire lung field.

Palpate for the point of maximal intensity and for thrills. Auscultate heart sounds for rate, rhythm, and character and for murmurs.

Abdomen. Inspect for shape and size. Check the umbilicus for color, discharge, inflammation, herniation, veins, and odor. Auscultate bowel sounds, and palpate to assess abdominal tone. Palpate the liver, spleen, kidney, and bladder for position and presence of masses. Check femoral pulses, palpate the inguinal and lymph nodes, and note any inguinal or femoral hernias. Percuss the entire abdominal area, checking organ size, percussion intensity, and pitch.

Genitalia. In a boy, inspect the penis for size, check the foreskin, note the position of the urethral meatus, inspect the scrotum for size and color, note testicle size and shape, and inspect for secondary sex characteristics. Palpate the testicles for position, hernias, and masses.

In a girl, inspect the labia and clitoris for size; check the vagina for edema, redness, discharge, and adhesions; note position of the urethra; and inspect for secondary sex characteristics. Palpate for Skene's and Bartholin's glands.

Anus and rectum. Inspect for position, and check for fissures, fistulas, hemorrhoids, prolapse, pilonidal dimple, and polyps. Palpate the sphincter for tone, and check for masses.

Musculoskeletal system. Inspect the hands for finger clubbing, polydactyly (extra fingers), and syndactyly (webbed fingers). Check the nails for shape, color, and condition; inspect palmar creases.

Check the patient's muscle strength and tone. To assess muscle strength, ask the child to grab the nurse's index and middle fingers and squeeze as hard as possible. Test flexor muscle strength by asking the child to pull the nurse's hands toward the child while the nurse resists the child's pulling. Test extensor muscle strength by asking the child to push away the nurse's hands while the nurse resists the pushing.

Inspect legs and feet for symmetry, ankle position, knock knees, bowed legs, and clubbed feet. Note the patient's gait, and assess arm and shoulder joints for mobility. Palpate for quality of popliteal and dorsal pulses and for brachial and radial pulses. Inspect hips for symmetry of the gluteal folds; inspect the back for shape and position of the spine.

Neurologic system. Check the child's speech articulation. In a child over age 5, assess cerebellar function by asking the child to hop, skip, walk heel to toe, and touch the finger to the nose with eyes closed. Use the Romberg test to evaluate coordination associated with cerebellar function. To perform the Romberg test, ask the child to stand still, with eyes closed and arms at the side; leaning indicates cerebellar dysfunction.

Assess the child's cranial nerve function. Check reflexes in infants; check deep tendon reflexes in children age 2 and over.

Check for neurologic signs in children over age 3, including short attention span, poor coordination, poor position sense, hyperactivity or hypoactivity, labile emotions, impulsiveness, distractibility, poorly defined hand preference, language and articulation difficulties, and learning problems (such as with reading, writing, and arithmetic), which may indicate brain dysfunction or other abnormality.

Environmental assessment

Because the child's environment plays an important part in shaping overall development, some health care practitioners recommend a home assessment for all high-risk children — children of adolescent mothers, those from low socioeconomic groups, and those who score poorly on developmental screening tests.

To assess the child's environment, the nurse may use the Home Observation for Measurement of the Environment (HOME), a test that assesses the quality of the home environment. Test results can help care-givers provide anticipatory guidance to help enrich the child's environment.

Summarizing assessment findings

After completing the child health assessment, document findings in the appropriate records. As appropriate, share assessment findings with parents (and possibly the older child), and identify any problem areas. Allow sufficient time to answer parents' questions. Then, together with the physician and family, devise a plan of care for managing or correcting identified problems.

STUDY ACTIVITIES

Short answer

1. What information should the nurse obtain when eliciting a mother's prenatal and childbirth history?

_____

_____

_____

2. Identify the developmental areas assessed by the DDST-R.

_____

3. Define the following terms: hypertelorism, ptosis, polydactyly, and syndactyly.

_____

_____

_____

4. Which part of the stethoscope should the nurse use to auscultate heart sounds?

_____

Multiple choice

5. Which type of sound does percussion over the stomach normally elicit?
  A. Tympany
  B. Resonance
  C. Dullness
  D. Flatness

6. A child's ability to walk heel to toe reflects:
  A. Reflex function
  B. Cerebellar function
  C. Motor function
  D. Strength

7. Craig, age 6 months, is sitting on his mother's lap. What should the nurse do before starting Craig's physical examination?
  A. Place him on the examining table.
  B. Measure his respiratory rate.
  C. Check his reflexes.
  D. Ask the mother to place him on his back.

ANSWERS   **Short answer**

1. When obtaining the mother's prenatal and childbirth history, the nurse should find out when the mother began prenatal care; how much weight she gained during pregnancy; if she experienced pregnancy complications; if she used drugs, tobacco, or alcohol during pregnancy; where labor and delivery took place; if labor was spontaneous or induced; length of labor and any medications used; delivery presentation and method; and the child's gestational age at birth.

2. The DDST-R assesses the child's personal-social, language, fine motor-adaptive, and gross motor development.

3. Hypertelorism refers to wide-set eyes. Ptosis is a condition in which the eyelid covers the pupil or lower part of the iris. Polydactyly refers to extra fingers. Syndactyly refers to webbed fingers.

4. The nurse should use the bell of the stethoscope to auscultate heart sounds.

Multiple choice

5. A. Tympany normally is heard over the stomach and gas-filled intestinal areas.

6. B. A child's ability to walk heel to toe reflects cerebellar function.

7. B. The nurse should measure the infant's respiratory rate first because the physical examination may cause discomfort that alters the respiratory rate.

CHAPTER 6

The infant and family

OBJECTIVES After studying this chapter, the reader should be able to:

  1. Identify norms for infant physical growth, gross motor development, fine motor development, language development, and social development.

  2. Describe psychosocial, psychosexual, and cognitive development in the infant.

  3. Discuss nursing interventions that promote infant growth and development.

  4. Describe how the nurse can promote optimal infant nutrition, dental health, elimination, sleep, and safety.

  5. Describe the causes and treatment of common infant skin disorders, and discuss related nursing responsibilities.

OVERVIEW OF CONCEPTS This chapter discusses major growth and developmental milestones during infancy — from birth to age 12 months. It describes the infant's psychosocial, psychosexual, and cognitive development, and explains how the nurse can help parents cope with separation anxiety. The chapter details the nurse's role in promoting infant health, such as by teaching parents about infant nutritional requirements, weaning, dental health, bowel and bladder elimination, sleep patterns, and safety. The chapter concludes by describing common infant skin disorders.

Growth and development The infant develops at an astonishing rate. Rapid physical growth is mirrored by development of motor, language, and cognitive skills. By the end of infancy, the child is capable of independent locomotion and of making needs known readily. (For physical growth and gross motor, fine motor, language, and social developmental milestones, see *Major growth and developmental milestones during infancy,* pages 47 to 49.)

Psychosocial development
According to Erik Erikson, the infant's developmental task is to acquire a sense of trust. Initially, trust develops through the relationship between infant and parent (or other caregiver). An infant whose physical and emotional needs are met consistently learns to trust that these

Major growth and developmental milestones during infancy

This chart details the major milestones a child should achieve during the first 12 months. Age parameters are based on the ages recommended for routine health and developmental screening.

AGE	PHYSICAL GROWTH	GROSS MOTOR DEVELOPMENT	FINE MOTOR DEVELOPMENT	LANGUAGE DEVELOPMENT	SOCIAL DEVELOPMENT
Birth to 1 month	*Weight:* • Birth weight averages 7 lb, 1 oz • Normal weight ranges from 5 lb, 8 oz to 9 lb, 4 oz • Typical monthly weight gain is 1 to $1\frac{1}{2}$ lb; weekly gain is 4 to 6 oz for first 6 months *Length:* • Birth length ranges from 18″ to 21″ • Typical monthly length gain is 1″ for first 6 months *Head circumference:* • Typically, head circumference increases $\frac{1}{2}$″ per month for first 6 months *Reflexes:* • Tonic neck, grasp, and Moro reflexes are present • Doll's eye and dance reflexes disappear	• Moves both sides of body equally • Momentarily lifts head off mattress • Moves head from side to side when prone • Head lags behind when infant is pulled to sitting position	• Follows object to midline	• Responds to bell • Cries when hungry or uncomfortable • Makes soft, throaty sounds	• Looks intently at people's faces
2 months	• Posterior fontanel closes	• Lifts head off mattress up to 45-degree angle • Head lag decreases	• Follows object past midline	• Makes distinct vocalizations (separate from crying), such as "ooh" and "aah"	• Exhibits social smile
4 months	• Moro and tonic neck reflexes disappear	• Lifts head off mattress up to 90-degree angle • Pushes chest off mattress using arms • Rolls over (at age 4 to 5 months) • Bears weight on legs when held in standing position • Holds head steady when in sitting position	• Follows an object through a 180-degree arc • Grasps rattle placed in hand • Brings hands to midline	• Laughs • Squeals • May demand attention by fussing • Turns to rattling sound (at 4 to 6 months)	• Stares intently at own hands • Recognizes familiar faces • Reaches out to people • Is aware of and interested in new surroundings

(continued)

Major growth and developmental milestones during infancy *(continued)*

AGE	PHYSICAL GROWTH	GROSS MOTOR DEVELOPMENT	FINE MOTOR DEVELOPMENT	LANGUAGE DEVELOPMENT	SOCIAL DEVELOPMENT
6 months	*Weight:* • Birth weight doubles by age 6 months • Average weight: 16 lb, 12 oz in boys; 15 lb, 13 oz in girls • Average monthly weight gain during first 6 to 12 months: $3/4$ lb (12 oz) *Length:* • Average length: $26\tfrac{3}{4}''$ in boys, 26″ in girls • Average monthly length gain during first 6 to 12 months: $1/2''$ *Dentition:* • Lower central incisors erupt at age 6 to 7 months, followed by upper central incisors at age 7 to 8 months)	• Sits leaning forward on hands (at age 6 to 7 months) • Bounces when held in standing position • Head lag absent when infant is pulled to sitting position	• Reaches for objects • Stares intently at objects, including small items • Has good hand-mouth coordination • Grasps feet and pulls them toward mouth • Transfers objects from one hand to other (at age 6 to 7 months) • Uses raking motion to pick up objects • Bangs objects on table	• Turns to voice • Babbles, using single syllables • Babbles in response to other's vocalizations	• Can feed self crackers • Holds bottle • Begins to fear strangers • Acquires likes and dislikes • Imitates simple activities (at age 6 to 7 months) • Plays peek-a-boo (at age 6 to 7 months)
9 months	*Dentition:* • Lower lateral incisors erupt at 9 to 10 months	• Sits with no support (at age 8 to 9 months) • Moves into sitting position from prone position (at age 9 to 10 months) • Stands while holding on to table • Pulls self to standing position from sitting position (at age 10 months) • Creeps and crawls	• Holds two objects simultaneously • Bangs objects together (at age 9 to 10 months) • Uses thumb-and-finger grasp to pick up small objects	• Babbles, combining two syllables • Imitates speech sounds • Responds to simple words, such as "no" • Responds to own name • Vocalizes "mama" and "dada" nonspecifically	• Waves good-bye • May fear going to bed and being left alone
12 months	*Weight:* • Birth weight triples by age 12 months • Average weight: 22 lb, 7 oz in boys; 9.6 g 21 lb, 2 oz in girls	• Stands unassisted briefly • "Cruises" well (walks short distances, from one piece of furniture to another)	• Puts objects in container • Holds spoon, but turns it over when bringing it to mouth	• Vocalizes "mama" and "dada" specifically • May say one word • Shakes head for "no"	• Indicates desires physically or verbally • Plays ball by rolling it to another person

Major growth and developmental milestones during infancy *(continued)*

AGE	PHYSICAL GROWTH	GROSS MOTOR DEVELOPMENT	FINE MOTOR DEVELOPMENT	LANGUAGE DEVELOPMENT	SOCIAL DEVELOPMENT
12 months *(continued)*	*Length:* • Birth length doubles by age 12 months • Average length: 30″ in boys; 29¼″ in girls *Reflexes:* • Babinski reflex disappears *Dentition:* • Upper lateral incisors erupt	• Shifts from standing to sitting position unassisted		• Responds to simple verbal commands, such as "Give it to me"	• Gives hugs • May acquire "security" object, such as blanket • Plays "patty-cake"

needs will be met. An infant whose needs are not always met, who lives in an unpredictable or disorganized environment, or who becomes frustrated with the caregiver grows mistrustful and insecure.

Psychosexual development

Sigmund Freud proposed that the infant is in the oral stage of psychosexual development, discharging tension and obtaining gratification through oral stimulation. The infant achieves oral gratification through sucking during the first 6 months and through sucking and biting during the next 6 months (after teething begins). Conflicts arise if the infant does not receive adequate oral stimulation or if biting results in food or nipple withdrawal and maternal displeasure.

Cognitive development

According to Jean Piaget's cognitive theory, the sensorimotor period of cognitive development starts at birth and ends at age 24 months. During this period, the infant learns simple coordination activities that enhance interaction with the environment. The infant takes an active role in learning by engaging others directly and manipulating the environment, and solves problems through sensory manipulation and motor activity rather than such symbolic processes as language and thought, which develop later.

The sensorimotor period is divided into substages; the discussion below focuses on the four substages that occur during infancy.

Stage 1 (birth to age 1 month): reflex use. During this stage, reflexive behavior (sucking, rooting, and grasping) establishes a pattern of infant experiences.

Stage 2 (ages 1 to 4 months): primary circular reactions. During this stage, voluntary behavior replaces reflexive behavior. The infant learns that certain behaviors elicit consistent environmental responses. For example, the infant voluntarily initiates sucking and grasping to elicit a desired response. However, the behavior itself brings more pleasure than the response it elicits.

Stage 3 (ages 4 to 8 months): secondary circular reactions. During this stage, primary circular reactions evolve into secondary circular reactions. Grasping behavior progresses to reaching, shaking, and banging. The response elicited (such as noise) brings as much pleasure as the behavior itself. The infant also develops the concept of object permanency, remembering that an object continues to exist even when out of sight.

Stage 4 (ages 9 to 12 months): coordination of secondary schemas and application to new situations. During this stage, behavior becomes intentional. The infant searches for hidden objects and tries to remove barriers that prevent goal achievement. The infant now associates certain words, such as "bye-bye" and "night-night," with specific events. Advancing motor development allows the infant to explore the environment actively.

Enhancing infant growth and development

To help parents provide an environment that promotes optimal infant growth and development, the nurse should offer anticipatory guidance. (See *Teaching parents to promote infant growth and development.*) The nurse also can help parents cope with such concerns as separation anxiety, fear of strangers, and thumb-sucking or pacifier use.

Coping with separation anxiety and fear of strangers

Fear of strangers begins at about age 6 months, when the infant is able to distinguish familiar people from strangers. Separation anxiety begins at about age 8 months, when the infant develops object permanence. Now realizing that the mother has not disappeared permanently when not in sight, the infant misses her and strongly protests her absence.

Teach parents that fear of strangers and separation anxiety are signs of a healthy parent-child relationship, indicating that the infant has learned to trust the parents to meet physical and emotional needs. If the parents are distressed about these new behaviors, reassure them that crying and clinging during separation are normal, healthy infant behaviors. Also teach parents the following strategies to help the infant cope with separation and minimize associated distress:

• Use a regular baby-sitter with whom the infant can become familiar. If this is not possible, limit the number of baby-sitters.
• Before leaving, hold the infant briefly and say, "I'm going out for a little while." Then say good-bye to the infant and go quickly. Do not return if the infant protests.
• Instruct the baby-sitter to reassure the infant after you leave.
• When you return, approach the infant with a hug or kiss.

With repeated short separations, the infant learns that the parents will return. Eventually, protest behavior subsides.

Teaching parents to promote infant growth and development

For optimal growth and development, the infant needs certain types of stimulation at appropriate ages. This chart presents anticipatory guidance the nurse can offer to help parents provide such stimulation.

GROWTH AND DEVELOPMENT AREA	AGE	PARENT TEACHING
Gross and fine motor development	• Birth to 1 month	• Place infant in various positions (such as prone and supine). Provide visual stimulation using mobiles and pictures of human faces.
	• 2 to 4 months	• Place infant in various positions, including upright in infant seat. Provide visual stimulation. Stimulate grasping behavior.
	• 4 to 8 months	• Provide play materials (such as rattles, brightly colored blocks, large ball, and unbreakable mirror). Stimulate weight-bearing and bouncing (such as by holding infant upright). Stimulate reaching by holding brightly colored objects in front of infant. Stimulate creeping by placing infant in prone position with brightly colored object just out of reach, and encourage infant to move toward object. Place infant on floor for unrestricted large motor activity.
	• 8 to 12 months	• Provide play materials (such as nesting blocks, jack-in-the-box, brightly colored blocks, or large balls). Place infant on floor for unrestricted large motor activity. Provide objects (such as low tables and chairs) that infant can use to pull self to standing position.
Language development	• Birth to 12 months	• Talk to infant, call infant by name, and repeat infant's laugh. • Laugh with infant. • Change voice inflections to reflect emotion. • Provide music box. • Name objects in environment. • Read to infant.
Social development	• Birth to 6 months	• Take infant along during household chores, social outings, and neighborhood errands. Respond positively to infant's smile and vocalizations.
	• 6 to 12 months	• Continue above activities. Play "peek-a-boo." Begin interactive play (such as playing with ball and playing "patty-cake"). Encourage infant to imitate activities; for example, allow infant to play with large spoon and bowl when parent is cooking.
Psychosocial-psychosexual development	Birth to 12 months	• Consistently meet infant's needs. • Respond to infant's cries. Learn to differentiate among types of infant cries (such as those that indicate wetness, discomfort, and hunger), and respond appropriately. • Provide sufficient sucking time (infant may need pacifier). • Provide teething ring for older infant. • Talk to infant. • Hold infant when distressed. • Swaddle, bundle, stroke, or rock infant.
Cognitive development	• Birth to 12 months	• Provide enriching environment.
	• Birth to 4 months	• Provide play activities using bells, rattles, mobiles, and unbreakable mirrors.
	• 4 to 8 months	• Provide play activities using rattles, bells, and squeaky toys. Play "peek-a-boo."
	• 8 to 12 months	• Provide play activities using push/pull toys and jack-in-the-box. Play "search for the hidden toy."

Teaching about thumb-sucking and pacifier use

Before attempting to provide anticipatory guidance, explore the parents' beliefs about thumb-sucking and pacifier use. For instance, some parents believe thumb-sucking causes crooked teeth or pacifier use is unattractive.

If parents are concerned about the dental effects of thumb-sucking, inform them that thumb-sucking during infancy will not damage teeth; however, if it persists beyond age 4, it may promote malocclusion. Some practitioners believe that allowing pacifier use during early infancy decreases the incidence of thumb-sucking. Also, because pacifier use can be interrupted more easily than thumb-sucking, it may be preferred.

Be sure to explain that sucking is an important activity during the first 6 months and should not be thwarted. If parents strongly disapprove of pacifier use, inform them they may discard the pacifier when the infant is 6 months old; at this age, the infant can obtain oral gratification by biting and eating solid foods.

Encourage parents to increase the infant's sucking pleasure by prolonging feeding times. For example, suggest that a breast-feeding mother allow the infant to suckle longer, even after the infant has emptied the breast. For a bottle-fed infant, suggest parents use stiff, small-holed nipples that require stronger sucking and prolong the feeding.

Also explore patterns of pacifier use. For example, if parents offer the pacifier every time the child whimpers, point out that this practice may lead to excessive or continuous pacifier use. Suggest alternate comfort measures, such as holding, to relieve the infant's distress.

Promoting infant health

Advise parents on how to maintain wholesome patterns of infant nutrition, dental health, elimination, and sleep. Also teach them how to ensure infant safety and how to manage common skin problems.

Providing nutritional guidance

Breast milk is the most desirable food during the first 6 months; the breast-fed infant requires no nutritional supplements except fluoride (0.25 mg/day). If the mother wishes to discontinue breast-feeding before the infant is 12 months old, instruct her to provide a commercial iron-fortified infant formula.

If the mother has chosen not to breast-feed, recommend an iron-fortified infant formula. Depending on the local water supply, the formula-fed infant may need fluoride supplements. (For fluoride recommendations, see Chapter 7, The toddler and family.)

Most practitioners recommend giving breast milk or infant formula until the infant is 12 months old. However, the American Academy of Pediatrics found no harmful effects associated with using cow's milk after six months. However, recent research has demonstrated significantly lower levels of serum ferritin at age 1 year in infants receiving whole milk when compared to those on iron-fortified formula.

Instruct parents and other caregivers to hold a bottle-fed infant during feedings. Caution them not to "prop" the bottle because this may lead to aspiration, promote middle ear infection, and contribute to dental caries after the teeth have erupted. Also, emphasize that bottle propping is not conducive to close human contact, which the infant requires to mature physically and emotionally.

Calorie and fluid requirements

During the first 6 months, the infant requires 110 calories/kg/day (50 calories/lb/day) and at least 130 ml water/kg/day. Full-term infants typically consume at least 24 oz of breast milk or formula daily; few need more than 32 oz. Because of gastrointestinal immaturity and the risk of developing food allergies, urge parents not to introduce solid foods until the infant is at least 4 months old.

Feeding schedule

Most practitioners recommend feeding on demand — when the infant shows signs of hunger. A breast-fed neonate may feed every 2 to 3 hours; a bottle-fed neonate, every 3 to 4 hours.

Recommend that parents feed the infant no more often than every 2 hours. Instruct them to offer a pacifier to soothe a fussy baby between feedings. By age 6 weeks, most infants settle into a schedule of feeding every 4 to 5 hours during the day and every 5 to 6 hours at night.

Introducing solid foods

Solid foods may be introduced when the infant is 4 to 6 months old, beginning with spoon-fed, iron-fortified infant rice cereal. Tell parents that before becoming accustomed to spoon feeding, an infant may thrust out the tongue with each spoonful.

Once iron-fortified cereal is established in the infant's diet, supplemental iron may be discontinued and fruits or vegetables may be added. Instruct parents to introduce new foods, one at a time, at 4- to 7-day intervals to help identify any food allergies. Commercially prepared or home-prepared infant food may be used. For home preparation, recommend steaming fresh fruits and vegetables in small amounts of water, then pureeing them in a blender or food processor. Soft foods, such as bananas, may simply be mashed with a fork. Instruct parents to refrigerate prepared food or to freeze serving-size portions for later use.

After cereal, fruits, and vegetables are established firmly in the infant's diet, parents may add cheeses, yogurt, egg yolk, and meats. Instruct them to avoid adding salt or sugar to infant food. (For details on an appropriate diet for an infant, see *Typical diet for an infant,* page 54.)

Weaning an infant from breast or bottle

The best time to wean an infant from the breast or bottle to cup feeding depends on both the infant's psychological readiness and the parents' wishes. Most infants show signs of readiness to wean between ages 6 and 12 months. Such signs include reluctance to lie still for an

Typical diet for an infant

During the first 6 months, the infant should receive breast milk (if possible) and fluoride supplements. Initially, the infant typically feeds 8 to 10 times daily, then progresses to 6 times daily.

If the mother chooses not to breast-feed, instruct parents to give the infant 24 to 32 oz of a commercially prepared, iron-fortified infant formula or evaporated milk formula (diluted with water and with corn syrup added to provide additional carbohydrates) daily, plus fluoride (in areas without fluorinated public water). The infant receiving evaporated milk also should receive iron and vitamin C supplements.

Infants ages 6 to 12 months should receive breast milk, commercial infant formula, or evaporated milk formula, along with a fluoride supplement, as prescribed. As the infant's solid food intake increases, milk should be limited to 24 to 30 oz/day. The infant also may receive fruit juice (4 to 6 oz/day), starting with infant apple juice at 4 to 6 months.

Solid foods should be introduced in serving sizes of 1 tablespoon, progressing to 3 to 4 tablespoons. Teach parents to introduce one new solid food at a time, at 4- to 7-day intervals. Solid foods may include:

- iron-fortified rice cereal, introduced at 4 to 6 months in one to two daily servings, mixed with breast milk, formula, or apple juice
- pureed fruits, introduced at 4 to 6 months in one to two daily servings, starting with bananas, applesauce, and pears
- pureed vegetables, introduced at 4 to 6 months in one to two daily servings, beginning with carrots, squash, and sweet potatoes
- egg yolk (boiled and mashed, or soft-cooked), introduced at 6 months, up to three weekly servings. Egg whites should be delayed until age 9 months because of possible food allergy.
- cheese (as a substitute for one meat serving), introduced after cereal, fruit, and vegetable consumption is established. Cottage cheese can be given until the infant's chewing is established; it may be mixed with fruit.
- yogurt, introduced after cereal, fruit, and vegetable consumption is established. Yogurt may replace one daily meat serving and may be mixed with fruit.
- meat, introduced in one to two daily servings after cereal, fruit, and vegetable consumption is established.

entire bottle feeding, desire to carry the bottle around the house instead of sitting and drinking, and desire to imitate adults by drinking from a cup.

Teach parents to begin weaning slowly — for example, first eliminating one bottle- or breast-feeding session daily (whichever one the infant seems least interested in). Over the next few weeks, parents may eliminate additional bottle- or breast-feeding sessions. Generally, the nighttime feeding is the last to be discontinued.

If parents wish to wean a breast-fed infant before age 6 months, instruct them to switch to bottle feedings rather than cup feedings to satisfy the infant's sucking needs and maintain nutrition. (Formula consumption decreases when an infant switches to cup feedings.) Infants over age 6 months can be switched to cup feedings if they also consume sufficient amounts of solid foods.

Ensuring dental health

Oral hygiene practices should begin as soon as the infant's first teeth erupt. Teach parents to clean the infant's teeth and gums by wiping them with a soft, damp cloth; toothbrushes and toothpaste are too harsh for an infant's tender gums.

The first primary teeth — the lower central incisors — typically appear at age 6 to 7 months, followed by eruption of the upper central incisors at ages 7 to 8 months. Usually, the lower lateral incisors erupt at ages 9 to 10 months, followed by the upper lateral incisors by age 12 months. However, be aware that timing of tooth eruption varies; the ages given above are approximate.

To help build caries-resistant teeth, make sure parents provide appropriate fluoride supplementation. Counsel them to avoid propping a bottle for feedings or putting the infant to bed with a bottle because the contents pool in the mouth and may cause dental caries.

Coping with teething pain

When teething, most infants display such behaviors as increased drooling, finger-sucking, and biting. Some tolerate teething well; others become irritable and may have trouble eating and sleeping.

Counsel parents to soothe the infant's tender gums by providing a frozen teething ring. Instruct them to administer acetaminophen if teething pain interferes with eating or sleeping.

Teaching about bowel and bladder elimination

The neonate's first stools (meconium) are dark green to black, sticky, and odorless. Meconium stools are present for the first 3 days after birth, then change to transitional stools (yellow-green) by the fourth day.

After 7 days, bowel elimination patterns depend on the diet. Breast-fed infants have bright yellow or light green stools that are soft but not watery, with no offensive odor. Some breast-fed babies have a bowel movement after every feeding; others, every other day. Both patterns are considered normal.

Formula-fed infants typically have pale yellow, semi-formed stools with a stronger odor. Generally, they have one to three bowel movements per day. Green, watery stools indicate diarrhea. Instruct parents to notify the physician if the infant has two or three such watery stools because dehydration may occur quickly. The physician may suggest substituting an oral electrolyte solution, such as Pedialyte, for infant formula until diarrhea subsides.

Urine elimination is considered adequate if the infant wets six to eight diapers per day. Urine should be pale yellow and odorless. Dark yellow urine with a strong odor indicates insufficient water intake and the need for supplemental water.

Teaching about infant sleep patterns

Counsel parents to be sensitive to the infant's developing sleep-and-awake cycle and urge them to schedule activities accordingly.

During their first few months, infants sleep about 20 hours per day. By age 6 months, sleep decreases to an average of 16 hours per day; by age 12 months, to 12 to 14 hours.

By age 4 months, most infants can sleep at least 6 continuous hours during the night and have settled into a pattern of two daytime naps — one in the morning and one in the afternoon. By age 12 months, most infants need only one daily nap.

Sleep patterns depend on both infant temperament and feeding pattern. Active infants seem to require less sleep than placid ones; formula-fed infants sleep longer than breast-fed infants.

Teach parents that infant sleep patterns vary. However, mention that by age 4 months, most infants should sleep 6 to 8 hours during the night without awakening. Nonetheless, some may continue to awaken during the night for feeding. After age 6 months, few infants need a nighttime feeding; those who do seem to have established a pattern of nighttime awakening. To overcome nighttime awakening, suggest parents use the following strategies:

• Feed the infant as late as possible at night to delay the time of awakening.

• When the infant awakens, enter the room and reassure the infant by patting the infant on the back — but do not take the infant out of the crib or give a bottle. After a few minutes, leave the room. If the infant cries, wait 5 minutes before reentering the room, then offer reassurance again. On subsequent nights, allow the infant to cry for progressively longer periods. By the end of the first week, most infants will sleep through the night. (This technique also may be effective for infants who begin to awaken during the night after achieving uninterrupted nighttime sleep.) This technique is considered controversial by some experts.

• Have the infant sleep in a separate room from the parents.

• To help teach the infant that the crib is for sleeping and that the infant can fall asleep without the parent's presence, place the infant in the crib while awake but ready for sleep. Do not rock the infant to sleep because this may result in refusal to fall asleep without being rocked and the need to be rocked again after awakening in the middle of the night.

Promoting safety

Most infant accidents occur in the home. The accident rate rises with progressive motor development. The leading cause of fatal injury during infancy is aspiration of foreign substances. Other causes include suffocation, falls, motor vehicle injuries, and burns. Instruct parents to anticipate — and avoid — such hazards. (For specific points to cover, see *Infant safety guidelines.*)

Infant safety guidelines

To help guard against injury and ensure infant safety, provide the following instructions to parents.

Preventing aspiration of foreign substances
- Keep small objects out of the infant's reach.
- Avoid using powder during diaper changes.
- Inspect all toys — especially stuffed animals — for loose, removable parts.
- Do not feed the infant raisins, grapes, seeded foods, hard candy, nuts, or sliced hot dogs.
- Place the infant in a semi-reclining position during feedings.
- Avoid propping the formula bottle or cutting large holes in the nipple.
- Do not let the infant handle balloons.

Preventing suffocation
- Keep plastic bags out of the infant's reach.
- Make sure crib slats are no more than $2\frac{3}{8}''$ apart and the mattress fits the crib tightly.
- Do not put the infant to sleep in your bed.
- Do not use down-filled comforters on the infant's bed.
- Keep all appliance doors closed.

Preventing drowning
- Do not leave buckets of water unattended.
- Keep bathroom doors closed to prevent the infant from drowning in the toilet.
- Do not leave the infant unattended during baths.

Preventing falls
- Keep the sides of the crib up and securely fastened. Once the infant can sit up, lower the crib mattress to the lowest position.
- Remove bumper pads and large toys from the crib when the infant reaches age 6 months because the infant can use these to climb out of the crib.
- Strap the infant securely in an infant seat. Place the infant seat on the floor — never on a table or counter (unless directly supervised).
- Never leave an unrestrained infant on a changing table.
- Restrain the infant securely in a high chair or stroller.
- Open windows no more than 4″ if the infant is capable of climbing onto the window sill.
- Use safety gates on stairwells.
- Avoid using infant walkers because these can tip easily.

Preventing motor vehicle injuries
- Use only a federally approved infant car seat. Position an infant weighing less than 17 lb (7.7 kg) facing the rear of the vehicle; position a heavier infant facing the front.
- Do not place the infant's stroller behind parked cars.
- Do not leave the infant unattended while outdoors.

Preventing burns
- Install smoke detectors in the home, and test batteries regularly.
- Set the hot water heater at a temperature no higher than 120° F (48.8° C).
- Use cool-mist, not hot-water, vaporizers.
- Do not drink coffee or other hot liquids while holding the infant.
- Do not warm infant bottles in a microwave oven because this may cause uneven heat dispersion.
- Check the temperature of warmed bottles before giving them to the infant.
- Place safety guards in front of hot radiators, fireplaces, and space heaters.
- Keep electrical appliances out of the infant's reach; dangling cords from hot irons or curling irons are especially dangerous.
- Place covers over unused electrical outlets.
- Apply sunscreen to the infant before going outdoors.

Managing common skin problems

Common skin problems in infants include diaper dermatitis, atopic dermatitis, and seborrheic dermatitis. The nurse should offer parents guidance to prevent or eliminate these conditions.

Diaper dermatitis

Commonly called diaper rash, diaper dermatitis most often results from prolonged skin contact with urine or feces or from sensitivity to plastic, rubber, disposable diapers, or laundry products. Irritation causes skin reddening, possibly with scaling and ulceration. Characteristic signs of diaper rash include erythema; papules, vesicles, or ulcerations; and burned or scalded appearance of the skin.

Diaper rash almost always can be eliminated and its recurrence prevented. First, obtain a careful history to help identify the cause of the infant's rash. For example, if the family recently switched to another brand of disposable diaper, laundry detergent, or fabric softener, the probable cause of the rash is contact irritation, which can be eliminated by avoiding the offending product.

If the probable cause of the rash is irritation from feces or urine, treatment depends on severity of the rash. For mild irritation, (indicated by erythema alone), suggest parents change the infant's diaper after each voiding or bowel movement and, if needed, gently clean the diaper area with warm water and mild soap (not commercial diaper wipes). Instruct them to apply a water barrier ointment (such as petroleum jelly or zinc oxide) with each diaper change.

For moderate irritation (indicated by erythema and papules), instruct parents to keep the diaper area meticulously clean and dry, using the measures described above; to apply 1% hydrocortisone cream three times daily to the diaper area; to expose the diaper area to air by leaving diapers off for 30-minute periods (for example, at nap time); and to use cloth diapers without rubber pants until the rash clears.

For severe irritation (indicated by erythema, vesicles, and ulcerations), instruct parents to keep the diaper area meticulously clean and dry and to apply Neosporin-G cream to the diaper area three times daily.

To prevent the rash from recurring, instruct parents to change diapers frequently, clean the diaper area thoroughly with each change, avoid commercial diaper wipes if they cause irritation, avoid powders and cornstarch, and apply a water barrier ointment. If detergents cause irritation, recommend a mild detergent (such as Ivory Snow) for laundering cloth diapers. Advise parents to avoid bleach, fabric softeners, and softening sheets if these cause irritation. Instruct them to rinse diapers twice.

If the infant wears disposable diapers, urge parents to switch brands if sensitivity develops. Instruct them to fold the plastic section away from contact with the infant's skin.

One form of diaper dermatitis results from *Candida albicans*. This fungal infection causes a shiny, bright red, beefy-looking rash with sharply defined edges and satellite papules or pustules. To eliminate this rash, instruct parents to apply Lotrimin or Nystatin ointment sparingly three times daily, keep the diaper area dry at all times, avoid using rubber pants and plastic-backed disposable diapers, avoid other ointments and powders until the infection clears, and wash their hands carefully after each diaper change. (*Candida* organisms may be transmitted by direct contact).

Atopic dermatitis

Also called infant eczema, atopic dermatitis is a collective term for a group of skin conditions with certain common characteristics. *Acute eczema* is characterized by pruritus, erythema, vesicles, exudate, and crusting. *Chronic eczema* is characterized by pruritus, dryness, scaling, and skin thickening.

Eczema appears in various forms in infants, children, and adolescents. *Infantile eczema* typically begins between ages 2 and 6 months; in about half the cases, it resolves by age 3. It is marked by acute exacerbation of skin lesions, most commonly on the cheeks, forehead, scalp, and extensor surfaces of the arms and legs.

Childhood eczema begins between ages 4 and 10, although it also may follow infantile eczema. The rash is less likely to be exudative and crusty than infantile eczema, and more often causes chronic symptoms. Common areas of involvement include the wrists, ankles, and antecubital and popliteal areas.

Adolescent eczema and *adult eczema* may follow childhood eczema or may develop as a new problem. In adolescent eczema, characteristics of chronic eczema predominate; lesions most commonly appear on the face, neck, back, upper portions of the arms, and dorsal areas of the hands, feet, fingers, and toes.

Roughly 70% of children with atopic dermatitis have a family history of allergies (such as allergic rhinitis or hay fever), asthma, or eczema. Children with eczema also are at greater risk for hay fever and asthma.

Although atopic dermatitis is not easily cured, it can be controlled with appropriate management. Treatment of acute eczema involves wet compresses, topical steroids, and systemic antihistamines. Cool, wet compresses help dry weeping lesions, aid removal of crusty lesions, and reduce itching. Instruct parents to soak thin strips of cloth (such as from bedsheets or handkerchiefs) in Burow's solution (available without prescription) or in cool, clean tap water, and then apply the wet cloths for 10 minutes over affected areas four times daily. To reduce inflammation and itching, instruct them to apply 1% hydrocortisone cream sparingly on affected areas three times daily. If prescribed, teach them to administer a systemic antihistamine (such as diphenhydramine hydrochloride [Benadryl] 5 mg/kg/day) to treat severe pruritus or pruritus that interferes with sleep. Minimizing pruritus is important because scratching may lead to secondary bacterial infection.

Treatment of chronic eczema involves skin hydration, lubrication, topical steroids, and avoidance of aggravating factors. Instruct parents to bathe the child at least three times weekly, using warm (not hot) water and mild soap (such as Aveena, Neutrogena, or Dove). Tell them to apply lubricating lotion (such as Lubriderm or Nutraderm) two to three times daily and after each bath. Advise them to apply topical steroid ointments, as prescribed, to thickened skin areas three times daily. Suggest humidifying house air to reduce skin drying. To prevent skin irritation and subsequent itching, caution against using harsh laundry detergents and dressing the infant in rough-textured, scratchy clothing.

Seborrheic dermatitis

Commonly called cradle cap, seborrheic dermatitis is an inflammatory, scaling rash of the scalp. The condition also may affect the eyelids (blepharitis), external ear canal, and inguinal region. The cause is unknown but may be related to accelerated epidermal growth. Incidence is highest during infancy and adolescence.

Clinical manifestations of seborrheic dermatitis include pruritus; yellowish, greasy scaling of the scalp or other body areas; dandruff-like flaking; and mild to severe erythema.

Treatment involves frequent lubrication and cleansing of the scalp or other affected area. Instruct parents to rub petroleum jelly into the infant's scalp to soften the crusts, leave the jelly in place for 30 minutes, and then clean the scalp and hair thoroughly with baby shampoo. Afterward, they should remove loose scales with a soft brush or fine-toothed comb. Teach parents to repeat this procedure once daily until the scalp is clear. Thereafter, they should shampoo the infant's scalp and hair at least once a week. Reassure parents that they can safely wash over the infant's "soft spot."

If inflammation is present, advise them to apply 1% hydrocortisone cream once daily to the child's scalp. If scaling is present on the eyelids, instruct them to apply warm, moist compresses to the eyelids three times daily and, if prescribed, to apply sulfacetamide sodium (Sodium Sulamyd) at night to remove scales and crusts.

STUDY ACTIVITIES

Short answer

1. Identify at least five behaviors or activities parents can use to foster the development of trust in their infant.

_____

_____

_____

2. What strategies can parents use to ease infant distress during separation?

_____

_____

_____

3. Discuss recommendations for weaning an infant from breast- or bottle-feeding to cup feeding.

_____

_____

_____

4. Identify at least five instructions the nurse should give parents to help prevent infant injury.

_____

_____

_____

5. To prevent recurrence of diaper rash, what measures should the nurse suggest to parents?

_____

_____

_____

Multiple choice

6. A neonate's first bowel movements are:
   A. Yellowish-green and soft
   B. Dark green to black and sticky
   C. Brown and semi-formed
   D. Yellow and seedy

7. Most infants can sit unsupported at what age?
   A. 4 months
   B. 6 months
   C. 8 months
   D. 10 months

8. An infant's birth weight should double by what age?
   A. 4 months
   B. 6 months
   C. 8 months
   D. 10 months

9. Which meal plan is most appropriate for a 6-month-old infant?
   A. Breakfast: rice cereal, apple sauce, 6 oz of infant formula
   Lunch: sliced hot dog, peas, 6 oz of infant formula
   Snack: cracker
   Dinner: carrots, 6 oz of infant formula
   P.M.: 6 oz of infant formula
   B. Breakfast: rice cereal, 8 oz of infant formula
   Snack: half a mashed banana
   Lunch: cottage cheese, peaches, 6 oz of infant formula
   Snack: 6 oz of fruit juice
   Dinner: squash, rice cereal, 6 oz of infant formula
   P.M.: 8 oz of infant formula
   C. Breakfast: half an egg, scrambled; pears; 6 oz of infant formula
   Lunch: Spaghettios, 6 oz of infant formula
   Snack: 6 oz of juice
   Dinner: rice cereal, green beans, 6 oz of infant formula
   P.M.: 8 oz of infant formula
   D. Breakfast: 8 oz of infant formula
   Snack: cracker, 8 oz of infant formula
   Lunch: rice cereal, plums
   Snack: 8 oz of infant formula
   Dinner: rice cereal, carrots, 8 oz of infant formula
   P.M.: 8 oz of infant formula

10. Marie Santorelli reports that Lorrie, her 5-month-old daughter, has diaper rash. After removing Lorrie's diaper, the nurse notes that the diaper area is red, with numerous small papular lesions. Which management strategy would be appropriate?
   A. Apply petroleum jelly to the lesions.
   B. Apply 1% hydrocortisone cream to the entire diaper area.
   C. Apply bacitracin ointment to the entire diaper area.
   D. Apply Lotrimin cream to the entire diaper area.

11. Where does infantile eczema most commonly appear?
   A. On the buttocks
   B. On the back
   C. On the cheeks
   D. On the scalp

12. During a clinic visit, Anne Peterson reports that her daughter Amanda, age 6 weeks, appears to have dandruff. During inspection, the nurse notes greasy, scaly patches on the top of Amanda's scalp. Which response by the nurse would be appropriate?

    A. "Infants don't get dandruff. Have you been washing the baby's hair?"

    B. "I see what you mean. This happens often in infants. I can tell you how to reduce the scaling."

    C. "That isn't dandruff, but it's nothing to worry about. Daily bathing should take care of the problem."

    D. "The baby does seem to have something wrong with her scalp. You can try rubbing petroleum jelly into her scalp to decrease flaking."

ANSWERS   Short answer

1. To foster trust in an infant, parents should meet the infant's needs consistently; respond to the infant's cries; learn to differentiate among the types of infant cries and respond appropriately; provide sufficient sucking time or offer a pacifier; provide a teething ring for an older infant; talk to the infant; hold a distressed infant; swaddle or bundle a young infant; stroke the infant; and rock the infant.

2. To reduce separation anxiety, parents should consistently use a baby-sitter with whom the infant is familiar or limit the number of baby-sitters; before leaving, hold the infant briefly and tell the infant the parent is going out for a short period, say good-bye to the infant, then quickly leave and avoid returning if the infant protests; have the baby-sitter reassure infant when the parent leaves; and hug or kiss the infant upon returning.

3. To wean an infant, parents should look for signs that the infant is ready to wean, such as reluctance to lie still for an entire bottle feeding, desire to carry the bottle around the house instead of sitting and drinking, and imitating adults by drinking from a cup. Parents should begin weaning gradually, eliminating one bottle- or breast-feeding session every few days (the one the infant is least interested in). Over the next few weeks, they should eliminate additional bottle- or breast-feeding sessions.

4. To help prevent infant injury, the nurse should teach parents to keep plastic bags out of the infant's reach; make sure crib slats are no more than $2\frac{3}{8}''$ apart; make sure the infant's mattress fits the crib tightly; avoid putting the infant to sleep in their bed; avoid using down-filled comforters on the infant's bed; keep appliance doors closed; never leave buckets of water unattended; keep bathroom doors closed; and stay with the infant during bath time.

5. To prevent diaper rash from recurring, parents should change diapers frequently; clean the diaper area thoroughly with each diaper change; avoid commercial diaper wipes if they cause irritation; avoid powders and cornstarch; apply a water barrier ointment; use a mild detergent; avoid bleach, fabric softeners, and softening sheets; rinse diapers twice; and keep plastic pants and plastic parts of disposable diapers away from the infant's skin.

Multiple choice

6. B. Meconium stools are dark green to black in color and sticky.

7. C. Most infants can sit unsupported at age 8 months.

8. B. Birth weight should double by age 6 months.

9. B. This meal plan includes appropriate foods and the correct fluid intake for a 6-month-old infant. A is an inappropriate meal plan because a hot dog should never be given to a 6-month-old infant because of possible aspiration. C is inappropriate because an infant of this age should not consume egg whites to minimize chances of allergy. D includes excessive formula intake.

10. B. Lorrie's signs suggest moderate diaper rash caused by chemical irritation, which can be treated with 1% hydrocortisone cream.

11. C. Infantile eczema most commonly appears on the infant's face, including the cheeks.

12. B. Amanda's signs indicate seborrheic dermatitis. Fairly common in infants, this condition can be treated effectively.

CHAPTER 7

The toddler and family

OBJECTIVES

After studying this chapter, the reader should be able to:

1. Identify the norms for a toddler's physical growth, gross motor development, fine motor development, language development, and social development.

2. Describe psychosocial, psychosexual, and cognitive development in the toddler.

3. Discuss nursing interventions that promote the toddler's growth and development.

4. Describe nursing interventions that enhance the toddler's health, including those related to nutrition, bowel and bladder elimination, dental health, sleep, and safety.

5. Describe the nurse's role in preventing lead poisoning.

OVERVIEW OF CONCEPTS

This chapter discusses major growth and developmental milestones during the toddler period — from age 12 to 36 months. It describes the toddler's psychosocial, psychosexual, and cognitive development, and discusses ways parents can establish discipline. Then, the chapter details the nurse's role in promoting the toddler's health, including nutritional guidelines and strategies to prevent iron-deficiency anemia, promote proper sleep patterns, and prevent lead poisoning.

Growth and development

During the toddler period, physical growth slows while motor, language, and cognitive development progresses rapidly. (For growth and developmental milestones attained during the toddler period, see *Major growth and developmental milestones in toddlers,* pages 66 and 67.)

Psychosocial development

According to Erik Erikson, the toddler's developmental task is to achieve autonomy while overcoming shame and doubt. The toddler strives to control body functions (such as by toileting), learns to do things unassisted, and differentiates self from others. Doing things unassisted and exploring the environment help the child develop a sense of autonomy. Shame and doubt develop if the toddler cannot perform self-

Major growth and developmental milestones in toddlers

This chart details the major milestones a toddler should achieve.

AGE	PHYSICAL GROWTH	GROSS MOTOR DEVELOPMENT	FINE MOTOR DEVELOPMENT	LANGUAGE DEVELOPMENT	SOCIAL DEVELOPMENT
15 months	• Steady growth: Average weight gain: 5 to 8 oz/month; average height gain: $1/2''$/month • Average weight: 24 lb (boys); $22\frac{1}{2}$ lb (girls) • Average height: 31" (boys); $30\frac{3}{4}''$ (girls) *Dentition:* • First-year molars erupt • 12 teeth total	• Walks well • Bends over to pick up objects • Creeps up stairs	• Scribbles • Places objects in containers	• Has vocabulary of 4 to 6 words • Understands simple commands • Asks for objects by pointing	• Starts to imitate others • Drinks well from a cup • May discard bottle • Shows less fear of strangers
18 months	• Steady growth continues • Average weight: $25\frac{1}{4}$ lb (boys); $23\frac{3}{4}$ lb (girls) • Average height: $32\frac{1}{2}''$ (boys); 32" (girls) *Dentition:* • Four cuspids erupt • 16 teeth total	• Walks backward • Begins to run • Walks up stairs with assistance	• Can build a tower of two cubes • Uses a spoon well	• Has a vocabulary of 6 to 10 words	• Imitates others • Uses spoon and cup when eating • May assist with undressing (shoes, socks) • May have temper tantrums
24 months	• Steady growth continues • Average weight: $27\frac{1}{2}$ lb (boys); $26\frac{1}{2}$ lb (girls) • Average height: $34\frac{1}{2}''$ (boys); 34" (girls) *Dentition:* • One or more second-year molars may erupt • 16 to 18 teeth total	• Jumps in place with feet together • Throws ball overhand • Walks up stairs unassisted • Runs fairly well	• Can build tower of six cubes • Turns doorknob • Unscrews simple lids	• Has vocabulary of up to 250 words • Points to pictures • Combines two words • Uses pronouns "I," "me," and "you" • States first name • Verbalizes physical needs (such as hunger, sleepiness, and toileting needs)	• Feeds doll • Can put on simple clothing unassisted • May have temper tantrums

Major growth and developmental milestones in toddlers (continued)

AGE	PHYSICAL GROWTH	GROSS MOTOR DEVELOPMENT	FINE MOTOR DEVELOPMENT	LANGUAGE DEVELOPMENT	SOCIAL DEVELOPMENT
30 months	• Steady growth continues • Birth weight quadruples • Average weight: $30\frac{1}{4}$ lb (boys); $28\frac{1}{2}$ lb (girls) • Average height: $36\frac{1}{2}''$ (boys); $36''$ (girls) *Dentition:* • Second-year molars complete • Primary dentition complete • 20 teeth total	• Can jump off surfaces close to floor	• Holds pencil or crayon with fingers rather than fist	• Has vocabulary of about 400 words • Can state first and last names • Uses plurals • Begins to ask questions • Combines three words	• Washes and dries hands • Brushes teeth with assistance • Has fewer temper tantrums

care independently, if exploration is thwarted, or if the child's efforts are ridiculed.

The toddler shows characteristic behaviors that represent attempts to control the environment. These behaviors include:
• negativism — saying "no" in response to requests
• ritualism — relying on routines, such as at bedtime
• defiance — refusing to follow commands
• willfulness — being stubborn and insisting on doing things the child's way
• dawdling — responding slowly and offering excuses.

Psychosexual development
According to Sigmund Freud, the toddler is in the anal/sensory stage, showing great interest in bowel and bladder functions and experiencing conflict during toilet training. The toddler must choose between the physical pleasure derived from involuntary bowel evacuation and the emotional reinforcement derived by the parents' approval when the child voluntarily evacuates the bowel into the toilet.

Cognitive development
According to Jean Piaget, from age 12 to 24 months, the toddler completes the last two substages of the sensorimotor phase of cognitive development — tertiary circular reactions and invention of new means

through mental combinations. During these substages, the toddler continues to learn through sensory interaction with the environment.

At age 2, the toddler progresses into the first substage of the preoperational phase of cognitive development. During this substage, called the preconceptual stage, the toddler begins to develop reasoning capacities. A toddler's thinking is concrete, based on what the toddler sees, hears, and experiences. At this time, the toddler also begins to function symbolically through the use of language. (For details about the stages of cognitive development, see Chapter 2, The nurse–child–family relationship.)

Promoting toddler growth and development

To promote a home environment conducive to optimal development, direct nursing interventions at the toddler's parents. Inform them that the toddler develops motor, language, and social skills largely by playing and by interacting with others. Point out that a positive environment also permits psychological development. (For information on providing parents with anticipatory guidance for growth and development, see *Teaching parents to promote toddler growth and development*.)

Establishing discipline

During the toddler years, parents must establish rules of behavior and impose appropriate discipline. Such rules can have positive, growth-producing effects and are necessary to help the toddler avoid injury, learn socially acceptable behavior, channel unacceptable behavior into constructive activity, and maintain self-esteem and a positive self-concept while learning to adapt to the rules of the larger group and society.

The best strategy for avoiding undesirable behavior is to structure the toddler's environment to minimize or prevent such behavior. For example, urge parents to remove breakable objects from table tops and remove knobs from television and stereo sets.

To help parents establish effective discipline, provide the following instructions:

- Establish rules clearly, explain the rules to the toddler, and then follow them consistently.
- Model desirable behavior. For example, to minimize screaming and shouting, use a normal speaking voice and tone when talking to the child.
- Phrase requests for behavior in a positive way. For instance, say "Please close the cupboard door" rather than "Don't open that door."
- Praise desirable behavior and call immediate attention to undesirable behavior.
- Teach and help the toddler to practice desired behavior. For instance, before taking the child to a restaurant, practice correct eating behavior at home.
- When correcting behavior, approve or disapprove of the action, not the child. For example, say "We don't allow people to throw a ball in

Teaching parents to promote toddler growth and development

Like an infant, a toddler needs proper stimulation for optimal growth and development. This chart presents anticipatory guidance the nurse should provide to help parents provide such stimulation.

GROWTH AND DEVELOPMENT AREA	PARENT TEACHING
Gross motor development	• Encourage play activities, such as riding toys, playing with swingset and slide, pounding a board, using small climbing toys and activities, and playing outdoors (for instance, running and jumping).
Fine motor development	• Encourage play activities, such as with play dough, blocks, push/pull toys, paper and crayons (supervised), and placing large beads on a string.
Language development	• Use simple, adult language when talking to child. • Read to child. • Talk to child when performing ordinary tasks.
Social development	• Encourage play activities with household items, such as broom, vacuum, shovel, pots and pans, and telephone. • Encourage child to help with appropriate household chores. • Expose child to larger environment and community, such as by taking child for walks, for visits to park and zoo, and on neighborhood errands (such as shopping).
Psychosocial-psychosexual development	• Avoid conflict over toilet training. • Encourage child to participate in self-care activities, such as feeding, toileting, washing, and dressing. • Praise self-care efforts. • Allow child to explore environment. • Accommodate child's attempts to control environment. For instance, ignore negativism, establish and follow desired rituals, allow extra time for dawdling, cajole a defiant toddler into obeying, and avoid using anger or force.
Cognitive development	• Encourage play activities, such as with simple puzzles or cloth picture books, water play, sand play, building blocks, fantasy play (such as a farm set or gas station set), simple games (such as "What does the kitty say?"), and searching for a hidden object. • Read to child.

the house" instead of "You're a bad boy because you play ball in the house."

Also discuss the following strategies with parents to help them control and modify undesirable toddler behavior.

• *Providing distraction.* When the child misbehaves, distract the child from the activity. For example, if the child interrupts the mother's telephone conversation, she may offer the child a toy or something to eat.

• *Ignoring undesirable behavior.* By ignoring the behavior, the parent avoids reinforcing it or giving in to the child's demands. Without such reinforcement, the child learns that such actions as screaming, crying, and kicking will not get demands met. This strategy is especially effective at halting temper tantrums. However, caution parents to use it only for behavior that would not harm the child physically if allowed to continue.

• *Calling a time-out.* This technique also avoids reinforcing undesirable behavior. When the child misbehaves, the parent calls a "time-out" and isolates the child in a nonstimulating area. The child soon becomes bored; deprived of the reinforcement of parental attention in response to misbehavior, the child agrees to improve behavior and thus is allowed to rejoin the family group.

To help parents use this technique effectively, instruct them to explain the time-out procedure to the child before using it for the first time and to acquaint the child with the designated time-out area, which should be quiet and without toys. When the child misbehaves, the parent should warn the child that continued misbehavior will cause a time-out. If the child continues to misbehave, the parent tells the child to sit or stand in the time-out area for a specified time; 2 minutes is long enough for young toddlers. (Some experts recommend 1 minute per year of the child's age.) If the child cries or otherwise protests, the parent should inform the child that the time-out will not start until the child is quiet.

Instruct parents to stay within view of a young toddler but avoid speaking to the child during time-out. After the specified time has elapsed, the parent should allow the child to leave the time-out area. For misbehavior away from home, if time-out cannot be implemented appropriately, parents should tell the child that time-out will be imposed as soon as the family returns home.

Discipline methods to avoid

Inform parents that physical punishment, such as spanking, may halt a toddler's misbehavior in the short run but can have many long-term negative effects. For instance, it conveys the impression that physical aggression and violence are acceptable. Also, if the child becomes accustomed to spanking, this method eventually becomes ineffective in preventing undesirable behavior. Finally, spanking may harm the child physically, especially when administered by an angry parent.

Scolding also may have negative consequences. A scolding parent may use demeaning remarks, such as "Why can't you ever do anything right?" or "You're a bad girl." Such comments rarely change behavior and eventually make the child feel unworthy and truly bad.

Reasoning, or explaining why certain behavior is undesirable, has little effect on toddlers. Because of their egocentricity, toddlers cannot see the parent's point of view. Explaining why the behavior is unacceptable makes little sense to a toddler who is enjoying it.

Enhancing toddler health

Provide parents with anticipatory guidance regarding the toddler's nutrition, iron-deficiency anemia, elimination (toilet training), dental health, sleep, and safety precautions.

Providing nutritional guidance

During the toddler years, physical growth slows. Thus, a toddler has lower nutritional requirements than an infant. This may manifest as physiologic anorexia. For instance, the toddler may become a picky eater, eating almost nothing on certain days or refusing all food except one or two favorite items.

Inform parents that such erratic eating patterns are normal in toddlers. Counsel parents to avoid forcing food, and reassure them that a toddler will eat when hungry. Because food preferences are established at this time, also encourage parents to offer a variety of foods, served on small plates and in appropriately small portions.

After age 12 months, a child's solid food intake should shift from pureed infant food to most types of adult table food, modified for toddlers. For example, parents may soften hard fruits and vegetables by steaming. For a toddler just starting to coordinate chewing and swallowing, soft foods may be mashed. Toddlers especially enjoy finger foods, but by age 18 months they can be expected to use a spoon for self-feeding and to drink liquids from a cup. Caution parents not to add salt and pepper to the toddler's foods.

Weaning from the bottle completely begins during the early toddler period and is accomplished by age 36 months. By this time, the toddler no longer requires breast milk or infant formula and can tolerate cow's milk. Whole milk is recommended for brain cell development. The toddler after age 2 can drink 2% milk to reduce fat intake, but should not be given 1% or skim milk because the protein concentration is too high for the toddler's immature kidneys. Daily milk intake should be limited to 18 to 24 oz because excessive milk intake reduces solid food consumption.

Calorie, protein, and fluid requirements

Inform parents of the toddler's daily calorie, protein, and fluid requirements:
- *Calories* — 100 calories/kg (46 calories/lb)
- *Protein* — 1.2 g/kg (0.5 g/lb)
- *Fluid* — 115 ml/kg (52 ml/lb; approximately 2 oz/lb).

Recommended diet

Inform parents that the toddler's daily diet should include the following:
- Breads, cereals, rice, and pasta: six to eleven servings (one serving equals ½ slice of bread, two crackers, or ¼ cup of cereal, rice, or pasta)

- Fruits: two to four servings, including at least one citrus fruit (one serving equals $\frac{1}{4}$ banana, $\frac{1}{2}$ other raw fruit, $\frac{1}{4}$ cup canned fruit, or $\frac{1}{2}$ cup juice)
- Vegetables: three to five servings, including at least one leafy, green or yellow vegetable (one serving equals two to three pieces of raw vegetables or 2 tablespoons of cooked vegetables)
- Meat, poultry, fish, dry beans, eggs, and nuts: two servings (one serving equals 1 oz of meat, 1 egg, 1 tablespoon peanut butter, or $\frac{1}{4}$ cup dry beans)
- Milk, yogurt, and cheese: two to three servings (one serving equals 1 cup [8 oz] of 2% milk, 1 oz of cheese, $\frac{1}{4}$ cup cottage cheese, or $\frac{1}{4}$ cup yogurt).

Preventing iron-deficiency anemia

Children under age 3 are at risk for iron-deficiency anemia — mainly from inadequate iron intake. Excessive consumption of cow's milk contributes to iron-deficiency anemia. The iron in cow's milk is poorly absorbed. Children who consume large amounts of cow's milk may not want to eat other iron-rich foods because they are full. Thus, lack of iron-rich foods contributes to iron-deficiency anemia.

To help prevent iron-deficiency anemia, instruct parents to limit the toddler's milk intake to 24 oz/day — never to exceed 32 oz/day — and to make sure the diet includes iron-rich foods (such as beef, prunes, apricots, creamed wheat, kidney beans, raisins, fortified cereals, egg yolks, and spinach). For a toddler who eats poorly, suggest giving a multiple vitamin supplement with iron.

Screening for iron-deficiency anemia should begin at age 6 months for high-risk infants, such as premature infants and formula-fed infants who do not receive iron supplementation. Low-risk toddlers should undergo screening at age 18 months; a low hemoglobin level (below 10 g/dl) indicates the need for iron supplementation.

The recommended dose of supplemental iron is 6 mg/kg/day. Instruct parents to mix iron elixir with water or fruit juice and to have the child take it with meals to prevent gastrointestinal (GI) upset. Giving the elixir with fruit juice may be preferred because vitamin C enhances iron solubility and absorption. Caution parents never to mix the elixir with milk because milk impedes iron absorption.

Inform parents that the iron supplement may darken the child's stools and cause constipation. Mention that increasing the child's fluid and fiber intake can relieve constipation. Instruct parents to have the child drink water or juice after taking the iron preparation, which can cause temporary tooth staining.

Promoting bowel and bladder elimination

Toilet training is a major concern for parents of toddlers. Many parents attempt toilet training before the child is ready, causing frustration for all involved.

To help prevent this problem, inform parents that a child cannot achieve bowel and bladder control until certain physiologic and psychological maturation processes have occurred. The required physiologic processes — voluntary control of bowel and bladder sphincters, ability to stay dry for at least 2 hours, ability to maintain a regular bowel elimination pattern, and ability to remove clothing — occur at age 18 to 24 months. The required psychological processes — desire to control bowel and bladder function, verbal ability to indicate toileting needs, ability to sit on a toilet or potty for 5 to 10 minutes without fussing, curiosity about toilet habits, desire to have wet or soiled diapers changed, and ability to cooperate with parental desires or demands — occur at age 18 to 30 months.

Research shows that the average age at completion of daytime toilet training is 28 months; at completion of nighttime toilet training, 33 months. Also, most children achieve bowel and bladder control at the same time; girls achieve control 2 to 3 months earlier than boys. Roughly 80% of children achieve daytime and nighttime control by age 3.

During the early toddler period, discuss with parents the child's readiness to begin toilet training. Instruct parents to look for signs of readiness to toilet train starting at age 18 months. At this time, parents also should start to describe the processes of urination and defecation to the child and allow the child to observe them during bathroom activities. After age 20 to 24 months, when the child shows readiness to train, parents may introduce the child to the potty chair. Depending on parental and child preference, the potty chair may be attached securely to the toilet or placed on the floor; some children feel more secure when it sits on the floor.

Initially, the parent may ask the child to sit on the potty for 5 to 10 minutes while still dressed. Once the child is comfortable just sitting, the parent should place the child on the potty at regular intervals, with diapers removed, for 5-minute periods. Instruct parents to tell the child to "go potty" (or whatever words the parents decide to use). If the child has established regular urination and defecation patterns (for example, urinating soon after awakening from a nap or defecating soon after eating), parents should place the child on the potty at these times as well.

Teach parents to praise all the child's efforts to use the potty (including sitting and grunting) as well as all elimination processes. Emphasize that several weeks may pass before the child can produce urine or stool voluntarily during potty use. Tell them to keep using diapers during this initial phase and to ignore wet or soiled diapers.

After successfully using the potty several times, the child may begin to use training pants. Until nighttime bowel and bladder control is established, the child may continue to wear diapers at night.

Teach parents that even after the child has achieved full bowel and bladder control, they should expect some accidents and should not scold or punish the child if these occur. Accidents are most common during the day, when the child may be too busy playing to notice the need to void or defecate. To help avoid such accidents, parents may remind the child to use the potty every few hours. If the child shows disinterest in or resistance to toilet training, instruct parents to discontinue the training for a few weeks, and then try again.

Enhancing dental health

To promote dental health in a toddler, cover the following teaching points with parents:
• Provide fluoride toothpaste and a child-size toothbrush.
• Assist the toddler with brushing his or her own teeth at least twice daily.
• To teach correct technique, supervise the child during brushing.
• Be sure the toddler spits out the toothpaste and rinses with water after brushing; swallowing fluoride toothpaste can lead to fluoride excess.
• Limit consumption of foods with a high sugar content.
• If sweet desserts are allowed, have the child eat them with meals. Discourage sweet snacks between meals.
• Limit foods that stick to the teeth, such as raisins, dates, and caramels.
• Avoid bedtime bottles, except those containing only water.
• Begin regular dental visits at age 2.

To help prevent caries, the American Academy of Pediatrics recommends fluoride supplementation as specified below.

For a child whose drinking water has a fluoride concentration below 0.3 parts per million (ppm):
• Birth to age 2 — 0.25 mg/day
• Ages 2 to 3 — 0.50 mg/day
• Ages 3 to 16 — 1 mg/day.
For a child whose drinking water has a fluoride concentration of 0.3 to 0.7 ppm:
• Birth to age 2 — no supplementation required
• Ages 2 to 3 — 0.25 mg/day
• Ages 3 to 16 — 0.5 mg/day.
A child whose drinking water has a fluoride concentration above 0.7 ppm does not need fluoride supplementation.

Promoting good sleep patterns

Toddlers require less sleep than infants. By age 2, nighttime sleep averages 8 to 12 hours. However, toddlers still require one afternoon nap, which averages 2 hours.

Most toddlers have a bedtime ritual. Because these rituals seem to enhance the toddler's sense of security, urge parents to permit them. Even with such rituals, however, toddlers commonly try to delay sleep by asking for one more story or another drink of water. To establish firm bedtime habits, teach parents to refuse such requests consistently.

To help parents overcome a toddler's resistance to going to bed or staying in bed, instruct parents to:
• adhere to all bedtime rituals
• provide a "wind-down" period before bed, such as a bath or telling a story
• avoid stimulation before bed, such as excessive physical activity or frightening stories
• provide sufficient interaction during waking hours to minimize demands for attention at bedtime
• refuse to acknowledge delaying tactics
• be firm and consistent in establishing the bedtime hour
• provide security items, such as a night-light, blanket, or toy
• return the child to bed if the child gets up after being tucked in, and firmly request that the child stay there.

Ensuring safety

The most common cause of death in toddlers, injuries typically result from burns, falls, choking or suffocation, poisoning, and motor vehicle injuries. The toddler's great curiosity and increased motor skills — which allow the toddler to explore the environment, climb, turn handles, and open drawers and cupboards — contribute to such injuries. To help prevent injury, be sure to teach parents appropriate measures. (See *Preventing injuries in toddlers,* page 76.)

Preventing lead poisoning

Among the most common preventable childhood health problems in the United States, lead poisoning occurs when abnormal amounts of lead are absorbed through the skin, lungs, or GI tract. Common sources of lead exposure include lead-based paint as well as contaminated soil, dust, and drinking water. In 1991, the Centers for Disease Control and Prevention (CDC) issued a policy that redefined lead poisoning, lowered the minimum serum lead level for initiating treatment, and emphasized primary prevention. The normal level of lead in the body is less than 9 µg per 100 ml of whole blood. Lead levels are categorized by the CDC into five classes of increasing risk of toxicity. These classes are Class I (low risk) lead level — less than 9µg/dl; Class IIA (rescreen) — lead level of 10 to 14 µg/dl; Class IIB (moderate risk) — lead level 15 to 19 µg/dl; Class III (high risk) — lead level 20 to 44 µg/dl; Class IV (urgent risk) — lead level 45 to 69 µg/dl; Class V — lead level more than 70 µg/dl.

Lead-based paint may be found in homes painted before the late 1970s. Thus, toddlers living in older homes may eat lead-containing paint chips that are peeling from the walls and woodwork. Toddlers also may inhale lead in the dust produced by sanding old paint during home renovation or in the exhaust from cars using leaded gasoline. Toddlers may be exposed to lead when playing in contaminated dirt

Preventing injuries in toddlers

To guard against toddler injuries, provide parents with the following instructions.

Preventing burns
- Set the hot water heater at a temperature no higher than 120° F (48.8° C).
- Turn handles of cooking pots toward the back of the stove.
- Remove gas stove knobs within the toddler's reach.
- Keep electrical cords out of the child's reach.
- Place safety guards on the front of radiators, fireplaces, and space heaters.
- Keep matches and lighters out of the child's reach.
- Cover electrical outlets with safety caps.
- Teach the child the concept of hot.

Preventing falls
- Use locked safety gates on all stairs until the child can navigate stairs safely.
- Use safety latches on screened windows. If screens cannot be installed, open windows no higher than 4" (10 cm).
- Place nonskid decals in the bathtub.
- Keep crib rails up and place the mattress at the lowest level. If the child can climb out of the crib, use a bed with a guard rail.
- Restrain the child in shopping carts.
- Use an effective child car seat consistently.
- Avoid using child walkers.
- Supervise the child's play at all times, especially during climbing.
- Keep chairs and other objects that could be used for climbing away from counters.

Preventing choking and suffocation
- Cut solid food into small pieces.
- Remove skin from hot dogs and sausages.
- Peel fresh fruit and remove pits.
- Do not give the child grapes (unless they are cut in half), hard candy, gum, nuts, or popcorn.
- Keep plastic bags and balloons (except mylar balloons) out of the child's reach.

Preventing drowning
- Keep the bathroom door closed and use a safety latch.
- Supervise the child closely during bath time.
- If the home has a swimming pool, enclose it in a fence and secure the gate with a lock.
- Have the child wear a safety jacket when playing in water.
- Closely supervise all water play.

Preventing motor vehicle injuries
- Use an effective car seat restraint system until the child weighs 40 lb or reaches 40" in height. Make sure to use the restraint system properly.
- Supervise the child during outside play at all times — especially when crossing the street.
- Teach the child to stay away from the street.
- Instruct the child not to play near the curb.

Preventing poisoning
- Store all medications and household cleaning products in their original containers, behind locked doors.
- Keep house plants off the floor and out of the child's reach.
- Supervise the child outdoors to prevent ingestion of poisonous plants.
- Teach the child to keep nonfood items out of the mouth.
- Refer to drugs as medicine, not candy.
- Teach the child to stay away from garbage and trash containers.
- Keep syrup of ipecac in the house.
- Post the telephone number for the poison control center near the phone.

If the child ingests a poison
Instruct parents to call the poison control center immediately for specific instructions. Most noncaustic poisons can be removed from the stomach by inducing vomiting with syrup of ipecac. The child should drink at least 8 oz of water after ingesting the syrup.

If the child has ingested a caustic poison, vomiting should *not* be induced. The poison control center may instruct parents to have the child ingest at least 8 oz of water to dilute the substance.

along roadways. Pica, the compulsive eating of unusual nonfood items, also increases the risk of lead ingestion.

Lead poisoning can cause severe central nervous system (CNS) effects. A serum lead level above 70 µg/dl may cause acute manifestations, such as seizures and encephalopathy. However, in most children, chronic lead exposure, resulting in lower serum levels, produces more subtle effects — hyperactivity, delayed fine motor development, cognitive deficits, and learning disabilities. Lead poisoning also affects heme synthesis, resulting in iron-deficiency anemia. A child may show CNS effects with chronic serum lead levels as low as 15 µg/dl.

The nurse's role in primary prevention includes early identification of children with lead poisoning. To determine if the child's environment contains lead sources and to help assess the child's risk for exposure, obtain an environmental history. Also, teach parents and the community about the risk of lead exposure and ways to decrease the risk, such as keeping children away from chipping and peeling paint and washing children's dirt-soiled hands and faces before eating. Instruct parents to remove paint chips by picking them up and discarding them in a garbage bag. Advise them to remove any small, remaining chips and dust by damp mopping, not by vacuuming (which tends to disperse lead particles into the air, where they may be inhaled).

Screening for lead poisoning by direct measurement of venous lead content should begin at age 18 months and should be repeated at ages 24, 30, and 36 months. Children with serum lead levels between 10 and 14 µg/dl are at risk for lead poisoning and should be retested every 3 to 4 months. A serum lead level above 14 µg/dl indicates lead poisoning; affected children require nutritional and risk-reduction counseling. Because dietary fat speeds GI tract absorption, advise parents of a lead-poisoned child over age 2 to provide a low-fat diet. Perform an environmental assessment to identify lead sources, so that they can be removed or avoided. Iron-deficiency anemia, commonly associated with lead poisoning, increases the rate of lead absorption. Therefore, arrange for a child with lead poisoning to be tested for iron deficiency.

STUDY ACTIVITIES

Short answer

1. Explain why spanking a toddler is an ineffective discipline method.

_____

_____

2. Describe effective strategies parents may use to control and modify a toddler's behavior.

_____

_____

3. List some activities parents can encourage in a toddler to promote fine motor development.

_____

_____

4. Identify at least five instructions the nurse should give to parents when explaining how to prevent poisoning in toddlers.

_____

_____

_____

5. Melanie, age 2, comes to the physician's office with her mother for a well-child visit. During the initial history, Ms. Cox reports that Melanie takes a bottle of formula in the morning and another one before bed (for a total of 16 oz), and drinks an additional 18 oz of milk by cup during the day. When obtaining a 24-hour diet history, the nurse notes that Melanie had cereal with milk for breakfast; a morning snack of graham crackers; Spaghettios with milk for lunch; fruit as an afternoon snack; and a hot dog with corn and French fries for dinner. Her height and weight are in the 50th percentile for her age.

Based on this diet history, the nurse determines Melanie is consuming too much milk and not enough fruits and vegetables. A child of her age should consume no more than 32 oz of milk every 24 hours (preferably, 24 oz every 24 hours) and at least two daily servings of fruits and three servings of vegetables.

To decrease Melanie's milk intake to the recommended amount, the nurse might suggest which dietary changes? To increase her intake of fruits and vegetables to the recommended amount, the nurse should instruct her mother to add which foods, and in what amounts, to Melanie's diet?

_____

_____

_____

Multiple choice

6. Which anticipatory guidance should the nurse provide the parents of a 15-month-old child?

    A. Use a safety gate to block the child's access to stairs.

    B. Keep the child in a playpen to prevent ingestion of poisonous substances.

    C. Begin instruction in toilet training.

    D. Move the child from a crib to a junior bed.

7. Most toddlers can master self-feeding with a spoon by what age?
  A. 12 months
  B. 15 months
  C. 18 months
  D. 24 months

8. At what age can most children begin combining two words?
  A. 15 months
  B. 18 months
  C. 24 months
  D. 30 months

9. Iron-deficiency anemia in toddlers is associated with:
  A. Excessive intake of cow's milk
  B. Insufficient milk intake
  C. Physiologic anorexia
  D. Limited fruit intake

10. At what age should children be screened for iron-deficiency anemia?
  A. 15 months
  B. 18 months
  C. 24 months
  D. 30 months

11. When and how should a supplemental iron preparation be administered to a toddler?
  A. Before breakfast, with milk
  B. After breakfast, with orange juice
  C. Before lunch, with water
  D. After dinner, with milk

12. The minimum serum lead level that indicates lead poisoning in a child is:
  A. 10 µg/dl
  B. 15 µg/dl
  C. 25 µg/dl
  D. 40 µg/dl

13. A 3-year-old child with lead poisoning should consume a diet that is:
  A. High in protein
  B. High in carbohydrate
  C. Low in fat
  D. Low in sugar

14. Belinda Norton tells the nurse that Curtis, her 2-year-old son, has several temper tantrums each week. Ms. Norton asks what she can do to decrease these episodes. Which statement represents the nurse's best response?

　　A. "Ignore the temper tantrums."
　　B. "Call a time-out when Curtis has a tantrum."
　　C. "Promise Curtis a cookie if he stops crying."
　　D. "Tell Curtis that crying will not get him what he wants."

ANSWERS　　**Short answer**

　　1. Spanking rarely improves behavior over the long run and may have such negative effects as conveying the impression that physical aggression and violence are acceptable; it accustoms the child to spanking, which eventually becomes ineffective in preventing undesirable behavior, and it causes physical harm.

　　2. Strategies parents may use to control and modify undesirable toddler behavior include providing distraction, in which parents distract the child from the misbehavior; ignoring undesirable behavior; and calling a time-out, in which parents isolate the misbehaving child in a nonstimulating area for a specified time.

　　3. To promote a toddler's fine motor development, parents should encourage play activities involving play dough, blocks, push/pull toys, paper and crayons (supervised), and putting large beads on a string.

　　4. To help prevent poisoning, the nurse should teach parents to store household cleaning products behind locked doors; keep medicines and cleaning products in their original containers; keep plants off the floor and out of the child's reach; supervise the child during outdoor play; teach the child to keep nonfood items out of the mouth; post the telephone number of the poison control center number near the phone; keep syrup of ipecac in the house; refer to drugs as medicine rather than candy; and teach the child to stay away from garbage and trash containers.

　　5. To reduce Melanie's milk intake, the nurse should suggest that Ms. Cox substitute 4 oz of fruit juice for one milk serving during the day and eliminate one 8-oz bottle. To increase Melanie's fruit and vegetable intake, the nurse should instruct Ms. Cox to add at least one more daily fruit serving, such as 4 oz of apple or orange juice, $\frac{1}{4}$ banana, or $\frac{1}{4}$ cup fruit cocktail. Also instruct her to include at least one more vegetable serving, such as carrots or green pepper sticks, in a snack or lunch.

Multiple choice

　　6. A. A 15-month-old child is capable of creeping up stairs, increasing the risk for falling; a safety gate blocking access to stairs minimizes this risk. A toddler should not be restricted to a playpen for a prolonged period because this impedes exploratory behavior. Toilet training should not begin until age 20 to 24 months. A 15-month-old child is safest in a crib, with the mattress placed in the lowest position.

7. C. Most children can feed themselves with a spoon by age 18 months.

8. C. Most children can combine two words by age 24 months.

9. A. Excessive consumption of cow's milk contributes to iron-deficiency anemia by discouraging intake of solid foods. The iron in milk is poorly absorbed.

10. B. Children should be screened for iron-deficiency anemia at age 18 months.

11. B. A child should take iron elixir on a full stomach (such as during or just after a meal) to prevent stomach irritation; taking iron with orange juice may aid iron absorption. Iron elixir should not be taken with milk because milk decreases iron absorption; it should not be taken on an empty stomach (such as before breakfast) because this can cause stomach irritation.

12. B. Children with chronic serum lead levels as low as 15 µg/dl show CNS effects.

13. C. This child should consume a low-fat diet because dietary fat increases the rate of lead absorption from the GI tract.

14. A. The nurse should advise Ms. Norton to ignore the child's behavior and thus avoid reinforcing it. Temper tantrums should decrease when the child realizes they are ineffective.

CHAPTER 8

The preschool-age child and family

OBJECTIVES

After studying this chapter, the reader should be able to:

1. Identify the norms for physical growth, gross motor development, fine motor development, language development, and social development in the preschool-age child.

2. Discuss psychosocial, psychosexual, and cognitive development in the preschool-age child.

3. Identify nursing interventions that promote growth and development in the preschool-age child.

4. Describe nursing interventions that promote optimal nutrition, elimination, dental health, sleep, safety, and school entry in the preschool-age child.

5. Discuss characteristics of communicable diseases in preschool-age children, and identify related nursing responsibilities.

6. Describe characteristics of common intestinal parasitic infections in preschool-age children, and identify related nursing responsibilities.

OVERVIEW OF CONCEPTS

This chapter discusses major growth and developmental milestones during the preschool-age years — ages 3 to 6. It explores the nurse's role in promoting the child's growth and development, then discusses ways the nurse can enhance the child's health. The chapter concludes by describing the nurse's role in preventing and managing communicable diseases and parasitic infections in the preschool-age child.

Growth and development

Physical growth continues to slow during the preschool-age years. (For details, see *Major growth and developmental milestones in preschool-age children.*)

Psychosocial development

According to Erik Erikson, the preschooler's developmental task is to gain initiative without experiencing guilt. The child strives to master the environment and gains a sense of accomplishment from successful-

Major growth and developmental milestones in preschool-age children

This chart presents the major milestones a preschooler should achieve.

PHYSICAL GROWTH	GROSS MOTOR DEVELOPMENT	FINE MOTOR DEVELOPMENT	LANGUAGE DEVELOPMENT	SOCIAL DEVELOPMENT
3 years				
• Growth is steady, but starts to slow • Average weight: $32\frac{1}{2}$ lb (boys); $30\frac{3}{4}$ lb (girls) • Average height: 38″ (boys); $37\frac{1}{2}$″ (girls)	• Can broad jump • Balances on one foot for 1 second • Can ride tricycle • Can throw ball overhand	• Builds tower of eight cubes • Builds bridge using three cubes • Attempts to draw straight line	• Has vocabulary of about 800 words • Combines four words • Can name one color • Uses adjectives • Describes pictures	• Can put on T-shirt • Can name friend • Can use toilet (needs help with wiping) • Helps set table • Pulls on shoes • May have fears, such as fear of the dark or of going to bed
4 years				
• Steady growth • Average weight: $40\frac{1}{2}$ lb (boys); $37\frac{1}{2}$ lb (girls) • Average height: 40″ (boys); 35″ (girls)	• Can balance on one foot for 2 to 3 seconds • Can hop on one foot • Can catch ball	• Imitates drawing of a circle • Uses scissors	• Averages five words per sentence • Can name four colors • Enjoys rhyming words • Asks many questions • Speaks with 90% intelligibility • Understands such concepts as "under" and "beside"	• Dresses self with minimal help • May have many fears • Is extremely independent
5 years				
• Steady growth • Average weight: $42\frac{1}{2}$ lb (boys); 40 lb (girls) • Average height: 43″ (boys); $42\frac{1}{2}$″ (girls)	• Balances on one foot for 4 to 5 seconds • Skates • Skips	• Draws person with at least three body parts • Copies a cross (+) • Copies a square (when demonstrated) • Prints several letters (typically, the child's name)	• Averages six words per sentence • Understands meaning of opposites • Can define ball, lake, desk, house, banana, curtain, fence, and ceiling • Uses all types of sentences	• Plays simple board games • Prepares own cereal • Is less fearful • Is eager to please

ly completing such tasks as dressing unassisted and helping out around the house.

The preschooler's need to master the environment may lead to overextending boundaries. Misbehavior causes anxiety and guilt, as may certain thoughts. The conscience, or superego, develops during the preschool years, and the child must learn right from wrong.

Psychosexual development

According to Sigmund Freud, the preschool-age child is in the phallic stage of psychosexual development, becoming aware of physical differences between the sexes and beginning the process of sex-role identification. For a boy, this process involves the Oedipal complex. He becomes very close to his mother, and may be jealous of the relationship she has with his father. He soon realizes that his father is much stronger than he is and that he cannot possibly "win" his mother away from him. He also notices that girls do not have penises and imagines that their penises were removed for some wrongdoing. His guilt over wanting to take over his father's role makes him fear that he, too, somehow will lose his penis. To resolve this conflict, the boy must identify with the father.

Freud proposed that a similar conflict, the Electra complex, occurs in the preschool-age girl. Wishing to marry her father and somehow get rid of her mother, the child develops penis envy (the desire to have a penis). To resolve this conflict, she must identify with her mother.

Cognitive development

According to Jean Piaget, the preschool-age child completes the preconceptual substage of preoperational thought from ages 3 to 4. Then, at age 4, the child enters the intuitive phase of preoperational thought, becoming less egocentric and slowly gaining an understanding of others' perspectives and views. The child also can understand simple explanations at this time.

During the preschool years, thought processes remain concrete and symbolic functioning improves. Symbolic functioning is evidenced in imaginative play. The child also may acquire an imaginary friend, who serves an important function. Under the child's complete control, the imaginary friend cannot threaten the child's sense of competency. The child may rehearse social interactions and replay situations with this friend, and may blame the friend for the child's own transgressions without fear of ridicule, shame, guilt, or scolding.

During the preschool years, the child's thinking is characterized by:
* *centration* — the ability to think of only one concept at a time
* *magical thinking* — the belief that thoughts are powerful and can cause events to occur
* *transductive reasoning* — the belief that events that occur at the same time have a cause-and-effect relationship.

Enhancing growth and development

The preschool-age child develops mainly through play and interaction with others. A supportive environment promotes optimal growth and development in the preschool-age child. The nurse directs teaching to the parents so they can provide learning opportunities for the child.

Teaching parents to promote the preschooler's growth and development

This chart presents anticipatory guidance the nurse should offer parents to help them provide proper stimulation for the preschooler's optimal growth and development.

GROWTH AND DEVELOPMENTAL AREA	PARENT TEACHING
Gross motor development	• Encourage play activities, such as simple physical games (kickball, catch, hopscotch, dodgeball, and tag). • Teach child how to ride a tricycle, roller skate, climb, and play on swings and slides.
Fine motor development	• Provide drawing materials, scissors, construction blocks, and finger paints. • Encourage child to practice printing letters.
Language development	• Read to child and respond to child's questions. • Play games that require language skills, such as "I see something red."
Social development	• Encourage child to play with other children. • Encourage child to complete simple chores, such as making the bed and setting the table. • Play simple board games.
Psychosocial and psychosexual development	• Encourage child to perform self-care tasks, such as dressing, brushing hair, and brushing teeth; praise the child's efforts. • Provide interaction with adults of same sex.
Cognitive development	• Encourage play activities, including imaginative play (such as playing with dolls and dollhouses; playing doctor, nurse, or policeman; using play kits; and wearing playclothes for dress-up). • Provide picture games. • Encourage counting games and simple games requiring dice.

(For more information, see *Teaching parents to promote the preschooler's growth and development*.)

Enforcing discipline   Discipline strategies are important in shaping the preschooler's behavior. Positive discipline also promotes a healthy self-concept. Encourage parents to use the time-out and distraction techniques (described in Chapter 7, The toddler and family), which continue to be effective during the preschool-age years.

Also suggest that parents establish a reward system for good behavior and clearly explain rules for good behavior to the child. Reward systems are based on reinforcement theory, which holds that a behavior that is rewarded will continue. In one commonly used reward system, parents give the child a stick-on star (which they may place on a chart) when the child behaves well. If the parents want to use this system, advise them to explain the desired behavior to the child in advance. For example, parents may say, "I will give you a star every time you pick up a toy." Advise parents to award the star immediately after the behavior is demonstrated and to praise the child verbally when awarding a star. Stars should represent something meaningful to the child. For example, parents may explain that if the child gains three gold stars by dinner, they will take the child to the park after dinner.

Preschool-age children are less egocentric than toddlers and can understand another's viewpoint. Therefore, encourage parents to use simple explanations to increase good behavior and minimize misbehavior. For example, if a four-year-old girl pushes another child out of the way to get to a slide, the parent should explain that the child has hurt the other's feelings, then ask her how she would feel if she were pushed. Or, if a child plays too noisily in the living room, the parent might say, "I can't talk with your father when you are so loud. Could you please play more quietly, or play upstairs in your room?"

Another effective discipline strategy with preschool-age children is "experiencing consequences." Suppose, for example, a four-year-old boy constantly jumps up from the table during dinner. First, parents explain the rule to the child — that all family members must sit at the table until dinner is over. The parents then tell the child that if he gets up from the table during a meal, his plate will be removed. When dinner starts, the parent reminds him of the rule. If the child gets up from the table, the parents warn him once; if he gets up again, they remove his plate from the table and inform him that he is finished eating and may leave the room. Because the child wishes to avoid the negative consequence of going without dinner, he soon learns he must remain seated during dinner.

Promoting health in the preschool-age child

Advise parents on nutrition, elimination, dental health, sleep, safety, sexuality, and school entry for the preschool-age child.

Enhancing nutrition

During the preschool-age period, growth slows and nutritional requirements decrease. The child may develop intense food preferences. Advise parents to continue to provide a variety of foods — but caution them not to force food on the child.

Calorie, protein, and fluid requirements

The preschooler's food requirements resemble the toddler's with some variations. Daily nutritional requirements include:
- *calories* — 90 cal/kg (41 calories/lb)
- *protein* — 1.2 g/kg (0.5 g/lb)
- *fluid* — 95 ml/kg (43 ml/lb; approximately 1.5 oz/lb).

Recommended diet

Inform parents that the preschooler's daily diet should included the following foods and beverages:
- Bread, cereal, rice, and pasta: six to eleven servings (one serving equals ½ slice to one slice of bread, two to three crackers, or ¼ to ½ cup of cereal, rice, or pasta)

- Fruits: two to four servings, including at least one citrus fruit (one serving equals $\frac{1}{2}$ banana, $\frac{1}{2}$ other raw fruit, $\frac{1}{4}$ to $\frac{1}{2}$ cup canned fruit, or 4 oz juice)
- Vegetables: three to five servings, including at least one leafy, green or yellow vegetable (one serving equals two to three pieces of a raw vegetable or 2 to 4 tablespoons of a cooked vegetable)
- Meat, poultry, fish, dry beans, eggs, and nuts: two servings (one serving equals 1 to 2 oz meat, one egg, 1 to 2 tablespoons peanut butter, or $\frac{1}{4}$ to $\frac{1}{2}$ cup dry beans)
- Milk, yogurt, and cheese: two to three servings (one serving equals 8 oz [1 cup] of milk, 1 oz hard cheese, $\frac{1}{4}$ to $\frac{1}{2}$ cup cottage cheese, or $\frac{1}{4}$ to $\frac{1}{2}$ cup yogurt).

Promoting bowel and bladder elimination

Most children achieve daytime bowel and bladder control by age 3 and nighttime control by age 6. By the end of the preschool-age period, most children are capable of independent toileting. However, occasional accidents may occur. Inform parents that the child can be responsible for changing clothes after an accident. However, caution them never to ridicule the child for accidents.

Ensuring dental health

By age 3, all deciduous (primary, or "baby," teeth) have erupted. Inform parents that the child needs supervision when brushing teeth. They may begin flossing the child's teeth at this time. Prophylactic dental care continues. (For recommendations on fluoride supplementation, see Chapter 7, The toddler and family.)

Promoting healthy sleep patterns

The preschool-age child needs an average of 8 to 12 hours of sleep per night. The younger preschooler still may require a nap (although nap length shortens to an average of 30 to 60 minutes). The older preschooler may not need to nap.

Sleep disturbances may emerge during the preschool years. Some children have difficulty falling asleep; others develop bedtime fears. Nighttime awakening, a common problem during this time, typically stems from nightmares (frightening dreams) or, less often, from night terrors. Nightmares typically occur during the second half of the night. They may cause the child to awaken; the child seems frightened and usually can describe the dream.

If the child has a nightmare and calls out to them, the parents should go to the child's room and provide reassurance. They should ask the child to describe the dream, reassure the child that it was a dream and that everything is all right, and then encourage the child to go back to sleep. To reassure the child, parents may leave a night-light on or offer a security item. The child may take 5 minutes or more to fall back to sleep.

If the child goes to the parents' room after a nightmare, a parent should accompany the child back to the child's room and stay until the child is reassured. Advise parents to avoid the temptation to let the child stay in the parents' room because this promotes the habit of going to the parents' room every time the child awakens at night.

Night terrors, episodes of crying, screaming or moaning which typically occur within 1 to 4 hours after the onset of sleep, do not occur during times of dreaming. During a night terror, the child may cry, thrash around the bed, and sweat profusely without awakening fully or being aware of others' presence. Advise parents to go to the child's room if they suspect a night terror and to observe but not try to comfort the child unless the child awakens fully. Inform them that crying and thrashing may continue for 10 minutes. Advise them not to hold or restrain the child because this may increase the activity. Inform them that when the night terror ends, the child will calm down and may or may not awaken fully. The child who awakens seems calm and not frightened. Typical sleep behavior follows soon after the night terror ends. In the morning, the child has no recollection of the incident.

Ensuring safety

Although preschoolers have fewer accidents than toddlers, motor vehicle injuries continue to be the major cause of death. Burns, recreational injuries, and drowning account for most other accidents in preschoolers. Teach parents how to prevent injury, as outlined below.

Preventing burns

In preschoolers, burns typically result from scalding water or direct flames. Instruct parents to set the hot water heater below 120° F (48.8° C) and to teach the child about the danger of matches, open flames, and hot objects.

Preventing recreational injuries

Many preschool-age children engage in group sports, ride bicycles, and use playgrounds and therefore may suffer recreational and sport injuries. Teach parents to monitor the safety of playground equipment. Mention that the preschool-age child requires supervision during playground use and bicycle riding. Advise parents to make sure the child wears shoes and a safety helmet when riding a bicycle and rides only on level ground.

Preventing drowning

Preschool-age children are less likely than toddlers to drown during unsupervised bathing — but are more likely to drown in swimming pools and lakes. Teach parents to supervise the child at all times during swimming and to make sure the child wears a safety jacket when playing in water. Instruct parents to ensure that pools are enclosed by a fence with a locked gate. If desired, the child may learn about water safety in organized swimming classes and take lessons in beginning swimming skills.

Preventing motor vehicle accidents

Advise parents to continue the use of a child restraint system in motor vehicles until the child weighs 40 lb (18 kg) or is 40″ (102 cm) tall. After that time, the child may be strapped into the car securely with an adult restraint system.

Inform parents that the preschool-age child should not be allowed to ride a bicycle in the street. Instruct them to reinforce street safety rules (discussed in Chapter 9, The school-age child and family) and to warn the child never to chase a ball or other object into the road.

Advise parents that young preschool-age children must be supervised when crossing the street. Teach parents to supervise street-crossing until the child consistently demonstrates safe street-crossing behavior. Make sure they inform the child which streets the child may cross alone. By age 5, some children can cross quiet roads safely.

Teaching parents about the preschooler's sexuality

The preschool-age child becomes increasing aware of the genitals and may begin to touch or fondle them. Inform parents that masturbation is normal and healthy as long as it does not interfere with the child's usual activities or cause tissue redness or soreness.

Be aware, however, that parents with certain beliefs about masturbation may be concerned about this behavior. If so, explore their beliefs further, then elicit information about the circumstances under which their child masturbates. For example, parents may report that the child seems to touch the genitals when tired and watching television. In this case, the child may masturbate not for sexual stimulation but because the child is tired or is using self-stimulation as a way to feel secure. Other children touch their genitals when bored or anxious or to make sure the genitals are still there. If the child's behavior upsets the parents, advise them to tell the child that masturbation is something that is done only in the privacy of the child's room.

Coping with school entry

Young preschoolers may enter nursery school; by age 5, most children are ready for kindergarten. School entry may cause stress for both the child and parents. Parents may be concerned with choosing the appropriate nursery school or kindergarten and may worry about the child's reaction to separation from them. Some parents are reluctant to turn the child over to the care and supervision of other adults. For the child, the greatest stress of school entry comes from separation from parents.

The nurse can help the parents choose an appropriate school environment. Inform them that the school's social climate, teacher qualifications, and teacher attitudes toward children are the most important features to evaluate. Advise them that the best way to evaluate social climate and teachers' attitudes is by observing teachers in the classroom setting. Suggest that they ask permission to observe a teacher in a classroom. If school administrators discourage such observation, urge parents not to enroll the child in the school.

Assessing the child's readiness

Besides necessitating separation from parents, nursery school and kindergarten entry cause a drastic change in the child's routine. To help parents determine if their child is ready to enter nursery school, discuss with them the following readiness indicators:

• capacity to separate from parents
• ability to sit for brief periods (indicating an adequate attention span)
• ability to tolerate frustration
• acquisition of such social skills as ability to wait, take turns, and share
• acquisition of such self-care skills as eating, toileting, hand washing, and dressing.

Inform parents that a child entering nursery school may benefit from attending a half-day program two or three days a week. This schedule works especially well for three-year-olds. By age 4, the child may be able to tolerate half-days for 5 days a week or even a full-day program.

Instruct parents to introduce the idea of nursery school to the child several weeks before school starts and to describe the school experience as pleasurable. Also, suggest that they describe school activities to the child.

Advise parents to act confidently on the first day of school; children can sense parental anxiety and may become anxious themselves. When they arrive at school, parents should introduce the child to the teacher, stay with the child briefly until the child seems comfortable, then say good-bye to the child and inform the child they will pick the child up when school is over.

To ease the transition to school, urge parents to tell the teacher about special home routines, such as quiet time; some home routines may be incorporated into the school routine. Also, parents can encourage the child to take a transitional object, such as a blanket or a favorite stuffed animal, to school.

Managing communicable diseases

With school entry, preschool-age children are exposed to a large number of children and adults. Consequently, the incidence of infectious diseases rises during the preschool-age years. Immunizations have reduced the incidence of such communicable diseases as rubeola (mea-

(Text continues on page 94.)

Common communicable diseases

This chart describes common communicable diseases seen in preschool-age children.

DESCRIPTION	SIGNS AND SYMPTOMS	TREATMENT	NURSING CONSIDERATIONS
Erythema infectiosum (Fifth disease)			
• Benign viral disease that primarily affects preschool- and school-age children • Cause: human parvovirus B19 • Transmitted via respiratory secretions • Incubation: 4 to 14 days • Communicable 1 to 2 days before onset of rash	• Facial rash on cheeks (looks as if child has been slapped in face); disappears in 1 to 4 days • Red maculopapular rash appears on upper and lower extremities 1 day after facial rash appears; progresses from proximal to distal areas; lasts approximately 7 days	• None needed	• Child need not be isolated. (Disease is not communicable once rash appears.) • Reassure parents that disease is benign.
Exanthem subitum (roseola)			
• Acute viral disease of infants and young children; most common in spring and fall • Cause: human herpesvirus 6 • Unknown transmission mode • Incubation: 5 to 15 days • Communicable period unknown	• Sudden onset of high fever (102° to 105° F [38.8° to 40.6° C]), which lasts 2 to 5 days • Irritability; otherwise, child appears healthy • After fever subsides, macular or maculopapular rash appears on neck and spreads to trunk and extremities; rash disappears within 4 to 48 hours • Posterior auricular and suboccipital lymphadenopathy	• Acetaminophen for fever	• Teach parents how to manage fever. • Reassure parents that disease is benign.
Hand-foot-and-mouth disease			
• Acute, highly contagious viral disease; occurs primarily in summer • Cause: Coxsackie A virus • Transmitted via respiratory secretions and stool • Incubation: 3 to 6 days • Communicable period unknown, but disease presumably is communicable during prodromal and acute phases	• Prodromal phase: sudden, low-grade fever (101° F [38.3 ° C]), sore throat, and anorexia • Acute phase: vesicles on tonsils, soft palate, and uvula (vesicles rupture, leaving shallow ulcers); maculopapular rash and vesicles appear on palms and soles and between fingers and toes	• Acetaminophen for fever	• Isolate child until 24 hours after fever subsides. • Encourage noncarbonated, nonacidic fluids; avoid giving fruit juices (acidity and carbonation irritate mouth ulcers). • Teach parents how to manage fever. • Suggest parents give warm saline mouth rinses to reduce oral pain and irritation. • Reassure parents that disease is self-limiting and full recovery is expected within 5 to 7 days. • Instruct child to wash hands after using toilet.

(continued)

Common communicable diseases *(continued)*

DESCRIPTION	SIGNS AND SYMPTOMS	TREATMENT	NURSING CONSIDERATIONS
Mumps			
• Acute viral disease; potential complications include meningo-encephalitis (in about 10% of cases) and orchitis (in about 25% of males contracting disease after puberty) • Cause: paramyxovirus • Transmitted via respiratory secretions • Incubation: 14 to 21 days • Communicable immediately before and after parotid gland swelling	• Prodromal phase: anorexia, headache, mild to moderate fever (101° to 103° F [38.3° to 39.4° C]) lasting 12 to 24 hours; ear pain during chewing • Acute phase: within 3 days, 10% of affected children develop pale pink, maculopapular rash (primarily on trunk), unilateral or bilateral parotid gland swelling, and pain and tenderness in parotid area	• Acetaminophen for pain and fever	• Isolate child during communicable period. • Teach parents how to manage fever. • Advise parents to encourage fluids and soft foods and to avoid giving foods that require excessive chewing. • Suggest parents apply hot or cold compresses to child's neck.
Rubeola (measles)			
• Acute, highly contagious viral infection; complications include otitis media, pneumonia, croup, and encephalitis (rare but potentially fatal) • Cause: measles virus • Transmitted via respiratory secretions and urine • Incubation: 10 to 20 days • Communicable 4 days before to 5 days after rash appears; most contagious during prodromal phase	• Prodromal phase: 3- to 4-day history of high fever, conjunctivitis, cough, rhinitis, and appearance of Koplik spots (small, red spots with tiny, bluish-white center) on buccal mucosa opposite molars • Acute phase: after 3 to 4 days, discrete deep red maculopapular rash appears on face and spreads downward; rash becomes more confluent over course of disease; by day 6, fever subsides and rash starts to fade, brownish discoloration may then appear and desquamation occurs over areas of heavy involvement	• Acetaminophen for fever • Antibiotics for secondary infections (such as otitis media and pneumonia)	• Isolate child until fifth day of rash. • Advise parents to give child fluids. Instruct them to encourage bed rest during febrile period. • Teach parents how to manage fever. • Instruct parents to dim lights and close blinds if child's eyes are sensitive to light. • Instruct parents to use cool-mist vaporizer for cough and cold symptoms. • Teach child to wash hands after using toilet.
Rubella (German measles)			
• Highly contagious viral infection causing little distress in children; however, if a woman is exposed to virus during first trimester of pregnancy, fetal infection may result, causing severe consequences	• Prodromal phase: absent in children • Acute phase: discrete, pink maculopapular rash starting on face and spreading to trunk and extremities, accompanied by tender postauricular and	• Acetaminophen for fever if present • Bed rest	• Isolate child from pregnant women. • Reassure parents that disease is benign in children.

Common communicable diseases *(continued)*

DESCRIPTION	SIGNS AND SYMPTOMS	TREATMENT	NURSING CONSIDERATIONS
Rubella (German measles) *(continued)*			
• Cause: rubella virus • Transmitted via respiratory secretions, stool, and urine • Incubation: 14 to 21 days • Communicable 7 days before to 5 days after rash appears	suboccipital lymph nodes; rash disappears in same order in which it appeared and generally disappears within 3 days		
Scarlet fever			
• Acute streptococcal infection; potential complications include otitis media, cervical adenitis, rheumatic fever, and acute glomerulonephritis • Cause: group A beta-hemolytic streptococci • Transmitted via respiratory secretions • Incubation: 1 to 3 days • Communicable during carrier phase (which can last weeks to months), during incubation period, and until 24 hours after antibiotic therapy begins	• Prodromal phase: sudden onset of high fever, vomiting, headache, chills, malaise, abdominal pain, and sore throat • Acute phase: strawberry tongue (red papillae on coated tongue), acutely erythematous and edematous tonsils and pharynx, possibly purulent yellowish exudate on tonsils, enlarged tender anterior cervical lymph nodes; 12 to 48 hours, bright red, discrete rash appears, first in skin creases, then spreads to trunk and extremities (less often to face); rash blanches with pressure (face appears flushed with circumoral pallor) and disappears within 7 days, leaving desquamation areas in skinfolds, palms, and soles	• 200,000 to 400,000 U of penicillin G q.i.d. for 10 days (erythromycin for penicillin-sensitive children) • Acetaminophen for fever	• Isolate child for first 24 hours of treatment. • Teach parents how to manage fever. • Instruct parents how to administer antibiotic. Stress importance of giving drug for full 10-day course. Instruct parents to administer penicillin 1 hour before or 2 hours after meals or to give erythromycin with meals. Teach parents that drug may cause nausea, vomiting, and diarrhea. • Inform parents that child may resume normal activity once fever is absent for 24 hours. • Instruct parents to give warm saline mouth rinses for throat pain. • Advise parents to give noncarbonated, nonacidic fluids.
Varicella (chicken pox)			
• Highly contagious viral disease; most common in children between ages 2 to 8; occurs primarily from January to May; potential complications include secondary bacterial infections (most commonly, cellulitis and abscesses) and encephalitis (rare)	• Prodromal phase: slight fever, malaise, anorexia, and headache lasting 24 hours • Acute phase: initially, several small red macules appear on trunk, followed by 3- to 4-day eruption of macules on trunk, face, scalp, extremities, and mucous membranes; macules	• Antihistamines (diphenhydramine hydrochloride or hydroxyzine) for pruritus • Acyclovir suspension (for children over age 2)	• Isolate child until lesions have dried (crusted). • Caution parents never to give aspirin products to child with chicken pox because of the risk of Reye's syndrome. • Teach parents that antihistamines may cause drowsiness or hyperactivity and insomnia. *(continued)*

Common communicable diseases *(continued)*

DESCRIPTION	SIGNS AND SYMPTOMS	TREATMENT	NURSING CONSIDERATIONS
Varicella (chicken pox) *(continued)*			
• Cause: varicella-zoster virus • Incubation: 10 to 21 days • Communicable from 1 day before rash appears until all vesicles have crusted over (approximately 6 days); crusty rash is not infectious	quickly progress to papules and then vesicles, which break and crust over (all three lesion types may be present during disease course); rash is highly pruritic		Instruct them to limit antihistamine use to 2 to 3 days and try giving them only at night. • Teach parents about adverse effects of acyclovir suspension, including diarrhea. • Encourage use of other methods to relieve itching — for example, cool compresses, calamine lotion, baking soda, or Aveeno oatmeal baths. • Advise parents that child should not scratch lesions. Instruct them to cut child's fingernails short, have child wear mittens or gloves to bed, and remind child to stop scratching during waking hours. Inform them that applying pressure to lesions may lessen itching.

sles), mumps, rubella (German measles), pertussis (whooping cough), polio, and diphtheria. However, these diseases recently have made a comeback because of the low immunization rates in many areas of the United States. (Only about 40% of poor rural and urban children are protected fully by immunizations.) Also, no immunizations are available for varicella (chicken pox), erythema infectiosum (Fifth disease), exanthem subitum (roseola), hand-foot-and-mouth disease, and scarlet fever. (For clinical manifestations and management of diseases occurring in preschoolers, see *Common communicable diseases.*)

Young children run an especially high risk for contracting intestinal parasitic infections from poor hand washing after bowel movements and frequent hand-to-mouth behavior. (For information, see *Common intestinal parasitic infections.*)

Common intestinal parasitic infections in children

Poor hand washing and hand-to-mouth behavior predispose young children to intestinal parasitic infections. This chart describes two common childhood intestinal parasitic infections.

DESCRIPTION	SIGNS AND SYMPTOMS	TREATMENT	NURSING CONSIDERATIONS
Giardiasis			
• Most common intestinal parasitic infection in United States; prevalent among children attending group day care or nursery school • Highly contagious • Cause: *Giardia lamblia* • Transmitted via stool, person-to-person fecal-oral route, contaminated water (including wading pools used by diapered children), contaminated food, and animals • Incubation: 7 to 14 days after ingestion of cysts • Communicable after incubation period, when cysts are excreted in stool	• Older children and adults may be asymptomatic • Children over age 5: abdominal cramps; intermittent, loose, malodorous, pale stools • Children age 5 and under: diarrhea, vomiting, anorexia, and failure to thrive	• Although infection commonly resolves spontaneously in 4 to 6 weeks, treatment is recommended because disease is highly contagious; treatment may include furazolidone (available in pleasant-tasting suspension) or quinacrine (available in bitter-tasting tablets at 10% of the cost of furazolidone)	• Teach parents that furazolidone causes few adverse effects and that quinacrine may cause nausea and vomiting. Emphasize that child must complete full course of drug therapy. Instruct parents to administer prescribed drug after meals. • Teach parents that giardiasis can be prevented by washing hands thoroughly after toilet use, disposing of soiled diapers appropriately, keeping dogs and cats away from play areas, and avoiding swimming in pools frequented by diapered children. • Instruct parents to disinfect toilet seats and diaper changing areas with a solution of 10% bleach or Lysol.
Pinworms			
• Typically a benign infection • Highly contagious • Cause: *Enterobius vermicularis* • Transmitted via stool, person-to-person oral-fecal route; inhalation of eggs in air; and from eggs on household surfaces (child picks up egg with hands and fingers and transmits it from hand to mouth) • Incubation: 3 to 6 weeks after egg ingestion • Communicable as long as viable worms are present in intestinal tract; eggs persist in environment for up to 1 week	• Perianal pruritus, especially at night; restlessness during sleep; on awakening, ova or white, threadlike worms may appear near rectum	• For child over age 2, chewable mebendazole tablets—100 mg immediately and 100 mg 10 days later; some physicians recommend treating all nonpregnant family members as well	• Teach parents that mebendazole may be chewed or crushed and mixed with food and may cause such adverse effects as abdominal cramps and diarrhea. Emphasize that they must administer second dose. • Advise parents to give child warm baths or apply Desitin ointment to relieve rectal irritation. • Stress personal hygiene to prevent autoinfection of child, including daily baths, hand washing after toileting and before eating, keeping child's fingernails short, changing child's underwear twice a day, having child wear snug-fitting underwear, changing child's bedding nightly, and washing bedding and underwear in hot water and drying in dryer set on high.

STUDY ACTIVITIES

Short answer

1. Explain how parents can use a reward system to encourage a four-year-old girl to play nicely with her two-year-old brother.

_____

_____

_____

2. Identify at least three ways parents can help the preschool-age child develop initiative.

_____

_____

3. To help prevent recreational injuries in a preschool-age child, list at least three instructions the nurse should provide parents.

_____

_____

4. Identify measures that can help prevent autoinfection with pinworms.

_____

_____

_____

Multiple choice

5. To help prevent scalding during a child's bath, the nurse should instruct parents to set the hot water heater below:

    A. 115° F
    B. 120° F
    C. 125° F
    D. 130° F

6. When can a child can begin using an adult restraint system in a motor vehicle?

    A. When the child reaches 35″ in height
    B. When the child reaches 40″ in height
    C. When the child reaches age 3
    D. When the child reaches age 4

7. Joan Wright tells the nurse she is concerned about her daughter Melissa, age 3. She says Melissa "is always touching herself in her private area." What would be the nurse's best response?
  A. "Melissa's behavior is normal for a three-year-old. But if it concerns you, explain to her how much her behavior upsets you."
  B. "Three-year-old girls usually don't masturbate. You may need to ask Melissa why she is touching herself."
  C. "This behavior is normal for a three-year-old. But if it upsets you, tell Melissa she should masturbate only in the privacy of her room."
  D. "This behavior is normal for a three-year-old. Don't you remember masturbating as a child?"

8. The physician prescribes quinacrine to treat *Giardia lamblia* infection in Jennifer, age 5. Which information should the nurse give Jennifer's mother?
  A. "Quinacrine may cause nausea or vomiting."
  B. "Quinacrine may cause diarrhea."
  C. "Quinacrine may cause drowsiness."
  D. "Quinacrine may cause insomnia."

9. Which maternal disease may cause defects in a developing fetus?
  A. Diphtheria
  B. Measles
  C. Rubella
  D. Scarlet fever

10. When is the child with chicken pox considered no longer contagious?
  A. Once the rash disappears completely
  B. Once all lesions have crusted over
  C. When no new lesions develop
  D. When the rash first appears

ANSWERS **Short answer**

  1. Parents can explain to their daughter that it is important that she be nice to her younger brother. To encourage this behavior, they would tell her that they will place a stick-on star on a chart every time she plays nicely with her brother. The parents would award the star immediately after the behavior is demonstrated and praise the child verbally when awarding a star. They would tell her that if she collects a certain number of stars, she will be rewarded in a predetermined way.

  2. To promote development of initiative, parents can encourage the child to dress unassisted, comb the hair, and brush the teeth; praise the child's accomplishments; and encourage the child to complete other appropriate tasks.

3. The nurse should instruct parents to monitor the safety of playground equipment, supervise the child during playground use and bicycle riding, make sure the child wears shoes and a safety helmet when riding a bicycle, and make sure the child rides the bicycle only on level ground.

4. To prevent pinworm autoinfection, parents should have the child bathe daily, wash hands after toileting and before eating, wear snug-fitting underwear, and change underwear twice a day. Parents should change the child's bedding daily, keep the child's fingernails short, and wash bedding and underwear in hot water and dry in a dryer set on high.

Multiple choice

5. B. The hot water heater should be set below 120° F (48.8° C).

6. B. A child can use an adult restraint system when he or she reaches 40″ (102 cm) in height or weighs 40 lb (18 kg). Age is not a valid criterion because it does not accurately reflect weight.

7. C. Masturbation is typical behavior in a preschool-age child. If it upsets the parent, the nurse should instruct the parent to tell the child to masturbate only in the privacy of the child's bedroom. Explaining that the behavior upsets the parent is inappropriate because it conveys the impression that masturbation is bad. The mother's experience with masturbation is irrelevant.

8. A. The nurse should tell Jennifer's mother that quinacrine may cause nausea or vomiting. Diarrhea, drowsiness, and insomnia are not adverse reactions to quinacrine.

9. C. Fetuses exposed to rubella have been born with birth defects. The other diseases are not associated with birth defects.

10. B. Chicken pox no longer is considered contagious when all lesions have crusted over.

CHAPTER 9

The school-age child and family

OBJECTIVES   After studying this chapter, the reader should be able to:

1. Identify the norms for physical growth, gross motor development, fine motor development, and social development in the school-age child.

2. Describe psychosocial, psychosexual, and cognitive development in the school-age child.

3. Discuss nursing interventions that promote growth and development in the school-age child.

4. Identify nursing interventions that enhance nutrition, elimination, dental health, sleep, exercise, and safety in the school-age child.

5. Describe characteristics of common pediatric skin infections in school-age children, and discuss the nurse's role in managing these disorders.

6. Discuss characteristics of selected pediatric emotional disorders, and identify related nursing interventions.

OVERVIEW OF CONCEPTS   This chapter describes psychosocial, psychosexual, and cognitive development during the school-age period — ages 6 to 12. It identifies major growth and developmental milestones attained during this time and describes the nurse's role in enhancing the school-age child's growth and development. The chapter also discusses how the nurse can promote the child's health. It includes nursing management of common pediatric skin infections and emotional disorders.

Growth and development   Physical growth is slow but steady during the school-age years. (For details, see *Major growth and developmental milestones in school-age children,* page 100.)

Psychosocial development
According to Erik Erikson, the school-age child's developmental task is to become industrious while overcoming a sense of inferiority. The child has a strong desire to achieve and to master fully whatever is undertaken — in school as well as in the personal and social spheres. The child achieves full self-care ability during this period. With strong likes

Major growth and developmental milestones in school-age children

This chart details the major milestones a school-age child should achieve.

PHYSICAL GROWTH	GROSS AND FINE MOTOR DEVELOPMENT	SOCIAL DEVELOPMENT
6 to 7 years		
• Slow, steady growth • Average weight: Boys—46 lb (age 6); 51 lb (age 7) Girls— 45 lb (age 6); 50 lb (age 7) • Average height: Boys— 45½" (age 6); 47 ½" (age 7) Girls— 45" (age 6); 47" (age 7) • Dentition: six-year molars (first permanent teeth) erupt; deciduous lower and upper central incisors fall out	• Rides two-wheel bicycle without training wheels • Uses knife to cut food • Ties a bow • Draws triangle and diamond • Prints letters legibly • Differentiates right and left	• Enjoys physical activity and games (may cheat to win) • May tattle • Bathes without supervision • Brushes and combs own hair
8 to 9 years		
• Slow, steady growth • Average weight: Boys—56 lb (age 8); 61 lb (age 9) Girls— 55 lb (age 8); 61 lb (age 9) • Average height: Boys— 49½" (age 8); 52" (age 9) Girls— 49" (age 8); 52" (age 9) • Dentition: deciduous upper lateral incisors and lower cuspids fall out	• Has good eye-hand coordination • Pounds nails • Hits ball with bat • Can sew, but needs help threading needle • Draws using the concepts of three dimensions • Can build models • Participates in team sports	• Has same-sex playmates • Helps with routine household tasks • Assumes responsibility for chores and pet care • Likes competitive games and sports • Is easy to get along with
10 to 12 years		
• Height gain is steady; weight gain accelerates • In girls, pubescent growth spurt begins at average age of 11 • Pubescent changes may appear, especially in girls • Average weight: Boys—67 lb (age 10); 77 lb (age 11); 87 lb (age 12) Girls—72 lb (age 10); 81 lb (age 11); 91 lb (age 12) • Average height: Boys—54" (age 10); 56" (age 11); 58" (age 12) Girls— 54" (age 10); 56" (age 11); 59½" (age 12) • Dentition: remaining deciduous teeth fall out	• Possesses all basic motor skills • Becomes clumsy during pubescent growth spurt	• Has acquired all self-care skills • May need reminders to bathe and change clothes • Begins to show interest in opposite-sex relationships • May be left at home for brief periods of time • Socializes more with friends

and dislikes in such areas as hair and clothing styles, the school-age child may refuse to wear clothing the child dislikes or may style hair according to "adult" norms.

Achieving mastery through accomplishments in academics and sports, the child strives to complete school tasks correctly and becomes increasingly competitive in sports. Failure causes a sense of inferiority. Through interaction with peers, the child gains a positive self-regard.

Psychosexual development

According to Sigmund Freud, the school-age years correspond to the latency period of psychosexual development. The child now focuses psychic and physical energy on acquiring new knowledge and achievement in school and play. No new psychosexual conflicts emerge during this time.

Cognitive development

According to Jean Piaget, the development of concrete operations begins during the school-age years. Reasoning changes from an intuitive, experienced-based process to a logical process. Interaction with others becomes less egocentric and more cooperative.

During this period, the child acquires cognitive operations to understand concepts related to objects. These cognitive operations include the following:

• *conservation skills* — the recognition that certain properties of an object (liquid, mass, number, length, area, and volume) remain the same despite changes in other properties of that object (such as shape). For example, suppose a round ball of clay is rolled into a log shape. The child who has acquired conservation skills will understand that the log and the ball both contain the same amount of clay, representing the conservation of mass. Or, suppose the water from a short, wide glass is poured into a taller and narrower glass, so that the liquid line is higher than in the shorter glass. A child who has acquired the concept of conservation of liquids understands that the second glass contains the same amount of water as the first. (In contrast, a preschool-age child who has not acquired this concept believes the short glass contains less water because it is not filled as high.) A child acquires conservation skills regarding liquids, mass, number, and length by age 6 to 7; area and volume, by age 9 to 10.

• *classification skills* — the ability to group objects according to shared characteristics. For example, a child age 6 to 7 can group marbles by color or size. As the child grows, classification skills become increasingly complex and may be based on abstract ideas rather than concrete, perceptual ideas.

• *combinational skills* — the ability to manipulate numbers and learn basic mathematics (such as addition, subtraction, multiplication, and division).

Teaching parents to promote growth and development in the school-age child

The school-age child needs proper stimulation for optimal growth and development. This chart presents guidance the nurse should provide to help the parents and the community provide such stimulation.

GROWTH AND DEVELOPMENTAL AREA	PARENT AND COMMUNITY TEACHING
Gross and fine motor development	• Provide opportunities for supervised bicycle riding. • Provide art materials, such as clay, paints, brushes, and paper. • Offer opportunities and supplies for model building, such as papier-mâché and commercial car and plane models. • Provide opportunities and supplies for crafts, such as sewing and jewelry making. • Allow opportunities and space for energetic play. • Provide outdoor play equipment, including balls, bats, and gloves.
Social development	• Provide opportunities for casual and organized sports activities. • Encourage board and card games. • Encourage responsibility for dressing and grooming. • Assign chores. • Promote opportunities for interacting with peers.
Psychosocial and psycho-sexual development	• Encourage realistic achievement goals to give the child a good chance for success. • Provide a variety of experiences to ensure that the child succeeds in at least some areas. • Provide positive feedback.
Cognitive development	• Play time-oriented games with young school-age children. • Tell stories about things that happened in the past or that may happen in the future. • Play word and number games. • Promote reasoning and decision-making; for example, ask the child, "What would happen if . . ."

The school-age child also develops the concept of time, learning to tell time early during this period, and begins to understand the concepts of past, present, and future. The older school-age child can use hypotheses in scientific problem-solving if the hypothesis is based on concrete evidence.

Enhancing growth and development

The school-age child acquires motor, social, and cognitive skills by interacting within the family and the larger community. Therefore, the nurse should direct interventions to the parents, the school, and the child's larger social community. (For anticipatory guidance that can enhance growth and development, see *Teaching parents to promote growth and development in the school-age child.*)

Enforcing discipline

For the school-age child, behavioral self-control is the goal of discipline. Through self-discipline, the child acquires a positive self-concept and learns to live in a complex environment without infringing on others' rights. The child also learns to live within the confines of family and social rules and boundaries. The child who fails to learn self-control feels inferior and develops a poor self-concept.

Effective discipline strategies for the school-age child include:

- explanation and problem solving — advise parents to give the child clear explanations regarding acceptable and unacceptable behavior; recommend that they give the older school-age child a chance to negotiate with parents in establishing behavioral rules acceptable to all family members.
- reasoning — the school-age child can see others' viewpoints and understand the effect of misbehavior on others
- experiencing consequences (see Chapter 8, The preschool-age child and family)
- withholding privileges
- imposing penalties, such as grounding
- demanding compensation — a child who breaks a window must pay to replace it
- using reward systems (see Chapter 8, The preschool-age child and family).

Promoting health in the school-age child

Teach parents ways to enhance the child's nutrition, dental health, sleep patterns, and exercise. Advise them on how to deal with sexuality issues, ensure the child's safety, and manage skin infections and emotional disorders.

Ensuring adequate nutrition

The school-age child is more willing than the preschooler to try new foods. Encourage parents to provide a variety of foods, in both snacks and meals. As the child enters school, eating patterns become increasingly independent of parental control. Therefore, to help the child learn sound eating habits, direct nutritional counseling at the child as well as the parents.

During the school-age period, caloric needs continue to decrease relative to body size. Food-group requirements for the school-age child resemble those for other children. However, the amount in a serving size increases. (For calorie, protein, and fluid requirements, see *Nutritional requirements for the school-age child,* page 104.)

Recommended diet

Inform the parents that the school-age child's daily diet should include the following foods and beverages:

- Bread, cereal, rice, and pasta: six to eleven servings (one serving equals one slice of bread, three to four crackers, or $\frac{1}{2}$ cup cereal, rice, or pasta)
- Fruits: two to four servings, including at least one citrus fruit (one serving equals one small banana or other raw fruit, $\frac{1}{2}$ cup canned fruit, or 4 oz juice)

Nutritional requirements for the school-age child

This chart presents daily calorie, protein, and fluid requirements for the school-age child.

AGE	CALORIE	PROTEIN	FLUID
6 years	90 cal/kg (41 cal/lb)	1.2 g/kg (0.5 g/lb)	95 ml/kg (43 ml/lb; approximately 1½ oz/lb)
7 to 10 years	70 cal/kg (32 cal/lb)	1.2 g/kg (0.5 g/lb)	80 ml/kg (36 ml/lb; approximately 1 oz/lb)
11 to 12 years	Boys: 55 cal/kg (25 cal/lb) Girls: 47 cal/kg (21 cal/lb)	1.2 g/kg (0.5 g/lb)	55 ml/kg (25 ml/lb; approximately ¾ oz/lb)

- Vegetables: three to five servings, including at least one leafy, green or yellow vegetable (one serving equals three to four pieces of raw vegetables or ½ cup cooked vegetables)
- Meat, poultry, fish, dry beans, eggs, and nuts: two servings (one serving equals 2 oz meat, one egg, 2 tablespoons peanut butter, or ½ cup dry beans)
- Milk, yogurt, and cheese: two to three servings (one serving equals 8 oz [1 cup] milk, 2 oz hard cheese, ½ cup cottage cheese, or ½ cup yogurt).

Promoting bowel and bladder elimination

By age 6, about 90% of children have gained complete bladder and bowel control. Most children also are capable of self-care in toileting (such as undressing, wiping, flushing, dressing, and hand washing) by age 6. However, some school-age children still have problems with bladder or bowel control.

Coping with enuresis

Enuresis is the involuntary release of urine in a child over age 6. *Primary enuresis* refers to involuntary urine release in a child who has never achieved full bladder control; *secondary enuresis* is involuntary urine release in a child who has achieved full bladder control for several months.

Most children with enuresis experience bed-wetting; *nocturnal enuresis* is involuntary bed-wetting that occurs at least once a month. Daytime wetting (diurnal enuresis) is less common.

Enuresis affects more boys than girls. An organic cause for enuresis rarely is found in children. The etiology of the disorder is unclear, but seems to involve a combination of factors. For example, enuresis is more common in children with a parent who had enuresis and in children who are deep sleepers (sleeping so soundly they cannot arouse themselves from sleep to respond to a full bladder). Other conditions that seem to promote enuresis include small bladder capacity and immature neurologic control of the bladder.

Most children with enuresis are embarrassed by their wetting episodes. Often teased by siblings and friends, many are reluctant to stay overnight at a friend's house because of the fear of wetting. Parents may become increasingly frustrated by the need to change and launder the child's sheets and nightclothes frequently.

Once an organic cause for enuresis has been ruled out, a management plan can be developed. Management strategies vary but may include: behavioral therapy, bladder-stretching exercises, drug therapy, and family and child support.

Nursing responsibilities. During treatment of enuresis, caution the family to avoid punishing, embarrassing, shaming, or diapering the child. Suggest that they restrict the child's fluids after dinner. Another strategy is to have the parents awaken the child to use the toilet before they go to sleep (if the child can be aroused). However, be aware that restricting fluids and awakening the child have had limited success when used alone without other proven management strategies.

Managing bowel incontinence

Some school-age children have problems with bowel continence. *Encopresis* refers to lack of bowel control in a child over age 4. Most children with encopresis reportedly do not feel the urge to defecate. Many are unaware when they have an accident; they seem immune to the odor of the bowel movement. Most bowel accidents occur in the late afternoon or early evening. Encopresis is more common in boys than girls.

The etiology of encopresis is unclear. The following factors appear to play a role in the disorder:
- constipation during infancy, accompanied by parental overconcern and aggressive treatment
- overaggressive or overpermissive toilet training
- pain during bowel elimination, commonly resulting from constipation
- fear of the toilet or of school bathrooms
- incomplete defecation
- psychosocial stressors
- a busy lifestyle (in older children).

Many children with encopresis live in fear of having an accident in school and may display symptoms of anxiety and depression. Parents commonly become frustrated because they do not understand why the child cannot feel the urge to defecate or does not clean up the mess after an accident has occurred.

Some children develop acquired megacolon with significant stool retention. Therefore, initial management entails emptying the large intestine, such as with enemas, suppositories, or laxatives. The child then starts a bowel training maintenance program, sitting on the toilet twice a day for at least 10 minutes, at the same time daily. (For most children, the best time is after a meal.) For the first 4 to 6 weeks, the child takes mineral oil and oral laxatives. Once the child achieves successful bowel elimination patterns, laxatives may be withdrawn gradually. Behavior modification also is an option for treatment.

Nursing responsibilities. Support the child and family, emphasizing that no one is to blame for the child's problem. Assure the family that most bowel control problems resolve with therapy.

Explain the prescribed therapeutic regimen to the child and family. Caution the parents that long-term enema and laxative use may complicate rather than alleviate the problem.

Enhancing dental health

The first permanent teeth erupt during the sixth year. Malocclusion (crooked teeth, gaps in teeth, overbite or underbite) may occur during the school-age years. Some children outgrow this problem, but others need orthodontic care.

To help the child maintain permanent teeth, advise parents to begin comprehensive dental supervision during the child's preschool-age years. To prevent dental caries and periodontal disease, make sure the child and family understand correct toothbrushing and flossing techniques. Recommend fluoride toothpaste; if the local water supply is not fluorinated, also recommend fluoride supplements. Counsel the parents to continue to monitor the child's toothbrushing. A younger school-age child may still need the parent's help in flossing.

Promoting healthy sleep patterns

Few school-age children need to nap. Nighttime sleep requirements vary greatly; most children require at least 8 to 10 hours of sleep. Nightmares and night terrors become less common. However, many school-age children walk or talk in their sleep. Inform parents that sleepwalking children normally return to bed on their own, so the best approach is to leave the child alone. If the child is in danger of self-injury, counsel parents to lead the child quietly back to bed. Assure parents that most children outgrow sleepwalking and sleeptalking.

Promoting exercise

Physical play enhances the development of strength, balance, and coordination. Most school-age children are physically active and are formally exposed to organized sports and group activities.

However, some children (especially those left home alone after school) spend much time indoors watching television — an activity linked to obesity. Advise parents to limit television watching to a maximum of 3 hours and to make sure the child engages in some form of physical activity daily.

Help parents explore ways for the child to channel physical energy. For instance, suggest that the child walk the family dog or play at a friend's house after school several times a week.

Teaching parents about the child's sexuality

The school-age child develops an interest in the biological nature of sexual function. The younger school-age child is curious about sex organs and their function. This child may engage in same-sex sexual play, which upsets some parents. To help parents understand the child's behavior, explain that the behavior is a normal result of sexual curiosity and in no way reflects the child's sexual orientation. Also help them understand the source of their concern. For example, some may view sexual play as "dirty."

Encourage parents to discuss sex organs and their functions with the child. Mention that a child's curiosity about sex organs and sexual play may decrease if parents display an open attitude and provide information about sex organs. Advise parents to avoid shaming or punishing the child for such behavior.

During the middle school-age years (ages 8 to 9), the child may be exposed to a formal sex education program. To minimize embarrassment and encourage an open atmosphere, these programs are offered to boys and girls separately. Information about sex organs, sexual maturation, and reproduction can be introduced at this time. Older school-age children (ages 10 to 12) need more detailed information about such matters as menstruation, wet dreams, erections, and ways to prevent pregnancy and sexually transmitted diseases.

Ensuring safety

Accidents, including motor vehicle injuries, account for nearly 20% of deaths in school-age children. Increased activity away from home and risk-taking behavior contribute to injuries in school-age children. To help prevent accidents, provide comprehensive instruction on injury prevention. (For specific teaching points, see *Preventing injuries in school-age children,* page 108.)

Managing common skin infections

Skin infections may result from bacteria, viruses, fungi, and parasites. Because school-age children are highly social and most skin infections are highly contagious, child-to-child transmission is extremely common. (For details on skin infections, see *Common skin infections in school-age children,* pages 109 to 112.)

Coping with emotional disorders

School-age children may experience school phobia, recurrent abdominal pain (RAP), and depression.

Managing school phobia

School phobia (sometimes called school avoidance syndrome) refers to resistance or refusal to go to school out of fear of the school situation or concern over leaving home. School phobia occurs in all socioeconomic classes, and is more common among girls. (Be aware that in the younger child just starting school, some separation difficulty is normal and is not classified as school phobia.)

Preventing injuries in school-age children

To help prevent injuries, review the following points with the parents of school-age children.

Preventing burns
- Teach the child what to do in case of fire, including how to use a fire extinguisher and matches safely.
- Directly supervise the young school-age child who is using the stove to prepare a meal. Parents should be home when the older school-age child cooks.
- Teach the child about the danger of firecrackers.

Preventing recreational injuries
- Instruct the child in proper use of play and sport equipment.
- Make sure that the child wears appropriate protective gear when engaging in contact sports and that a trained coach supervises all contact sports.

Bicycle riding
- Have the child demonstrate safe bicycle-riding behavior (including rules of the road) before letting the child ride alone.
- Make sure the child wears a bicycle helmet and proper shoes. Equip the bicycle with reflectors.
- Teach the child to watch for cars exiting driveways.
- Let the child cross the street only at the corner. Teach the child to ride single file when riding in a group of bicyclists.

Skateboarding
- Make sure the child wears a helmet and protective knee pads and elbow pads.
- Instruct the child to skateboard in driveways or unused parking lots — never on the street.
- Do not allow the child to skate on ramps.

Water sports
- Teach the child how to swim.
- Make sure the child knows water safety rules: always wear a life jacket while on a boat; do not swim alone; swim only at supervised beaches or pools; dive only in designated areas.

Preventing motor vehicle injuries
- Make sure the child wears a lap belt and shoulder harness at all times when in a motor vehicle.
- To ensure safe street crossing, tell the child to cross only at the corner, to observe traffic lights when crossing the street, and to walk on sidewalks (or on the side of the road and facing traffic if no sidewalks are available). If the child must walk in the street at night, make sure the child wears light-reflective clothing.

The child with school phobia experiences anxiety — possibly bordering on panic — at the prospect of going to school. Typically, the child has somatic complaints, such as stomachache, headache, and dizziness, which disappear quickly if parents let the child stay home.

Several factors have been linked to the development of school phobia. These include:
- fear of some aspect of school, such as fear of teachers, fear or failing, or fear or threats or harassment by peers
- fear of abandonment
- a dependent mother-child relationship
- an overprotective, overinvolved mother.

The short-term goal of managing school phobia is to promote the child's immediate return to school; the longer the child stays home, the more difficulty the child has returning to school.

Nursing responsibilities. Advise parents that the child must return to school immediately. Suggest they emphasize that the child must go to school every morning. In some cases, parents may need to take the child to school. Once in the school environment, most children calm down and can go to their classroom. If the child is extremely anxious,

(Text continues on page 112.)

Common skin infections in school-age children

This chart describes pediatric skin infections and related nursing responsibilities.

DESCRIPTION	SIGNS AND SYMPTOMS	TREATMENT	NURSING CONSIDERATIONS
Impetigo contagiosa			
• Highly contagious bacterial infection characterized by honey-colored, crusted lesions • Most common in toddlers and preschool-age and school-age children • Poor hygiene is a predisposing factor • Caused by group A beta-hemolytic streptococci or *Staphylococcus aureus* • Transmitted by direct contact • Incubation period is 1 to 3 days • Communicable before treatment starts and for 48 hours after treatment begins	• Reddish macules, seen mainly around mouth and nares, progress to clear vesicles, which rapidly progress to pustules; honey-colored crust forms after pustules rupture • Lesions are pruritic; scratching causes infection to spread	• Topical antibiotic ointment (Neosporin or bacitracin) • Systemic antibiotic (penicillin or erythromycin) for severe cases	• Teach parents to remove crusty lesions by gently washing child's skin with antibacterial soap, such as Dial. • Advise parents to have child complete full course of drug therapy (even if skin clears). • Instruct parents to have child use separate washcloth and towel to prevent transmission to other family members. • Instruct parents to cut child's fingernails to minimize scratching. • Have parents keep child out of school until 48 hours after therapy begins. • Reassure parents and child that skin will heal without scarring.
Verruca (warts)			
• Caused by human papillomavirus • Transmitted by direct contact with virus (presumably) • Incubation period unknown • Communicable as long as lesion is present (presumably) • Small warts may disappear spontaneously	• Small, brown, benign lesions, which may appear anywhere on body but are most common on face, fingers, hands, and soles • Lesions may be singular or multiple	• Electrocautery • Cryotherapy • Caustic solutions	• Instruct parents to apply caustic solution (commerical wart remover) to surface of wart, cover with provided adhesive, remove adhesive after 24 hours, and rub with abrasive brush provided; repeat until wart is gone.
Herpes simplex virus type 1			
• Recurrent viral infection seen primarily on lips or in mouth; virus remains latent and may reappear, causing lesions during times of stress, sun exposure, menses, trauma, febrile illness, and systemic infection • Caused by herpes simplex virus type 1 • Transmitted by direct contact with saliva	• Burning or tingling sensation before lesion appears • One or more vesicular lesions, which dry and form a crust; lesions last 8 to 14 days	• Idoxuridine ointment every hour during the day, then q.i.d. until lesions heal • Oral acyclovir	• Isolate child from newborns, children with eczema or burns, and persons with depressed immunity. • Teach child to avoid picking at lesions because this may cause secondary infection. • Inform parents that recurrence is likely.

(continued)

Common skin infections in school-age children *(continued)*

DESCRIPTION	SIGNS AND SYMPTOMS	TREATMENT	NURSING CONSIDERATIONS
Herpes simplex virus type 1 *(continued)*			
• Incubation period is 2 to 12 days • Communicable as long as lesion is present			
Dermatophytoses (ringworm)			
• Highly contagious, superficial fungal infection • May appear on nonhairy skin surfaces (tinea corporis), on scalp (tinea capitis), in groin area (tinea cruris), or between toes (tinea pedis) • Caused by various fungi, depending on site • Transmitted by direct or indirect contact with infected person or animal, or from clothing • Incubation period is 4 to 10 days • Communicable as long as lesions are present	• Tinea corporis: flat, small papules forming a circular lesion, which clears centrally; develops into scaling lesion, with advancing borders • Tinea capitis: similar to tinea corporis but found on scalp; hair loss around lesion is common • Tinea cruris: reddened, sore, raw-looking skin in groin area; chafing from clothing may cause pain and pruritus; most common in adolescents and adults • Tinea pedis: causes cracks between toes; with deep fissures, infection is pruritic and painful; may involve widespread fine scaling extending to sole and toes	• Antifungal creams, such as clotrimazole (Lotrimin), miconazole (Micatin), or tolnaftate (Tinactin) • Oral griseofulvin for persistent tinea capitis	• Emphasize that treatment must continue for 1 week after lesion disappears. • Teach parents to monitor for adverse effects of griseofulvin: headache, nausea, fatigue, insomnia, and photosensitivity. • Tell parents that child should not share unlaundered clothing or bedsheets. Advise them to launder clothing and bedsheets in hot water and dry in dryer on hot setting. • Teach parents to keep child's skin dry, and to cover lesions on nonhairy areas of the skin with clothing or adhesive bandages. • Instruct parents to have child avoid wearing tight, constricting clothing. • Advise the child with tinea capitis to avoid sharing hat or combs with other people. • Advise parents that improvement may take 5 to 7 days and that lesion may take up to 3 weeks to disappear. • Inform parents that child's hair will grow back eventually. • Encourage parents to examine household pets for evidence of infection, and to have pets treated.
Scabies			
• Highly contagious parasitic infection seen in persons of all ages; most common in crowded urban areas	• Linear, threadlike, grayish burrows, 1 to 10 mm long; may become vesicles	• Children under age 2: Bathe thoroughly, scrubbing entire body with rough, soapy towel, and then dry. Apply Eurax cream	• Teach parents to eliminate mite from environment by laundering clothing and bedding in hot water and drying in dryer on high

Common skin infections in school-age children (continued)

DESCRIPTION	SIGNS AND SYMPTOMS	TREATMENT	NURSING CONSIDERATIONS
Scabies (continued)			
• Occurs in 30-year cycles, each cycle lasting 15 years • Caused by female mite, *Sarcoptes scabiei* • Transmitted by direct or indirect contact with infected person or infested clothing, bedding, or household items • Incubation period is 1 to 3 weeks • Communicable until 24 hours after treatment ends	• Highly pruritic • Most common in finger webs, on flexor surface of wrists, and in antecubital area; less commonly seen in popliteal folds, inguinal region, on axillae, and on waist • Papules also may develop; skin may appear excoriated • Pustules indicate secondary infection	(60 mg) to entire body (except face and scalp, unless infested); repeat application after 24 hours. Bathe 48 hours after last application. Change clothing, bedding, and towels after each application and at end of therapy • Children over age 2: Bathe thoroughly, scrubbing entire body with rough, soapy, towel, and then dry. Apply Kwell or Elimite lotion over entire body (except face and scalp, unless infested); leave on for 12 hours; then bathe thoroughly. Change clothing, bedding, towels after Kwell application and final bathing. Repeat application in 1 week • Neosporin or bacitracin ointment t.i.d. after treatment (for secondary infections) • 1% hydrocortisone cream t.i.d. after treatment, or Benadryl (5 mg/kg/day) q.i.d. for pruritus • Prophylactic treatment of all immediate family members	setting; by changing clothes daily until treatment is complete; by using R & C spray on rugs and upholstered furniture; and by damp-mopping floors, table tops, and counters. • Caution parents not to let medication get in child's eyes or mouth. Warn them not to let child ingest medication (it is poisonous). Instruct them not apply it to badly inflamed skin or raw, weeping areas. • Teach parents about adverse drug effects, such as skin irritation and excoriation. • Teach parents not to touch or hold child until treatment is complete. • Inform parents that pruritus may last for 2 to 3 weeks.
Pediculosis capitis (head lice)			
• Highly contagious infestation of scalp; occurs in persons of all ages; most common in crowded urban areas • Caused by *Pediculus humanus capitis* • Transmitted by direct or indirect contact • Incubation period: 8 to 9 days • Communicable as long as lice are present on scalp	• Pruritus of scalp • Lice may be visible on scalp—most commonly behind ears and at base of hairline • Ova look like whitish-gray flecks; are firmly attached to hair shaft	• Nix creme rinse: Shampoo, rinse, and towel dry hair. Apply Nix, thoroughly saturating hair and scalp; allow Nix to remain on hair for 10 minutes; then rinse. Nits need not be combed out of hair. (Nix is ovicidal and is ffective for 14 days after initial treatment.) • Kwell shampoo (contraindicated in pregnant women and children under age 2): Thoroughly wet hair and scalp with Kwell;	• Teach parents to prevent transmission by not sharing or borrowing combs, hair ornaments, or hats; by not sharing pillows; by laundering bedsheets and hats in hot water and drying on hot dryer setting; by changing bedsheets and clothing daily; by spraying rugs and upholstered furniture with R & C spray; and by damp mopping and dusting floors, countertops, and table tops. (continued)

Common skin infections in school-age children (continued)

DESCRIPTION	SIGNS AND SYMPTOMS	TREATMENT	NURSING CONSIDERATIONS
Pediculosis capitis (head lice) (continued)			
		add small amount of water and lather; shampoo for 4 minutes; rinse thoroughly and towel-dry hair. Using a fine-toothed comb, remove nits from hair. Repeat in 7 days (Kwell is not ovicidal.)	• Teach parents about medication, including following directions closely. If using Kwell, stress importance of combing nits from hair and repeating application in 7 days. • Inform parents that lice cannot jump or fly from person to person; however, they may crawl from one place to another. • Inspect immediate family members for infestation.

parents may need the assistance of the school nurse or psychologist in helping the child to separate from the parents.

Both parents and child may benefit from counseling to determine the cause of school phobia. Certain causes are dealt with more easily than others. For example, fear of failing may be managed through parental and teacher support and assistance with study habits. If school phobia results from family and marital difficulties, the child and family should be referred to a family therapist or psychologist. Other nursing responsibilities include explaining the management plan to the child and family and providing ongoing family support.

Coping with RAP

RAP refers to abdominal pain with no organic cause that is severe enough to interfere with normal activity and occurs at least once a month for at least 3 months. Located in the periumbilical region, the pain may be cramping, dull, or sharp. It typically lasts 1 to 3 hours.

Approximately 15% of school-age children experience RAP. Characteristically, the child with RAP is a high achiever.

Some experts blame RAP on a colicky, spastic colon. Others suggest RAP results from the interaction of many factors, including:
• lifestyle patterns, such as daily routines, diet, and elimination patterns
• temperament
• behavioral style
• learned coping skills
• home and school environment
• stressful events
• somatic predisposition.

Nursing responsibilities. Teach the child and parents about the nature of this disorder and provide ongoing support. Inform them that the child's abdominal pain is real and is *not* just "in the child's head." Reassure them that the pain is not related to disease but probably results from gastrointestinal spasms, such as from lifestyle patterns or personality factors. Advise them to avoid school absences.

Teach the parents and child about mineral oil, if prescribed, and recommend a high-fiber diet to prevent constipation. To relieve the pain, instruct parents to apply a heating pad to the child's abdomen.

If RAP results from psychosocial or environmental factors, advise parents on how to modify these. For example, explain that undue parental attention to the painful episodes may contribute to both the onset and duration of abdominal pain.

Dealing with depression

Depression is common in children, adolescents, and adults. However, its manifestations vary with the child's developmental level. Depression affects about 5% of children and accounts for roughly 10% to 20% of children treated for psychiatric disturbances. Depression presumably results from a combination of genetic factors, biochemical abnormalities, and stress.

The following signs and symptoms indicate depression in a child:
- depressed mood (sadness)
- loss of interest or pleasure in activities
- significant changes in weight or appetite
- sleep difficulties
- motor agitation or retardation
- fatigue or loss of energy
- feelings of worthlessness or excessive guilt
- diminished ability to think or concentrate
- recurrent thoughts of death.

Clinical depression is diagnosed if the child exhibits a depressed mood or loss of interest, in addition to at least four of the other signs and symptoms listed above, during a 2-week period.

Nursing responsibilities. The nurse plays an important role in recognizing signs and symptoms of depression and making appropriate referrals. Management of childhood depression may involve tricyclic antidepressants (such as imipramine) and monoamine oxidase (MAO) inhibitors (such as phenelzine). Psychosocial interventions, such as modeling, role-playing, and positive reinforcement, can enhance social behavior and decrease the incidence of depression. Psychotherapy has been tried with depressed children, but its effect has not been proven.

STUDY ACTIVITIES

Short answer

1. Define conservation as it relates to cognitive development in the school-age child.

_____

_____

2. List at least four strategies parents can use to discipline the school-age child.

_____

_____

3. Define encopresis.

_____

Multiple choice

4. Which statement accurately describes physical growth in school-age children?
   A. In boys, the growth spurt begins, on the average, at age 11.
   B. Weight gain is steady until age 10 to 12; after this time, it accelerates.
   C. Boys and girls are approximately equal in height and weight throughout the school-age period.
   D. Height increases an average of 4″ (10 cm) per year.

5. Which statement about young school-age children is *not* true?
   A. They can clean themselves adequately after using the toilet.
   B. They can brush and comb their own hair.
   C. They can brush their teeth unassisted.
   D. They can choose their own clothes and dress unassisted.

6. Warts are caused by:
   A. Viruses
   B. Parasites
   C. Bacteria
   D. Fungi

7. The child with impetigo typically has which of the following symptoms?
   A. A fine, red papular rash
   B. Honey-colored, crusted skin lesions
   C. Linear-shaped skin lesions
   D. Circular skin lesions, which clear centrally

8. How is RAP characterized?

A. Acute, stabbing pain felt under the rib cage

B. Cramping pain felt near the umbilicus

C. Continuous pain felt near the left lower abdominal quadrant

D. Dull, throbbing pain felt near the right upper rib margin

9. To diagnose clinical depression in a child, which sign or symptom must be present?

A. Irritability

B. Sadness

C. Weight gain

D. Fatigue

ANSWERS

Short answer

1. Conservation refers to the child's ability to understand that certain properties of an object remain the same despite changes in other properties.

2. Effective discipline strategies for the school-age child include explanation and problem-solving, reasoning, experiencing consequences, withholding privileges, imposing penalties, demanding compensation, and using reward systems.

3. Encopresis is lack of bowel control in a child over age 4.

Multiple choice

4. B. The growth spurt begins at age 11 for girls — not boys. By the end of the school-age period, girls typically are taller and heavier than boys. Height increases an average of 2″, not 4″, per year.

5. C. School-age children still need to be monitored during toothbrushing.

6. A. Warts are caused by viruses.

7. B. In impetigo, honey-colored crusted lesions develop once the pustules rupture.

8. B. RAP is characterized by cramping pain in the periumbilical region.

9. B. A diagnosis of clinical depression in a child hinges on the presence of a depressed mood (sadness). The child also may gain weight and report fatigue, but these are not essential to the diagnosis. Irritability does not occur in depression.

CHAPTER 10

The adolescent and family

OBJECTIVES After studying this chapter, the reader should be able to:

1. Describe physical growth patterns during adolescence.

2. Discuss psychosocial, psychosexual, and cognitive development in the adolescent.

3. Describe the nurse's role in promoting the adolescent's growth and development.

4. Identify nursing interventions that promote nutrition and ensure the safety of adolescents.

5. Discuss the nurse's role in dealing with sexuality issues for the adolescent.

6. Describe the causes, signs and symptoms, and treatment of acne, and identify related nursing interventions.

7. Discuss the causes of eating disorders, and describe the nurse's role in their management.

8. Describe the personality, behavioral, and family characteristics of suicidal adolescents.

OVERVIEW OF CONCEPTS This chapter explores physical, psychosocial, psychosexual, and cognitive development during the adolescent period — ages 13 to 19. After discussing ways to set limits and enforce discipline, the chapter details the nurse's role in promoting the adolescent's health. It highlights nursing interventions that enhance nutrition, address sexuality issues, ensure safety, manage acne, cope with eating disorders, and deal with suicidal tendencies in adolescents.

Growth and development

Adolescents of both sexes experience growth spurts and puberty (the development of secondary sex characteristics and the capacity to reproduce sexually).

Physical growth patterns

During adolescence, the release of hormones causes a rapid increase in physical growth and spurs the development of secondary sex characteristics. In females, the growth spurt begins during the late school-age period (at approximately age 11) and continues into early adolescence (about 3 years later). During this time, a girl may grow up to 8" (20 cm) taller and may gain up to 50 lb (23 kg). In males, the growth spurt begins at approximately age 13 and ends 3 to 4 years later. During this time, a boy may grow up to 12" (30.5 cm) taller and may gain up to 60 lb (27 kg).

J. M. Tanner developed a classification system, also known as a sexual maturity rating scale, consisting of five stages. The scale rates the development of pubic hair and breasts in girls, and pubic hair and genitals in boys, from 1 to 5 (1 being the least developed; 5 being the most developed).

Puberty begins earlier in girls than in boys, starting at any time between age 8 and 14. Developmental changes associated with puberty in girls are complete within 3 years; secondary sex characteristics develop in stages. Menstruation occurs approximately $2\frac{1}{2}$ years after the onset of puberty. In boys, puberty may begin at any time from age 10 to 16. Related developmental changes are complete within 4 years.

Psychosocial development

According to Erik Erikson, the adolescent's developmental task is to establish a personal identity while overcoming identity or role confusion.

The adolescent searches for trust within the peer group and the larger community, and strives for autonomy by asserting independence. Displaying initiative, the adolescent plans for the future and achieves a sense of industry by successfully undertaking steps toward an occupational goal.

The adolescent struggles to fit the past role and the desired future role with the current role the adolescent is playing. Another struggle centers on the desire to integrate personal values and ideas with those of the larger society. The teenager develops a sense of identity by defining the self favorably in relation to others. Role confusion occurs if the adolescent has continued conflicts with the family and society over the current role and anticipated future role. As the adolescent strives to define a self-identity, relationships with parents and peers change.

Early adolescence (ages 11 to 14)

During this period, the child develops close ties with members of the same sex. Within the safe confines of the supporting peer group, the adolescent practices new behaviors. Despite the teenager's initial attempts to gain independence from parents, major conflicts over parental authority are rare during early adolescence.

The teenager may seem moody and have intense mood swings, and may get angry when frustrated. Parental requests or restrictions may induce loud protests.

Nursing responsibilities. The nurse must support the adolescent and family through the changes experienced during this early period. Encourage parents to acknowledge the importance of the child's peer group, to become acquainted with the child's friends, and to maintain an open, welcoming home environment in which the child and friends feel comfortable. Advise them to give the child "space" and privacy and to ignore moodiness.

Middle adolescence (ages 15 to 17)

The peer group now becomes increasingly important as the teenager strives to develop a self-image. The teenager now has an intense need to be accepted by peers, and the peer group becomes the major influence on behavior. The parent-child relationship is stormy and may be marked by major conflicts over rules, boundaries, independence, and control. The adolescent may prefer to be alone and may use the bedroom to escape from the demands and scrutiny of family life.

Nursing responsibilities. Counsel the parents and child to keep lines of communication open. Encourage them to discuss and negotiate both the rules for behavior and the consequences of breaking the rules. Advise parents to choose their battles wisely. For example, conflict over the child's clothing may not be worth the effort — and may be less important than rules governing more serious issues, such as forbidding the child from riding in a car driven by an inebriated friend. Urge parents to get acquainted with the child's friends. Counsel them to recognize the teenager's need for privacy, and suggest that they encourage — but not command — the child to engage in family activities.

Late adolescence (ages 17 to 19)

During this period, the peer group becomes less important as the child develops individual friendships and relationships. By this time, the teenager and parents generally have negotiated rules for behavior. As the child gains increasing independence, parent-child conflict decreases. Although spending increasing amounts of time away from the home, the adolescent typically is pleasant when at home and willing to engage in "adult" family conversation.

Nursing responsibilities. For some parents, late adolescence is stressful because it marks the child's physical and emotional independence. Counsel parents to recognize that teenagers need to separate from their parents. Suggest that parents become involved in recreational or occupational interests to substitute for the self-fulfillment previously attained though child care.

Psychosexual development

According to Sigmund Freud, adolescence corresponds to the genital stage of psychosexual development, which starts at puberty and lasts through old age. During this stage, the genital organs become the major source of sexual tension and pleasure.

During early adolescence, sexual energy focuses on self-exploration and self-evaluation. The child may become interested in opposite-sex relationships but prefers group activities to one-on-one dating.

Heterosexual dating takes on greater importance during middle adolescence. During this period, many homosexual adolescents first realize that heterosexual dating relationships do not arouse the same feelings in them that they arouse in heterosexual teenagers.

By late adolescence, most children are aware of their sexual identity, whether heterosexual or homosexual. Energy now focuses on developing close relationships, courting, and eventually becoming committed to one partner. Conflict may arise if the child meets social disapproval when seeking sexual identity and finding acceptable outlets for sexual desires.

Cognitive development

At about age 12 (later in some children), the child moves into the period of formal operations, as described by Jean Piaget. Acquiring the capacity for abstract thought, the child now can think about things that do not exist. Able to work with hypotheses, the child can entertain various solutions to a problem simultaneously, without manipulating the variables.

The adolescent also develops an orientation to the future and can delay immediate gratification to obtain future gain. Idealistic, the adolescent may become frustrated with the world.

Enhancing growth and development

Although adolescents gain increasing independence from their parents, most still live with their families. The parents and child must negotiate rules that allow the child to gain independence within the structure of the family and the larger community.

Setting limits and enforcing discipline

Family conferences have proven to be effective in defining the limits of adolescent behavior and in negotiating rules for conduct and the consequences for misbehavior. During such a conference, the child and parents separately list desired behaviors and responsibilities, along with undesirable behaviors or activities for which either the child or parent no longer wishes to be responsible. The parents and child then share their lists, and label each behavior and responsibility as "very important," "important," or "less important."

Next, parents and child negotiate a list of rules; preferably, the list includes only those rules deemed important by either the parents or child. The child and parents then discuss realistic penalties for rule-breaking. Rules and penalties must be made clear to all parties, so that the child who breaks a rule understands the consequences beforehand. This strategy minimizes conflict over confronting the child with misbehavior. For example, suppose a 16-year old boy stays out past curfew. The next day, the parents simply inform him that he came home late the previous night and must come home 1 hour earlier (or whatever the agreed-on penalty is) the next night he goes out.

Besides helping the adolescent gain a sense of control over discipline, such negotiation gives the child experience in solving problems and making decisions.

Promoting health

Advise the teenager and parents on health-related matters, including nutrition, sexuality, and safety.

Enhancing nutrition

Nutritional needs during adolescence vary with the timing of the growth spurt. Nutrient needs peak during the growth spurt; poor nutritional intake at this time can slow growth and sexual maturation. Sports participation also increases nutrient and energy needs.

Many teenagers — especially those with hectic schedules — skip meals, eat on the run, frequent fast-food restaurants, and substitute snacks for one or two meals a day. This can cause obesity and other problems, especially if snacks and fast foods are high in sugar, calories, fat, or sodium content.

Nutritional requirements

Because the nutritional needs of adolescents vary widely, nutritional allowances are flexible, providing for more calories for rapidly growing or physically active teenagers and fewer calories for inactive teenagers and those who have reached full growth potential. (For details, see *Nutritional requirements for the adolescent.*)

Recommended diet

Food-group requirements for adolescents are essentially the same as for school-age children. However, adolescents need the upper limits of the ranges provided below for each food group:
- Breads, cereals, rice, and pasta: six to eleven servings (one serving equals one slice of bread, three to four crackers, or 1 cup of rice, cereal, or pasta.)
- Fruits: two to four servings, including at least one citrus fruit (one serving equals one small banana, one medium-sized other raw fruit, $\frac{1}{2}$ cup canned fruit, or 4 oz fruit juice.)
- Vegetables: three to five servings, including at least one leafy, green or yellow vegetable (one serving equals three to four pieces of raw vegetables or $\frac{1}{2}$ cup cooked vegetable)
- Meat, poultry, fish, dry beans, eggs, and nuts: two servings (one serving equals 1 to 2 oz meat, one egg, 1 to 2 tablespoons peanut butter, or $\frac{1}{4}$ to $\frac{1}{2}$ cup dry beans)
- Milk, yogurt, and cheese: two to three servings (one serving equals 8 oz [1 cup] milk, 1 oz hard cheese, $\frac{1}{4}$ to $\frac{1}{2}$ cup cottage cheese, or $\frac{1}{4}$ to $\frac{1}{2}$ cup yogurt).

Dealing with sexuality issues

Although most children receive some sex education during their school-age years, many adolescents are ill-prepared for the physical and emotional impact of puberty. Much of the information they re-

Nutritional requirements for the adolescent

This chart presents daily calorie, protein, and fluid requirements for adolescents.

AGE	CALORIE	PROTEIN	FLUID
11 to 14 years	Girls: 33 to 66 cal/kg (15 to 30 cal/lb); average of 2,200 cal/day Boys: 44 to 81 cal/kg (20 to 37 cal/lb); average of 2,700 cal/day	1.2 g/kg (0.5 g/lb)	55 ml/kg (25 ml/lb; approximately 1 oz/lb)
15 to 18 years	Girls: 33 to 66 calories/kg (15 to 30 calories/lb); average of 2,100 cal/day Boys: 44 to 81 cal/kg (20 to 37 cal/lb); average of 2,800 cal/day	1.2 g/kg (0.5 g/lb)	45 ml/kg (21 ml/lb; approximately 0.66 oz/lb)

ceive comes from peers and the media and may be incomplete or inaccurate.

Teenagers need information about the normal body functions of both sexes as well as sexual activity, including intercourse and its consequences. Required teaching topics include pregnancy (such as how it occurs and how it can be prevented) and sexually transmitted diseases [STDs] (such as transmission modes, signs and symptoms, and how to get treatment). Teenagers also need to discuss their feelings about their sexuality, establish values regarding sexual behavior, and discuss issues concerning relationships.

Nursing responsibilities. Besides teaching the adolescent about sexual activity, pregnancy, and STDs, promote primary prevention of STDs by teaching about abstinence, condom use, and the need to avoid indiscriminate sexual practices. Be sure to emphasize the need for persons with active disease to abstain from sex. (For information about STDs, see *Sexually transmitted diseases,* pages 122 and 123.)

Ensuring safety

Accidents are a common cause of death and injury among adolescents. Increasing independence, obtaining a driver's license, risk-taking behavior, and the need for peer-group conformity and acceptance contribute to the accident rate in adolescents. Motor vehicle accidents are more common in this age group, while other types of accidents decrease. (For information on preventing motor vehicle injuries and other accidents, see Chapter 9, The school-age child and family.)

Firearm use is a leading cause of death in teenagers. Typically, accidental injury from firearms occurs at home from accidental discharge or risk-taking, such as accepting a dare. To help prevent such accidents, advise parents never to keep loaded guns in the home and to keep all guns and ammunition in locked cupboards. Inform them that

Sexually transmitted diseases

The chart below describes sexually transmitted diseases (STDs) that are common in adolescents.

DESCRIPTION	CLINICAL MANIFESTATIONS	TREATMENT
Genital herpes		
• One of most common STDs; presents as an acute infection or as recurrence of latent herpes • Typically caused by herpes simplex virus type 2, less commonly by herpes simplex virus type 1 • Transmitted by close sexual contact with person who has active herpes lesions • Incubation period is 3 to 12 days after exposure • Communicable for 15 to 42 days during primary infection, for 6 days during recurrences; also communicable during prodromal phase, which precedes recurrence; both primary infection and recurrences are highly contagious	• Multiple vesicular lesions, which subsequently erode • Vulvar edema and erythema • Vaginal or penile discharge • Inguinal lymphadenopathy • Dysuria • Headache, fever, and malaise • Prodromal symptoms: Intense burning, tingling, and itching of vulva or penis • Primary disease lasts 2 to 6 weeks; recurrences last 1 to 10 days	• Topical or oral acyclovir • Sitz baths followed by thorough drying of lesions • Benzocaine spray or lidocaine jelly to relieve pain • Betadine ointment t.i.d. to prevent secondary infections • For females with dysuria, instructions to void while taking a bath to reduce pain on urination
Syphilis		
• Caused by *Treponema pallidum* • Transmitted by close sexual contact with infected person • Incubation period is 10 to 90 days • Communicable from time primary chancre appears until treatment begins; most contagious during first year of disease	• Fever, malaise, and lymphadenopathy • Shallow, firm, nontender lesion (chancre) with raised border and scant yellow discharge; lesion most commonly appears on penis, vulva, or cervix	• Penicillin G or tetracycline
Genital warts		
• Caused by human papillomavirus • Highly contagious • Transmitted by close sexual contact with infected person • Incubation period is 30 to 90 days • Communicable once lesions appear	• Single or multiple firm, gray, rough-surfaced lesions on vulva, vagina, cervix, perineum, anus, or penis	• Topical podophyllum resin (which must be rinsed off after 4 hours) • Cryosurgery • Surgical excision
Gonorrhea		
• Most commonly reported STD among adolescents • Caused by *Neisseria gonorrhoeae* • Transmitted by close sexual contact with infected person • Incubation period is 3 to 14 days • Communicable during period of active infection, which begins when symptoms appear and ends when infection is eradicated)	• Cervical erythema • Urethritis (in both males and females) • Thick, creamy vaginal or penile discharge • If pelvic inflammatory disease is present: lower abdominal pain, fever, and mucopurulent cervical discharge	• For uncomplicated gonorrhea: ampicillin or amoxicillin, as well as probenecid and tetracycline • For a less compliant patient: intramuscular penicillin G and probenecid

Sexually transmitted diseases *(continued)*

DESCRIPTION	CLINICAL MANIFESTATIONS	TREATMENT
Chlamydia		
• Caused by *Chlamydia trachomatis* • Transmitted by close sexual contact with infected person • Incubation period is 5 to 12 days • Communicable during period of active infection, which begins when symptoms appear and ends when infection is eradicated	• Urethritis (in both males and females) • Thick, creamy vaginal or penile discharge • If pelvic inflammatory disease is present: lower abdominal pain, fever, and mucopurulent cervical discharge	• Tetracycline or erythromycin
Trichomoniasis		
• Caused by *Trichomonas vaginalis* • Incubation period is 3 to 28 days • Communicable during period of active infection, which begins when symptoms appear and ends when infection is eradicated	• Males: May lack symptoms • Females: Heavy, yellowish-green or thin, gray vaginal discharge; vulvar and vaginal inflammation; vulvar pruritus; dysuria; and dyspareunia	• Oral metronidazole (except in pregnant females), with instruction to avoid alcohol during treatment • For pregnant females: intravaginal clotrimazole
Acquired immunodeficiency syndrome (AIDS)		
• Caused by human immunodeficiency virus type 1 • Transmitted by direct contact with contaminated blood or blood products, sharing intravenous needles with an infected drug user, or intimate sexual contact with an infected person • Also transmitted transplacentally from an infected mother to her unborn child • Incubation period: as long as 2 years in transplacental transmission; as long as 8 years via the other modes of transmission • Communicable when infected with HIV	For older children and adolescents • Prodromal phase: weight loss, fever, malaise, and lymphadenopathy • Opportunistic infections • Encephalopathy • Thrombocytopenia • Nephrotic syndrome • *Pneumocystis carinii* pneumonia	• No cure currently exists; however, drug therapy — zidovudine (AZT), trimethoprim or sulfamethoxazole and pentamidine, and gamma globulin — appears to slow disease progression

air rifles and BB guns also can cause injury and should not be available for recreational use.

Managing acne

Acne is a common skin condition that primarily affects adolescents. Up to 85% of teenagers experience acne, although the severity of the condition varies considerably. Acne peaks in late adolescence.

Many factors seem to contribute to acne: androgen secretion, emotional stress, hereditary factors, a humid environment, and menstruation. No evidence suggests that certain foods play a role.

Clinical manifestations of acne depend on the severity of the condition. Mild acne may cause closed comedones (whiteheads), open comedones (blackheads), and occasional pustules. Moderate acne is characterized by open and closed comedones, papules, and pustules. Severe acne typically causes open and closed comedones, erythematous papules, pustules, and cysts. The skin and hair may appear oily.

Acne lesions are most common on the face, but also may appear on the chest, back, and buttocks. Scarring may occur during any stage.

During the history, ask the adolescent to describe the skin condition, including what factors seem to make it worse, what the child does when a pimple occurs, how the acne responds to remedies, whether the acne bothers the child, and whether the child wants treatment.

Treatment for mild acne involves topical agents — keratolytic gels (Benzagel, Persa-Gel) applied once daily. If the condition does not respond to this therapy, advise the child to apply the agent twice. Alternatively, the physician may prescribe tretinoin 0.05% cream (Retin-A), applied once daily.

For moderate acne, treatment may involve the topical agents described above, in addition to hot soaks to pustules and tetracycline 250 mg P.O. q.i.d. Treatment for severe acne includes topical agents, hot soaks to pustules or cysts, and tetracycline 500 mg P.O. q.i.d.

Nursing responsibilities. Support the child and family during acne treatment. Inform the adolescent that although acne cannot be cured, it can be controlled. Teach the patient about prescribed treatment. Mention that treatment initially may cause facial irritation and redness. Advise the patient to apply topical creams lightly to the entire face and to rub them gently into the skin. Mention that these creams initially may cause minor tingling and warmth.

Review good hygiene practices: avoiding abrasive over-the-counter acne creams, shampooing the hair frequently, changing the pillowcase after shampooing, washing the skin with warm water and mild soap at least twice a day, and never picking or squeezing acne lesions because this delays healing and causes scarring. Teach girls to use water-based rather than oil-based cosmetics, which may promote acne.

If the physician prescribes tetracycline, instruct the adolescent to take the medication on an empty stomach (1 hour before or 2 hours after meals). Mention that tetracycline therapy may take up to 1 month to produce results. Caution the adolescent not to take tetracycline during pregnancy. Mention that the drug may cause moniliasis in females. Because both tretinoin and tetracycline may cause photosensitivity, advise the patient to apply sunscreen with a skin protection factor (SPF) of at least 15 before sun exposure.

Coping with eating disorders

Anorexia nervosa and bulimia are eating disorders that typically begin during adolescence and may persist into young adulthood.

Anorexia nervosa

A complex psychological disorder, anorexia nervosa is characterized by a pathologic fear of weight gain leading to faulty eating patterns, malnutrition, and, possibly, extreme weight loss. Commonly starting during early adolescence, it affects more girls than boys. Although the disorder occurs in all socioeconomic groups, it is more common in the middle and upper classes.

Anorexia nervosa results in severe malnutrition if allowed to continue. An estimated 5% to 20% of anorexic teenagers die from physiologic consequences of malnutrition or from suicide.

The disorder presumably has both developmental and psychological underpinnings. Experts speculate that it reflects a disturbance in the separation-individuation process inherent in adolescent development. Self-starvation gives the teenager a sense of self-control over what is happening to her body.

The classic anorexic is a high achiever in school, a perfectionist, and a "model" child with low self-esteem. The parents typically are overprotective and demanding, and the child may feel unable to live up to their expectations.

Clinical manifestations of anorexia nervosa include:
• loss of 20% or more of body weight
• morbid fear of gaining weight
• self-description or self-concept as fat and unattractive
• unreasonably low food intake (the patient may push food around the plate during meals, consuming little)
• preoccupation with food and dieting, including denial of hunger
• preparation of food for others but refusal to eat
• excessive exercising
• laxative use
• self-induced vomiting after eating
• decreased pulse rate, blood pressure, and temperature
• dry, flaky skin with fine hair covering the arms
• amenorrhea
• constipation
• abdominal pain
• cold intolerance
• fatigue
• insomnia
• increasing social withdrawal as preoccupation with weight, eating, and exercise grow.

Nursing responsibilities. The nurse plays a primary role in identifying the anorexic teenager and conducting the initial assessment. To avoid grave consequences, the anorexic must be referred for psychiatric consultation; a severely malnourished patient requires hospitalization.

Treatment involves both family and individual therapy. Behavior modification has proven helpful in changing the eating patterns of anorexics. Most anorexic adolescents respond positively to therapy, although treatment and counseling may take 2 to 3 years to achieve results.

Bulimia

This eating disorder is characterized by episodes of binge eating followed by self-induced vomiting. Typically, it begins during late adolescence and primarily affects girls. Psychological factors seem to contribute to the development of bulimia, although a specific cause has not been identified.

Clinical manifestations of bulimia include:
- weight typically within the normal range but with frequent fluctuations
- recurrent episodes of rapid consumption of high-calorie foods (which may be hard to detect because most bulimics binge in private)
- self-induced vomiting after binge eating
- abdominal pain after binge eating
- laxative use
- preoccupation with weight and body image
- excessive exercise
- poor impulse control
- constant dieting
- awareness of abnormal eating patterns but lack of a sense of control in modifying the binge-purge pattern.

Bulimia may lead to tooth enamel loss (from repeated vomiting of acidic gastric contents); chronic sore throat; esophageal irritation; and electrolyte imbalances, including hyponatremia, hypokalemia, hypochloremia, and metabolic alkalosis.

Nursing responsibilities. The nurse plays a crucial part in identifying bulimic patients and performing the initial assessment. Refer a teenager with suspected bulimia for psychiatric counseling.

Therapeutic strategies for bulimic patients resemble those used for anorexics. Goals of therapy include resolving psychological issues, restoring normal eating patterns, increasing self-esteem, and promoting self control.

Dealing with suicidal tendencies

Nearly everyone recognizes that adolescence is a time of tremendous stress. The teenager with inadequate coping mechanisms and support systems may see suicide as the only way to manage this stress.

In some cases, suicidal tendencies represent a maladaptive response to adolescent depression. (For more information about depression, see Chapter 9, The school-age child and family). However, many suicidal teenagers do not exhibit characteristic behaviors associated with depression.

Because adolescents have higher suicide rates than other age groups, some theorists suspect that developmental issues play a part in suicidal tendencies during adolescence. These issues include the search for an identity, the drive to separate from the parents and become independent, dramatic physical and physiologic changes, and development of close interpersonal relationships.

Identifying the suicidal adolescent

Many suicidal adolescents exhibit the traits detailed below. An asterisk (*) indicates that the person is at high risk for suicide.

PERSONALITY TRAITS	BEHAVIORAL TRAITS	FAMILY TRAITS
• Pronounced depression • Feelings of hopelessness, worthlessness, self-hatred, or guilt • Desire to be punished for unidentified wrongdoing • Social withdrawal (may become a loner) • High intelligence • Poor problem-solving ability • Tendency to make excessive demands on oneself • Unwillingness or inability to use support systems	• Recent changes in appetite, school behavior (such as emotional outbursts or failing grades), peer-group relationships, and appearance • Loss of energy (may always be tired) • Sleep disturbances (such as excessive sleeping or difficulty falling asleep or getting out of bed) • Increased irritability • Increased somatic complaints (such as recurrent abdominal pain and headaches) • Frequent accidents • Increased drug or alcohol use • Changes in school attendance pattern (such as delinquency or refusal to attend) *• Desire to give away cherished possessions *• Preoccupation with death, such as talking about death frequently, focusing on morbid thoughts and events, and expressing thoughts of suicide (such as "This place would be better off without me")	• Severe parent-child conflict • Family history of suicide • Absence of one or both parents from the home due to separation, divorce, or death • Unrealistic parental expectations • Parental indifference toward or rejection of the child • Frequent residence changes • Physical or sexual abuse

Certain factors commonly precipitate adolescent suicide — loss of a close friend, enrollment in a new school, failure to achieve important personal goals, and the breakup of an important relationship. Researchers have discovered that adolescents who contemplate suicide share certain characteristics. (See *Identifying the suicidal adolescent*.)

Nursing responsibilities. The nurse must be able to recognize suicidal risk factors early and intervene swiftly. If a teenager exhibits any personality, behavioral, or family traits indicative of suicide, do not hesitate to ask, "Have you ever felt like hurting or killing yourself?" Refer the high-risk teenager to a mental health specialist for complete evaluation and therapy.

STUDY ACTIVITIES **Short answer**

1. Which assessment findings suggest that a boy is in the second stage of secondary sex characteristic development?

_____

_____

2. Describe characteristics of the parent-child relationship during middle adolescence.

_____

_____

3. List at least three features of cognitive development during adolescence.

_____

_____

_____

4. Identify at least three factors that may affect nutritional intake in adolescents.

_____

_____

5. Jason, age 15, has mild acne. To address this problem, the nurse formulates the following nursing diagnoses: _Impaired skin integrity related to increased androgen secretions_ and _Knowledge deficit related to self-management of acne._ The expected outcomes are that Jason will exhibit fewer acne lesions, exhibit skin healing with minimum scarring, and verbalizes self-care practices consistent with proper acne management. List five nursing interventions that would help achieve these outcomes.

_____

_____

_____

Multiple choice

6. When do adolescent boys reach the peak of their growth spurt?
  A. At about age 15
  B. When axillary hair develops
  C. One year after pubic hair first appears
  D. During the same year the scrotum starts to enlarge

7. Which emotional pattern is typical during early adolescence?
  A. Frequent anger
  B. Cooperativeness
  C. Moodiness
  D. Combativeness

8. Acne has been linked to:
   A. Hereditary factors
   B. Consumption of greasy foods
   C. Squeezing of facial lesions
   D. Excessive sweating

9. Which statement about genital herpes is accurate?
   A. It is relatively uncommon in adolescents.
   B. During a primary episode, lesions may last over a month.
   C. Once the lesions are treated, recurrence is rare.
   D. It is accompanied by white, cheesy vaginal discharge.

10. In males, *Trichomonas* infection commonly causes:
   A. Painful urination
   B. No symptoms
   C. A vesicular lesion on the penis
   D. A thick, yellow penile discharge

11. Which trait typifies the adolescent with anorexia nervosa?
   A. High academic achievement
   B. High self-esteem
   C. Disruptive family relationships
   D. History of school failure

12. Which metabolic disturbance is associated with bulimia?
   A. Hypoglycemia
   B. Metabolic alkalosis
   C. Metabolic acidosis
   D. Hyperkalemia

13. What is the most serous risk factor for suicide in an adolescent?
   A. Depression
   B. Increased sleep requirements
   C. Cocaine abuse
   D. Talking about death frequently

ANSWERS **Short answer**

   1. During stage 2, the scrotum, testes, and penis enlarge; scrotal skin reddens and changes in texture; and long, straight, sparse, lightly pigmented pubic hair appears at the base of the penis.

   2. During middle adolescence, the child and parents may have major conflicts over rules, boundaries, independence, and control. The child may prefer to be alone and may use the bedroom to escape from the demands and scrutiny of family life.

   3. Moving into the period of formal operations, the adolescent acquires the capacity for abstract thought; is able to work with hypotheses; can entertain multiple solutions to a problem simultaneously without manipulating the variables; develops an orientation to the future and can delay immediate gratification to obtain future gain; and is idealistic and may become frustrated with the world.

4. Factors that may affect an adolescent's nutritional intake include spending more time away from home; participating in sports; skipping meals, eating on the run, frequenting fast-food restaurants; and substituting snacks for meals.

5. Teach Jason about prescribed treatment; teach him to apply topical creams to the entire face, gently rubbing them in. Review good hygiene practices with Jason, instructing him to avoid abrasive over-the-counter creams and soaps, shampoo his hair frequently, change his pillowcase after shampooing, wash his skin with warm water and mild soap at least twice a day, and never pick or squeeze his acne lesions. If the physician prescribes tretinoin or tetracycline, advise Jason to apply sunscreen with an SPF of at least 15 before sun exposure.

Multiple choice

6. B. The peak of the male growth spurt occurs during stage 4 of sexual development — the stage during which axillary hair appears. Age is a poor indicator of adolescent growth patterns.

7. C. During early adolescence, the child may be moody. Anger and combativeness are more typical of middle adolescence; cooperative behavior typifies late adolescence.

8. A. Hereditary factors play a role in the development of acne in teenagers. Greasy food and excessive sweating do not contribute to acne development. Squeezing may lead to inflammation and scarring but does not cause the initial lesion.

9. B. The initial genital lesion may last 2 to 6 weeks. Herpes is common among promiscuous adolescents. Recurrences are common; vaginal discharge is rare.

10. B. Males infected with *Trichomonas* commonly are asymptomatic.

11. A. The typical anorectic teenager is a high academic achiever with low self-esteem and parents who typically are overprotective and demanding.

12. B. Metabolic alkalosis may occur secondary to hydrogen losses caused by vomiting. The blood sugar level commonly is within the normal range. Hypokalemia (resulting from potassium loss caused by vomiting) is more common than hyperkalemia.

13. D. An adolescent who talks of death frequently should be considered at high risk for suicide. Although depression, increased sleep requirements, and cocaine abuse are seen in suicidal adolescents, they also occur in adolescents who are not suicidal.

CHAPTER 11

The infant with disturbances in physical development

OBJECTIVES After studying this chapter, the reader should be able to:

1. Describe typical parental responses after the birth of a newborn with a congenital malformation.
2. Describe the etiology, the pathophysiology, and the signs and symptoms of Type C tracheoesophageal fistula, cleft lip and palate, and imperforate anus.
3. Discuss medical and nursing management of infants with Type C tracheoesophageal fistula, cleft lip and palate, and imperforate anus.
4. Identify the causes, the pathophysiology, and the signs and symptoms of myelomeningocele and hydrocephalus.
5. Discuss medical and nursing management of infants with myelomeningocele and hydrocephaly.
6. Describe the causes, the pathophysiology, and the signs and symptoms of congenital hip dysplasia and clubfoot.
7. Discuss medical and nursing management of infants with congenital hip dysplasia and clubfoot.

OVERVIEW OF CONCEPTS Congenital structural abnormalities (abnormalities present at birth) contribute significantly to infant mortality and morbidity. However, many of these abnormalities can be repaired or corrected surgically. To provide optimal care for affected infants, the nurse must possess expert skills in preoperative and postoperative management and must help the family deal with the crisis. This chapter describes the causes and pathophysiology of selected disturbances in physical development and discusses medical and nursing management of infants with these disturbances.

Parental responses During pregnancy, parents fantasize about their unborn child. Their fantasies may center on such traits as the child's sex, hair color, and eye color. Of course, all parents hope for a healthy, normal baby. Yet at the same time, many fear something will be wrong with their child.

If the infant has a congenital abnormality, the gap between the fantasized child and the actual child may be large enough to jeopardize the parent-child relationship. The parents experience a grief response similar to the one that follows the death of a loved one, progressing through such stages as shock, disbelief, and denial; adjustment; and acceptance.

Gastrointestinal disorders

This chapter discusses three congenital gastrointestinal (GI) disorders: Type C tracheoesophageal fistula (TEF), cleft lip and palate (CLP), and imperforate anus.

Tracheoesophageal fistula

TEF is a congenital defect in which the esophagus fails to develop as one continuous passage. TEF affects boys and girls equally. About half of infants with TEF have other congenital defects.

Etiology

Genetic factors seem to play no role in the development of TEF, but little else is known about the cause of the disorder. The mother's antepartal history may be positive for polyhydramnios (excessive amniotic fluid). Typically, the newborn is premature and has a lower than average weight at birth.

Pathophysiology

TEF occurs in at least five different forms. This chapter focuses on the most common form, Type C. In this defect, the proximal end of the esophagus ends in a blind pouch. A fistula links the distal end of the esophagus to the trachea, and the proximal and distal ends of the esophagus are not connected. The newborn's oral secretions accumulate in the blind pouch instead of being swallowed into the stomach. Also, the reflux of gastric secretions can enter the trachea via the fistula.

Assessment

The newborn has increased oral secretions accompanied by continuous drooling, and may choke and cough frequently. During attempts at feeding, infant formula returns through the newborn's mouth and nose, and the newborn has forceful coughing and cyanosis. The risk for aspirating saliva or formula is high.

Air from the trachea enters the newborn's stomach through the fistula, resulting in abdominal distention. GI secretions may flow backward through the fistula into the trachea and bronchial tree, leading to chemical pneumonitis. With aspiration or chemical pneumonitis, expect signs of respiratory distress, such as tachypnea, retractions, crackles, and cyanosis.

The physician orders diagnostic tests for any newborn with excessive oral secretions, continuous drooling, or choking during feeding. Inability to pass a suction catheter into the stomach also calls for further evaluation. A suction catheter is passed through the oropharynx into the child's esophagus until resistance is met; radiography reveals the catheter curled in the blind pouch of the proximal esophagus. To determine the form of TEF, radiographic studies are performed.

Medical management

The newborn with TEF is placed on a radiant warmer and given nothing by mouth (NPO); a peripheral intravenous (I.V.) line is inserted for hydration. A #8 or #10 gavage tube is passed through the oropharynx into the blind esophageal pouch and connected to wall suction; this serves as a nasopharyngeal (NP) tube. Because of the risk of aspiration and subsequent pneumonia if accumulated oral secretions enter the oropharynx, the head of the radiant warmer is raised to promote downward drainage of secretions and prevent gastric reflux.

The newborn then undergoes a gastrostomy. The gastrostomy tube is connected to suction to remove accumulated air and gastric secretions and thus help prevent gastric reflux into the trachea. A newborn with pneumonia also receives I.V. antibiotics.

Once the newborn's respiratory status is stable, the TEF is corrected surgically. (The NP tube is discontinued just before surgery.) In most newborns, TEF can be corrected completely at this time. Surgery involves anastomosis (connection) of the proximal and distal ends of the esophagus, as well as ligation (severing) of the fistula.

Postoperatively, the newborn returns to the unit and is placed on a radiant warmer; the gastrostomy tube is connected to wall or gravity suction. Once bowel sounds return (in 3 or 4 days), the gastrostomy tube is elevated at a point above the level of the stomach and gastrostomy feedings begin. Until then, the newborn receives all nutritional intake via parenteral nutrition. The chest tube, inserted during surgery to restore negative pressure and remove collected pleural fluids, is connected to a closed chest drainage system.

Nursing management

Preoperatively, the goal of nursing care is to stabilize the newborn in anticipation of surgical correction of TEF. Be aware that aspiration of saliva or gastric contents poses the greatest risk. Monitor the NP and gastrostomy tubes for patency. If either tube becomes occluded, gently irrigate with 5 to 10 ml of air. (Do not irrigate with 0.9% normal saline [sodium chloride] solution because this may cause aspiration.)

Be sure to keep the gastrostomy site dry. Clean the site at least twice daily with half-strength hydrogen peroxide and a sterile water solution. Monitor I.V. therapy and administer antibiotics and pain medications, as prescribed.

Postoperative nursing care resembles that for any newborn who has undergone surgery. (See Chapter 16, Management principles, for details.) Goals of care during this period include:
• providing fluid and electrolytes
• promoting comfort
• preventing injury to the surgical site

• providing sufficient calories to promote growth
• supporting the newborn's parents.

Administer and monitor the medical management plan. Monitor the chest tube for patency and leakage. Protect the anastomosis site from injury by limiting suctioning to the oropharynx and nasopharynx. Be aware that pacifier use may be contraindicated because sucking causes excessive production and swallowing of saliva, which may damage the surgical site.

Keep the gastrostomy tube patent. Clean the insertion site and keep it dry. Once bowel sounds return (about 3 to 4 days postoperatively), initiate gastrostomy feedings, as prescribed. Begin oral feedings, as prescribed, once the anastomosis site heals completely (10 to 14 days postoperatively).

Because the esophagus narrows after surgery, the newborn may have trouble swallowing. With continued practice of oral feeding, most infants can progress to complete bottle- or breast-feedings.

Once the newborn can take all feedings orally, the gastrostomy tube is removed and the child can be discharged. To help identify esophageal strictures (a potential and long-term complication), teach the parents to observe for difficulty swallowing or choking and to report this problem promptly.

Cleft lip and palate

CLP is a congenital anomaly characterized by an abnormal fissure, or division, between the lip and nares (cleft lip) and another fissure in the midline of the palate (cleft palate). Some infants have a cleft in the lip only or in the palate only.

The most common facial malformation, CLP affects more males than females. It is more common in Native Americans and Asians than in Caucasians or African-Americans.

Etiology

CLP stems from a multifactorial inheritance pattern.

Pathophysiology and assessment

Cleft lip is readily apparent at birth. The cleft may appear as a mere notch in the vermilion border, or it may extend completely to the nares. Cleft lip may be unilateral (one cleft, involving only one nares) or bilateral (two clefts, involving both nares). Nasal distortion of varying degrees accompanies the cleft.

Cleft palate is apparent on inspection and palpation of the palate. Like cleft lip, it may be unilateral or bilateral. Cleft palate results in a continuous opening between the mouth and nasal cavity. The newborn cannot establish negative pressure in the mouth for effective sucking, and has difficulty feeding. Formula or breast milk leaks into the nasal cavity and may leak out of the nares, causing breathing problems during feeding.

Complications
CLP may lead to recurrent otitis media (middle ear infection), dentition problems (such as severe malocclusion of the teeth), speech impairment, and facial scarring and distortion (with an imperfect repair).

Medical management
Cleft lip is repaired surgically during early infancy. The surgeon approximates the lip and skin borders, then sutures them closed. To prevent tension on the incision, a Logan bow may be applied on either side of the suture line.

Cleft palate is surgically closed later, between ages 1 and 2, but before speech patterns develop.

Nursing management
Preoperative nursing goals include providing nutrition to the infant and providing emotional support to the child's parents. Because CLP is a facial malformation clearly visible to others, it may be particularly devastating to the parents. To ease their distress, show them pictures of children whose clefts have been repaired surgically and introduce them to other parents of children with CLP.

Also teach the parents special feeding techniques to help the infant establish an effective sucking and swallowing pattern. Inform them that nipple feedings are preferred over medicine dropper or syringe feedings because sucking provides oral satisfaction and promotes oral muscle development, essential for later speech development. If adaptive feeding devices are prescribed, teach parents how to use them. Such devices cover the cleft palate to minimize fluid leakage into the nasal cavity and maximize sucking efficiency.

Breast-feeding may be possible; the soft breast tissue may occlude the cleft palate sufficiently and thus promote sucking. Advise the mother to place her entire nipple in the infant's mouth. If the infant cannot establish an effective sucking pattern, advise parents to deliver formula or breast milk though an irrigating syringe and a soft, short catheter to the back of the infant's mouth. To minimize formula or milk leakage into the infant's nasal cavities, instruct parents to keep the infant upright during feedings.

The infant with CLP swallows large amounts of air during feeding. To prevent abdominal distention and regurgitation, teach parents to burp the infant frequently.

Nursing care after cleft lip repair. Goals at this time include preventing injury to the incision, promoting comfort, providing sensory-perceptual stimulation, and providing adequate nutrition.

Postoperatively, place the infant on the back or side. The prone (face-down) position is contraindicated because friction with bedsheets may disturb the incision. Apply elbow restraints to prevent the infant from touching the incision. Clean the incision site with half-strength hydrogen peroxide and sterile water solution at least three times daily. To minimize scarring, keep the incision meticulously clean.

Take measures to minimize crying, which may produce tension on the incision. To promote comfort, administer analgesics, as prescribed, use distraction techniques, hold the infant, and provide comfort measures. Pacifiers are contraindicated until the incision is healed fully.

Oral feedings can begin once the infant recovers from anesthesia. Use an irrigating syringe and a short, soft catheter to deliver fluids to the back of the infant's mouth. Give clear fluids first, and progress to formula or breast milk, if tolerated. Place the infant in a side-lying position if oral secretions are excessive. After a feeding, clean the infant's oral cavity with water.

Teach parents how to feed the infant with the irrigating syringe. Also teach them how to keep the incision clean and dry. Once the incision heals completely, bottle- or breast-feeding may resume.

To provide sensory-perceptual stimulation, place mobiles and music boxes in the crib and take the infant for walks in the hallway. Be sure to take the time to hold, cuddle, and talk to the infant.

Nursing care after cleft palate repair. Goals include preventing injury to the incision, promoting comfort, and providing nutrition. Place the child on the stomach to promote drainage of secretions from the oral cavity and to allow the child to breathe entirely through the nose (unlike the breathing pattern established before surgery).

Apply elbow restraints to prevent the child from placing anything in the mouth and thus damaging the incision. Be sure to avoid putting anything — including suction catheters and thermometers — in the child's mouth.

Once the child recovers from anesthesia, give clear fluids from a cup, resuming formula feedings when tolerated; straws are contraindicated. Provide a soft diet, using a large spoon, when the child can tolerate this. Do not feed with a fork to prevent trauma to the suture line. Rinse the infant's oral cavity with water after feeding.

Ability to tolerate a full, soft diet indicates that the child is ready for discharge. Before discharge, teach the parents to keep the child in arm restraints until the palate heals fully, to provide a soft diet until the palate heals completely (4 to 6 weeks), and to rinse the child's oral cavity with water after feedings.

Imperforate anus

In imperforate anus, the anus has an abnormal closure. The disorder is equally common in both males and females and in children of all ethnic backgrounds.

Etiology

Imperforate anus is caused by persistence of the membrane that separates the lower rectum from the lower aspect of the large intestine.

Pathophysiology and classification

Imperforate anus occurs in two forms. In the simple form, structural components of the rectum and anus are intact and an anal membrane may be present. In the complicated form, the rectum and anus fail to meet or the anus is absent.

Because the large intestine does not connect to the anal opening, bowel contents cannot be excreted, unless the defect is accompanied by a rectoperineal, rectovaginal, or rectourethral fistula. If a fistula is present, bowel contents are excreted onto the floor of the perineum (with a rectoperineal fistula), into the vagina (with a rectovaginal fistula), or into the urethra (with a rectourethral fistula).

Assessment

Inspection of the newborn's perineum reveals a thin membrane covering the anus. In some cases, the anal opening is absent completely. Occasionally, however, the anal opening appears to be present because the defect is found higher in the rectum; this situation may delay diagnosis until failure to pass meconium alerts the health care team to the need for further evaluation.

Medical management

Simple imperforate anus can be corrected through surgical excision of the anal membrane followed by daily anal dilation. For complicated imperforate anus, surgical correction is more involved. The surgeon reconstructs the anus in the proper position, then performs a pull-through anastomosis, connecting the rectum to the anus. A child with a defect high in the rectum may require a temporary colostomy. A child born without an internal anal sphincter, an external anal sphincter, or both may never be able to establish bowel control and may need a permanent colostomy.

Nursing management

Preoperatively, prepare the infant for surgery and discuss the procedure with the parents. Keep the infant NPO and administer I.V. fluids, as prescribed. As prescribed, assist with insertion of a nasogastric (NG) tube for gravity drainage.

After surgical repair in an infant without a colostomy, the primary nursing goal is to prevent trauma to the surgical site. To prevent pressure on anal sutures, place the infant either on the side, with hips elevated, or supine, with legs positioned at a 90-degree angle to the trunk.

The infant may pass stool continuously. Be sure to keep the perineal area clean, such as by giving sitz baths or wiping gently with gauze pads soaked in sterile water. Be sure to monitor patency of the NG tube, which is reconnected to gravity drainage after surgery.

Once bowel sounds return, initiate oral feedings, as prescribed. The infant is ready for discharge once oral intake is adequate. Teach parents to observe the infant's stool patterns and to report signs of anal stricture, such as ribbon-like stools accompanied by straining.

If the infant has a colostomy, perform colostomy care. Inspect the stoma to detect problems with stoma perfusion. Prevent irritation to abdominal skin by keeping the area free of feces. (For details on colostomy care, see Chapter 19, Gastrointestinal dysfunction.) Before the infant is discharged, teach the parents about colostomy care and refer them to appropriate support groups.

Central nervous system disorders

The following discussion focuses on two congenital central nervous system (CNS) disorders — myelomeningocele and hydrocephalus.

Myelomeningocele

Myelomeningocele (sometimes called meningomyelocele) is a neural tube defect in which part of the meninges and spinal cord protrude through the vertebral column. The defect may occur anywhere along the vertebral column but is most common in the lumbar or lumbosacral area.

Etiology

Myelomeningocele results from failure of the neural tube to close during embryonic development. A multifactorial inheritance pattern is suspected as the cause. Researchers have identified such environmental factors as radiation, maternal hyperthermia, vitamin A deficiency or excess, valproic acid deficiency, and folic acid deficiency in the development of this anomaly.

Pathophysiology

Normally, the spinal cord is encased in a protective covering of bone (vertebrae) and meninges. In myelomeningocele, contents normally encased within the neural tube escape through an opening. Typically, a cystlike sac filled with nerves, spinal cord, meninges, and cerebrospinal fluid protrudes through the opening. The sac may be covered by a translucent membrane or by dura, meninges, or skin. The membrane is fragile and prone to tearing. A torn membrane permits leakage of cerebrospinal fluid (CSF) and provides an entry route for bacteria, possibly leading to meningitis.

Hydrocephalus — abnormal accumulation of CSF within the cranial vault — occurs in roughly 90% to 95% of infants with myelomeningocele. Hydrocephalus may not be apparent at birth but almost always develops shortly thereafter. (For information on assessing hydrocephalus, see the section on "Hydrocephalus" later in this chapter.)

Myelomeningocele also is associated with Arnold-Chiari deformity, a congenital anomaly in which the cerebellum and medulla oblongata protrude down into the spinal canal through the foramen magnum. This deformity leads to obstructed CSF flow.

The degree of neurologic impairment in a child with myelomeningocele depends on the anatomic level of the defect and the nerves involved. The affected extremities have sensory deficits. The prospects for future ambulation depend on the location of the defect. Typically, a child with a defect at or above L2 is confined to a wheelchair. With a defect between L2 and L5, the child may learn to walk using braces and crutches. A sacral defect permits walking, although the child may need braces for support. For the older child, bowel and bladder incontinence and ambulation problems may cause emotional distress and low self-esteem.

Prognosis. Surgical intervention, aggressive antibiotic therapy to prevent meningitis, and treatment of hydrocephalus have improved survival dramatically for infants with myelomeningocele. However, surgery does not correct associated physical disabilities. Complications related to bowel and bladder dysfunction and hydrocephalus management persist throughout life. Also, most children with myelomeningocele require numerous hospitalizations, causing additional stress for the child and family.

Assessment

Myelomeningocele is apparent at birth, with the protrusion of the cystlike sac through the skin along the vertebral column. Regardless of the location of the defect, interrupted nerve supply to the bladder and anus impairs bladder and bowel elimination. Some newborns dribble urine constantly. Others have overflow incontinence, in which a urine stream is present but the bladder does not empty completely; residual urine greatly heightens the risk for urinary tract infection (UTI). Poor anal sphincter tone interferes with bowel control and may cause rectal prolapse. The child may ooze stool constantly or may have severe constipation.

Some children with myelomeningocele have orthopedic deformities — most commonly, hip dislocation and clubfoot. Presumably, such deformities occur in utero as a result of denervation of muscles in the lower extremities.

Myelomeningocele may be detected prenatally through ultrasonography, which visualizes the protruding sac. Elevated maternal serum levels of alpha-fetoprotein (AFP), a fetal gamma globulin found in amniotic fluid, also may indicate myelomeningocele. Amniotic fluid sampling for AFP is recommended for women with elevated serum AFP levels.

Medical management

Because myelomeningocele affects multiple body systems, management calls for a multidisciplinary approach. Typically, pediatric neurology and neurosurgery, orthopedic, and urology services are involved.

Myelomeningocele is repaired surgically within a few days after birth. The surgical goal is to replace the contents of the sac within the neural tube and to close the defect without disturbing neural contents further.

Clinicians differ on optimal timing of surgery. Some recommend early closure — within the first 12 to 18 hours after birth — to reduce the risk of infection and trauma to the sac and to avoid stretching of nerve fibers from sac enlargement, which could lead to further motor impairment.

Other physicians advocate delaying closure for up to 72 hours after birth to allow epithelialization of the sac, which they believe reduces the risk for infection. The delay also allows the infant to adapt more fully to extrauterine life and thus better tolerate surgery.

Orthopedic deformities that may affect later ambulation are evaluated early and corrective therapy initiated (as discussed in the sections on "Congenital hip dysplasia" and "Clubfoot"). The child also will need pediatric rehabilitation and occupational and physical therapy to deal with motor and sensory deficits from irreversible nerve damage.

Frequent UTIs and the risk of hydronephrosis (urine collection in the renal pelvis, which cause distention) may result in renal failure. To help prevent UTI and hydronephrosis and to help the child achieve continence, the physician typically orders regular bladder emptying, with intermittent bladder catheterization. Such medications as oxybutynin (Ditropan) or propantheline (Pro-Banthine) may be prescribed to increase bladder size and reduce pressure, thus decreasing the risk of hydronephrosis. If these measures fail to achieve continence, the child may require a urinary diversion procedure, such as ureterostomy.

Many children with myelomeningocele achieve bowel continence through a bowel training program that involves dietary modification, prevention of constipation, regular physical activity, and regular bowel emptying through the use of laxatives, stool softeners, and enemas.

Nursing management

Nursing care begins during the neonatal period and continues throughout life. Long-term nursing management includes working with the multidisciplinary team to help the child and family deal with the chronic effects of the myelomeningocele. The following discussion focuses on measures the nurse carries out during the neonatal period.

Preoperative care. Before surgery, place the newborn on a radiant warmer and assist the physician in conducting a comprehensive neurologic assessment. After the assessment is completed, the newborn may be moved to an Isolette (preferred over a radiant warmer because the warmer's heat source may cause excessive drying of the sac, thereby promoting tearing.)

Major nursing goals before surgery include preventing trauma to the sac, preventing infection, and providing emotional support to the family. To protect the membrane covering the sac, position the newborn prone, with the head slightly lowered. This position reduces CSF pressure in the sac, thus reducing traction on the sac. Flex the child's hips slightly and abduct the legs. To support the sides of the sac, the nurse may construct a protective doughnut from foam. Inspect the sac for tears and abrasions. If surgery will be delayed, initiate feeding with the newborn lying prone and the head turned to the side.

Be sure to monitor the newborn for signs of CNS infection, such as elevated temperature, irritability, high-pitched crying, vomiting, lethargy, and seizures.

If the sac is in the lower lumbar or sacral region, its proximity to the anus may cause fecal contamination, contributing to the risk of infection. To help keep feces and urine away from the sac, leave the newborn undiapered and place a protective drape near the anus, proximal to the sac. If prescribed, cover the sac loosely with a moist, sterile dressing, taking care to avoid putting pressure on the sac. Keep the dressing moist by applying sterile sodium chloride solution periodically. Never allow the dressing to dry because this may make the dressing adhere to the sac, causing damage or tearing of the sac when the dressing is removed. As prescribed, administer I.V. antibiotics.

Allow sufficient time to answer parents' questions about the child's condition and anticipated surgery. Also review the postoperative course of recovery with the parents.

Postoperative care. Nursing goals during this period include:
• preventing infection
• preventing increased intracranial pressure (ICP)
• avoiding perineal skin breakdown
• establishing routine bladder emptying
• minimizing further musculoskeletal deformity.

After surgery, place the newborn in a prone or side-lying position. To prevent fecal contamination of the surgical site, apply protective drapes between the surgical incision and anus. Do not apply diapers until the surgical incision heals completely. As prescribed, administer prophylactic I.V. antibiotics to reduce the risk of infection of the CNS or the incision site.

To detect hydrocephalus, which indicates CSF accumulation, measure the child's head circumference daily. Palpate the fontanels; if they are tense and bulging, suspect increased ICP caused by abnormal accumulation of CSF. Other signs of early ICP include irritability, high-pitched cry, poor feeding, and distended scalp veins.

Constant dribbling of urine and stool predisposes the perineal skin to breakdown. Be sure to clean the perineal area with warm water after each bowel movement, dry the area carefully, and, as needed, apply a protective ointment, such as A & D or zinc oxide.

Also monitor the efficiency of the child's bladder emptying. To determine if residual urine remains after spontaneous voiding, catheterize the bladder after each voiding, as prescribed. A residual volume below 25 ml reflects effective bladder emptying. Consistent residual volumes above 25 ml call for a bladder training program. If residual urine persists, implement an intermittent catheterization schedule, as prescribed.

To help prevent further musculoskeletal deformities, position the child appropriately for sleeping. To keep the hips in proper alignment, place the child prone, with the hips flexed slightly and legs abducted. Place small log rolls under the ankles to keep ankles and feet in the proper position. To prevent contractures, perform gentle range-of-motion (ROM) exercises to the lower extremities.

Before discharge, teach the parents proper newborn positioning and ROM exercises. Also teach them how to perform the Credé maneuver and intermittent catheterization techniques, if prescribed. Instruct them to report signs of UTI, such as elevated temperature, cloudy urine, and mucus shreds in the urine.

Hydrocephalus

Hydrocephalus, or abnormal accumulation of CSF within the cranial vault, is caused by an imbalance in the production and absorption of CSF within the ventricular system. An imbalance may occur when too little CSF is absorbed or when CSF circulation is obstructed.

When caused by decreased CSF absorption, hydrocephalus is called communicating hydrocephalus. An example is the hydrocephalus that follows meningitis; exudate produced during the infectious process causes fibrosis and impaired CSF absorption within the subarachnoid spaces. Hydrocephalus caused by obstructed CSF circulation is called noncommunicating hydrocephalus. This form of hydrocephalus may result from Arnold-Chiari deformity or brain tumors.

Pathophysiology

Hydrocephalus results in increased ICP and passive dilation of the ventricles. Ventricular dilation causes displacement of brain tissue outward, toward the skull. With sufficient displacement, brain damage occurs. Cranial sutures and fontanels do not close fully, and passive ventricular dilation causes progressive skull enlargement.

Prognosis. The prognosis for an infant with hydrocephalus depends on the cause of the disorder, the rate at which it develops, the duration of increased ICP, and any complications that occur. Infants with myelomeningocele who subsequently develop hydrocephalus have a fairly good prognosis; because skull enlargement accommodates the accumulation of CSF, they typically do not have high ICP. Prompt surgical intervention also improves their prognosis.

The prognosis is less certain for infants who experience prolonged periods of increased ICP. CNS infections also worsen the prognosis.

Assessment

Inspection reveals dilated and prominent scalp veins. Scalp palpation reveals tense, bulging fontanels and causes separation of the cranial sutures. The frontal area of the skull may be displaced outward. The infant's eyes are displaced downward. The iris also is displaced downward, and the sclera appears above the iris ("setting sun" sign).

As ICP increases, the infant becomes lethargic and irritable and may have a high-pitched cry. Opisthotonos (neck and spinal hyperextension) and lower limb spasticity may occur. Infants with Arnold-Chiari deformity and subsequent brain-stem involvement may have difficulty breathing and swallowing. If ICP increases rapidly, vomiting and seizures may occur.

Once the fontanel closes, signs and symptoms of hydrocephalus directly reflect the consequences of increased ICP. In an older child, ICP increases more rapidly because the skull cannot enlarge further; signs and symptoms of increased ICP include headache accompanied by vomiting, lethargy, irritability, papilledema, and strabismus.

In an infant, hydrocephalus is diagnosed using head circumference measurements that are inconsistent with typical growth patterns. The diagnosis is confirmed by computed tomography scan.

Medical management

Hydrocephalus generally requires surgery. If the disorder stems from an obstructive lesion, the lesion is removed. Commonly, a drainage catheter (shunt) also is placed within the obstructed ventricle and threaded into an extracranial compartment (typically the peritoneum); such a shunt system is called a ventriculoperitoneal (VP) shunt. Excess CSF fluid drains from the obstructed ventricle to the peritoneum, resolving the effects of increased ICP caused by the obstruction. Valves in the catheter system are designed to open at a preset ICP and to close when ICP falls below that point. Thus, CSF always flows outward, away from the ventricles.

Potential complications of a VP shunt include infection and malfunction. CNS infections, such as meningitis, may develop at any time but are most common 1 to 2 months after shunt insertion or revision. Because CNS infections may impair the child's cognitive development, they warrant aggressive treatment with I.V. (and sometimes intraventricular) antibiotic therapy. Peritonitis also may occur. Signs of peritonitis include a tender and distended abdomen, irritability, and fever.

The shunt also may become obstructed or displaced — this is a serious complication because without adequate drainage, CSF accumulates quickly in the ventricles, causing ICP to rise. An obstructed or displaced shunt must be removed and replaced with a new one.

Nursing management

Preoperatively, prepare the infant for surgery. Maintain and monitor I.V. therapy and keep the infant on NPO status. Explain the infant's condition to the parents, and discuss with them the surgical procedure and postoperative recovery period.

Postoperatively, nursing goals include:
• preventing injury
• preventing infection
• promoting comfort
• monitoring for increased ICP
• providing nutrition.

After surgery, position the child on the side opposite the shunt insertion site to prevent pressure on the shunt valve and injury to the incision site. Keep the head of the bed flat to help prevent too-rapid drainage of intracranial fluid, which may cause the cortex to tear away from the dura, resulting in a subdural hematoma.

As prescribed, administer prophylactic antibiotics. Monitor the infant closely for signs of CNS infection. Check the incision site for redness and drainage, which may indicate infection.

Monitor I.V. therapy closely, and document fluid intake and output carefully. Be aware that fluid overload can have especially grave consequences for the infant with hydrocephalus because it may lead to or exacerbate increased ICP. Monitor for signs of increased ICP, which indicates shunt malfunction.

Pain medications may be contraindicated if CNS depression is suspected because of their sedative effect. As appropriate, use alternative comfort measures, such as offering a pacifier. Gentle stroking may help calm the infant.

Withhold all oral intake until bowel sounds return. Offer clear fluids initially. When tolerated, the child may be bottle- or breast-fed.

The family needs education about the shunting procedure and need for follow-up care. Instruct parents to watch for signs of shunt malfunction and CNS infection and to report these to the physician immediately.

Musculoskeletal deformities

This section discusses two congenital musculoskeletal deformities — hip dysplasia and clubfoot.

Congenital hip dysplasia

Congenital hip dysplasia refers to a condition in which the femoral head does not sit properly in the acetabulum. It can range from a minimal lateral displacement to complete dislocation of the femoral head. This disorder (also called congenital dislocated hip) is more common in females than males. Typically, only one hip is involved — the left hip more often than the right.

Etiology

The cause of congenital hip dysplasia is unclear. However, its increased incidence in identical twins suggests that hereditary factors play a role. Also, it is more common in newborns with a frank breech presentation at delivery.

Pathophysiology

Varying forms of congenital hip dysplasia exist. The degree of deformity ranges from mild, in which the femoral head remains within the acetabulum, to the most severe, in which the femoral head does not touch the acetabulum and a complete dislocation exists.

Assessment

Thorough assessment of the newborn reveals the presence of this anomaly. During assessment, health care personnel perform Ortolani's sign and Barlow's sign. Further testing may be performed with the infant in the supine position and the hips and knees flexed. The examiner observes the level of the infant's knees; uneven knees suggest hip dislocation. The examiner also holds the infant upright, with legs suspended, then observes the infant from the back. Unequal gluteal and thigh folds may indicate hip dislocation.

If congenital hip dysplasia escapes diagnosis during infancy, typically it is not identified until the child begins to stand and walk, at which time the leg on the affected side appears shorter. If dislocation is suspected in an older child, the child is asked to stand on each leg alternately; weight-bearing on the affected hip makes the opposite hip appear lower (positive Trendelenburg sign) rather than higher, as would be expected.

Prognosis. With early diagnosis and treatment, the prognosis for normal hip function is excellent.

Medical management

Treatment for an infant up to age 6 months, treatment involves the use of devices that maintain the hips in flexion. The most common device is the Pavlik harness, which the infant wears continuously for 3 to 6 months or until the hip is stable (as determined by X-rays).

Hip contractures may develop if congenital hip dysplasia goes untreated. Older children (age 6 to 18 months) who develop contractures require reduction by Bryant's traction, which requires hospitalization. Once the dislocation is reduced, a spica cast is applied. The child is discharged when the cast is dry; the cast is kept on until the hip is stable.

In children older than 6 months who have been diagnosed late or for whom early treatment has been unsuccessful, treatment is more complicated. Surgical reduction commonly is necessary, followed by casting for immobilization.

Nursing management

The nurse may play an important role in detecting congenital hip dysplasia. During routine newborn assessment, note any deviation in the gluteal or thigh folds. If trained in eliciting Ortolani's and Barlow's signs, also perform these tests.

After diagnosis, teach parents how to apply the Pavlik harness. Stress that the harness must remain in place continuously. Demonstrate diapering and sponge-bathing techniques with the harness in place. If the physician approves occasional tub bathing, demonstrate tub-bathing techniques. Because the infant's hips must be kept flexed and in midline position, inform parents that bathing requires two people — one to stabilize the infant's hip, the other to bathe the infant.

Clubfoot

In this deformity, the metatarsal bones of the forefoot deviate, and the foot appears to be twisted out of shape. Clubfoot may be unilateral or bilateral, and may appear by itself or in combination with other malformations. It affects more males than females.

Etiology

Because the incidence of clubfoot is greater in identical twins than in fraternal twins, hereditary factors appear to play a role in the disorder. Abnormal positioning in utero also has been implicated.

Pathophysiology and classification

Clubfoot may take various forms. In *talipes varus,* the ankle appears to be twisted inward, with the foot pointing inward. In *talipes valgus,* the ankle appears to be twisted outward, with the foot pointing outward. In *talipes equinus,* the foot is plantarflexed, with toes pointing downward. In *talipes calcaneus,* the foot is dorsiflexed, with toes pointing upward. **Prognosis.** With early treatment, the prognosis for complete correction is good.

Assessment

Clubfoot is apparent at birth. To differentiate true clubfoot from positional deformities, the examiner attempts to return the newborn's ankle and foot passively to a normal position. In true clubfoot, ankle and foot positions are fixed and resistance is met when the foot is manipulated.

Medical management

Manipulation and successive casting are used to correct the deformity and maintain correct positioning until the child gains muscle balance. During infancy, when the child grows rapidly, manipulation and casting may be required every few days initially. If these techniques fail, surgical correction may be necessary. Following correction, some type of splint, such as a Denis-Browne splint with corrective shoes, is necessary.

Nursing management

Use measures similar to those required by any child in a cast. After cast application, instruct parents to watch for complications and teach them how to protect the cast from damage. Also review with them the overall plan of care.

STUDY ACTIVITIES

Short answer

1. Identify the typical stages of grief that parents go through after the birth of a child with a disturbance in physical development.

_____

_____

2. Which prenatal tests can identify myelomeningocele in the fetus?

_____

_____

3. Compare the cause of communicating hydrocephalus with the cause of noncommunicating hydrocephalus.

_____

_____

4. List two potential complications of VP shunt insertion.

_____

_____

5. Brendan, age 2 weeks, has undergone VP shunt insertion to treat hydrocephalus. To address related problems, the nurse formulates the following nursing diagnosis: _Parental knowledge deficit related to monitoring the child for shunt complications._ The expected outcome is that Brendan's parents will verbalize the ability to recognize signs of shunt obstruction and CNS infection. Identify at least three nursing interventions that would help achieve this outcome.

_____

_____

_____

Multiple choice

6. The health care team suspects that Michael, born several hours ago, has TEF. During the initial assessment, what would the nurse expect to find?

  A. Continuous drooling
  B. Diaphragmatic breathing
  C. Slow response to stimuli
  D. Passage of frothy meconium

7. Joan is born by cesarean delivery when her mother's labor fails to progress. The health care team discovers a meningomyelocele measuring 3″ × 3″ over her lower lumbosacral region. Joan is scheduled for corrective surgery 18 hours after birth. What is the most important goal of her preoperative nursing care?

  A. To prevent infection.
  B. To provide adequate hydration.
  C. To ensure adequate nutrition.
  D. To prevent contracture deformities.

8. Postoperatively, the nurse monitors Joan for signs of hydrocephalus. What is the earliest indication of increased ICP in an infant?

  A. Vomiting
  B. Papilledema
  C. Headache
  D. Increasing head circumference

9. Insertion of a VP shunt may cause all of the following complications *except*:

    A. CNS infection

    B. Peritonitis

    C. Shunt obstruction

    D. Myocarditis

10. The signs and symptoms of hydrocephalus reflect:

    A. Inadequate oxygenation of the cerebral cortex.

    B. Accumulation of toxic cellular metabolites.

    C. A pronounced increase in ICP.

    D. Slow destruction of brain cells.

ANSWERS

Short answer

1. The parents progress through the stages of shock, disbelief, and denial; adjustment; and acceptance.

2. Ultrasonography, maternal serum AFP tests, and amniocentesis can identify myelomeningocele prenatally.

3. Communicating hydrocephalus results from insufficient CSF absorption. Noncommunicating hydrocephalus results from obstructed circulation of CSF.

4. Complications of VP shunt insertion include CNS infections (such as meningitis) and shunt obstruction or displacement.

5. The nurse should instruct Brendan's parents to observe for signs of shunt obstruction, such as irritability, a high-pitched cry, vomiting, and a bulging, tense fontanel; to observe for signs of CNS infection, including fever, a high-pitched cry, irritability, vomiting, lethargy, and seizures; and to notify the physician immediately if any signs occur.

Multiple choice

6. A. The signs and symptoms of TEF include excessive oral secretions and continuous drooling as well as choking and coughing, which are especially pronounced during feeding. Slow response to stimuli and passage of frothy meconium are not seen in infants with TEF.

7. A. Preventing infection is the nurse's primary goal during the preoperative period. Options B, C, and D also are relevant during the preoperative period, but are less important.

8. D. Increasing head circumference is the first sign of hydrocephalus in an infant. Vomiting occurs later. Papilledema may not be evident because increased ICP may be a late sign of hydrocephalus in an infant. Because the infant cannot speak, the nurse would have trouble determining if the infant had a headache.

9. D. Myocarditis is not a complication of VP shunt insertion.

10. C. Increased ICP causes hydrocephalus. Increased ICP results in cerebral hypoxia and brain cell destruction. Cellular metabolite accumulation does not cause signs of hydrocephalus.

CHAPTER 12

The high-risk infant

OBJECTIVES

After studying this chapter, the reader should be able to:

1. Define the following terms: appropriate for gestational age (AGA), small for gestational age (SGA), and large for gestational age (LGA).

2. Define premature, full-term, and postmature as these terms relate to gestational age.

3. Compare and contrast the physical characteristics of a premature neonate, a full-term neonate, and a postmature neonate.

4. Identify the causes of and physiologic risks associated with prematurity, post-maturity, SGA status, and LGA status.

5. Discuss the nurse's role in caring for the premature neonate and family.

6. Describe medical and nursing management for the neonate with respiratory distress syndrome or hemolytic disease.

7. Describe how maternal diabetes affects the developing fetus and the neonate's adaptation to extrauterine life.

8. Discuss the effects of maternal substance abuse on the fetus and on the neonate.

9. Identify medical and nursing management for neonates exposed to alcohol or cocaine in utero.

OVERVIEW OF CONCEPTS

The high-risk neonate is one who has an increased chance of dying during or shortly after delivery, or who has a congenital or perinatal problem necessitating prompt intervention. High-risk infants are most commonly classified according to size, gestational age, and predominant pathophysiologic problems. Variations of gestational age (prematurity being the most common) and birth weight predispose the neonate and infant to various problems.

Better understanding of pathophysiologic events during the neonatal period has significantly reduced mortality and morbidity in high-risk infants. High-quality nursing care can influence the survival, general status, and future development of these children. To provide the most effective care, the nurse must recognize the implications of birthweight and gestational-age variations on the neonate's well-being. The nurse also must understand the causes of neonate high-risk status.

The premature neonate

The premature neonate is at risk for respiratory distress syndrome, asphyxia, intracranial hemorrhage, patent ductus arteriosus, hyperbilirubinemia, impaired thermoregulation, poor nutrition, hypoglycemia, hypocalcemia, and central nervous system immaturity (which may cause apnea). Causes of prematurity include various maternal factors, as well as antepartal and fetal or neonatal conditions that necessitate early delivery.

Maternal factors include poverty, malnutrition, age under 16 or over 35, closely spaced pregnancies, pregnancy-induced hypertension, and tobacco, alcohol, or narcotic use during pregnancy.

Antepartal conditions include placenta previa or placentae abruptio, premature rupture of membranes, intrauterine infection, and incompetent cervix.

Fetal or neonatal factors include multiple gestation, hemolytic disease of the neonate, a nonreactive stress test, and intrauterine growth retardation.

Assessment

The premature neonate who is appropriate for gestational age has a head that is large in comparison to body length. Lanugo is abundant, and the skin appears thin, with many veins visible. Skin cracking is minimal.

Plantar creases may be absent or may cover only the anterior third of the sole. Breast tissue and subcutaneous fat are minimal. The pinna (external ear) is soft and may appear flattened to the skull. Hair is fine, with a patchy distribution.

Genitalia are immature. A boy has fewer-than-normal scrotal rugae and may have undescended testes. In a girl, the labia majora may not cover the labia minora and the clitoris may be prominent.

This chapter defines birth-weight and gestational-age variations. It then discusses the nurse's role in caring for the premature neonate and family, including ways to support thermoregulation and respiratory effort, manage jaundice, prevent infection, and help parents cope with their child's condition. Next, the chapter discusses common perinatal problems in high-risk neonates.

Birth-weight and gestational-age variations

Birth-weight and gestational-age variations may cause a wide range of problems in a neonate. To plan the care of the high-risk neonate, the nurse must understand the significance of these variations.

Some neonates have variations in both gestational age and birth weight. They exhibit a combination of physical characteristics, as well as alterations in physiologic function that reflect each variation. (For causes, possible complications, and assessment of conditions causing high-risk status for different types of neonates, see *The premature neonate; The postmature neonate; The small-for-gestational-age neonate,* page 152; and *The large-for-gestational-age neonate,* page 153.)

Gestational-age variations

In terms of gestational age, a neonate may be full-term, premature (preterm), or postmature (postterm). The full-term neonate is born be-

The postmature neonate

The postmature neonate is at risk for birth asphyxia, meconium aspiration, and hypoglycemia. The cause of postmaturity is unknown.

Assessment
Signs of postmaturity include absence of vernix caseosa; dry, cracking skin; long nails; and an abundance of subcutaneous fat and long, silky hair.

---

tween 38 and 42 weeks' gestation. A premature neonate is born before 38 weeks' gestation; a postmature neonate, after 42 weeks.

The health care team assesses the neonate's gestational age soon after birth using the Dubowitz tool or another standard gestational age assessment instrument. (Birth weight is not a factor in determining gestational age.) Using the Dubowitz tool, the examiner evaluates 11 external and 10 neurologic signs and plots the results on a graph to identify the neonate's gestational age.

Birth-weight variations
A birth-weight variation occurs if the neonate's weight is inappropriate for the estimated gestational age. The small-for-gestational-age (SGA) neonate is one whose birth weight falls below the tenth percentile for gestational age. SGA status typically results from intrauterine growth retardation.

A neonate whose birth weight falls between the 10th and 90th percentile for gestational age is classified as appropriate for gestational age (AGA). One whose weight exceeds the 90th percentile for gestational age is classified as large for gestational age (LGA).

Nursing care for the premature infant and family

Because multiple body systems are immature in the premature infant, the health care team must provide for the infant's physiologic needs. Nursing goals include:
• providing a neutral thermal environment
• maintaining fluid and electrolyte balance
• providing adequate nutrition
• preventing skin breakdown
• supporting respiratory effort
• preventing infection
• supporting the infant's psychosocial needs.

Ensuring thermoregulation
Because of immature thermoregulation, the premature infant has trouble maintaining body temperature. A large body surface area relative to size, minimal subcutaneous tissue, and lack of brown fat (adipose tissue) predispose this infant to hypothermia.

The small-for-gestational-age neonate

The full-term, small-for-gestational-age (SGA) neonate is at risk for meconium aspiration, birth asphyxia, intracranial hemorrhage, hypoglycemia, and polycythemia and related hyperbilirubinemia. SGA status results from various factors.

Maternal factors include advanced age, advanced parity, underweight before pregnancy, inadequate weight gain during pregnancy, and alcohol use.

Maternal conditions that interfere with placental blood flow also may cause a full-term SGA neonate. These conditions include heart disease, renal disease, hypertension, tobacco or cocaine use, sickle cell anemia, preeclampsia, placental lesions, multiple gestation, and diabetes mellitus.

Assessment

Physical characteristics of the full-term SGA neonate include a thin, wasted body; minimal subcutaneous fat; and loose, peeling, cracked skin.

Guarding against heat loss is a priority. As discussed in Chapter 6, The infant and family, the infant, like anyone, can lose heat through convection, radiation, evaporation, and conduction. Convective heat loss occurs when heat is transferred from the body to cooler environmental air; causes of convective heat loss include inadequate Isolette temperatures and drafts near an open radiant warmer. Radiant heat loss occurs when heat is transferred from the body to a cooler solid surface not in direct contact with the body; proximity to a cool Isolette wall can cause radiant heat loss in an infant. Evaporative heat loss occurs when liquid is converted to a vapor; it may occur after the infant is bathed or when environmental humidity is low. Conductive heat loss occurs when heat is transferred from the body to a cooler solid surface that is in direct contact with the body; such heat loss may occur if a caregiver handles the infant with cold hands, weighs the infant on a cool scale, or uses unwarmed bed linens.

Hypothermia (defined as a rectal temperature below 35.5° C [95.9° F] or a skin temperature below 36.5° C [97.7° F]) can cause cold stress (heat loss and inability to maintain thermoregulation) in the neonate. Cold stress stimulates heat-generating processes, which expend the neonate's calories and oxygen. Because oxygen demands increase during periods of heat generation, the infant experiencing cold stress may become hypoxic. Continued cold stress interferes with growth by diverting calories to thermoregulation. Also, because glucose is metabolized during heat production, cold stress quickly depletes the infant's glucose reserves, leading to hypoglycemia. Without sufficient oxygen, anaerobic glycolysis occurs, resulting in metabolic acidosis.

The large-for-gestational-age neonate

The full-term, large-for-gestational-age (LGA) neonate is at risk for birth trauma and hypoglycemia. LGA status may result from a genetic predisposition or from maternal diabetes mellitus. Certain fetal factors also may contribute to LGA status, including transposition of the great vessels and hemolytic disease of the newborn.

Assessment

Physical features of the LGA neonate include a head circumference and length that is larger when compared to the average-for-gestational-age neonate. The weight of a diabetic mother's LGA neonate is disproportionately heavier, and this weight is not in proportion to the neonate's head circumference and body length.

Maintaining a neutral thermal environment

The nurse's challenge is to maintain a neutral thermal environment — a narrow range of environmental temperatures at which the least amount of energy is needed to maintain a stable core temperature. With a neutral thermal environment, the infant maintains a normal body temperature (a rectal temperature of 35.5° to 37.5° C [95.9° to 99.5° F] and a skin temperature of 36° to 37° C [96.8° to 98.6° F]), with minimal oxygen consumption and the lowest possible metabolic rate.

To ensure a neutral thermal environment, the neonate should be wiped dry after delivery. Place the premature neonate on a radiant warmer, starting immediately after delivery, until the rectal temperature stabilizes at 35.5° C to 37.5° C. Once stable, the neonate may be moved to an Isolette. Adjust Isolette temperature to maintain a skin temperature of 36° to 37° C.

Make sure always to use prewarmed bed linens and to wipe the infant dry after bathing. If the nurse's hands are cool, warm them under warm tap water. Keep the infant's warmer or Isolette away from drafty areas, cool windows, and air conditioners. If the neonate is extremely small, use heat shields to prevent drafts. Place a knitted or stockinette cap on the neonate's head to prevent heat loss through the scalp and skin on the head, which can be substantial.

Maintaining fluid and electrolyte balance

With a body composition of 90% water (compared to 75% in the full-term neonate), the premature neonate has trouble maintaining fluid and electrolyte balance. This neonate may lose up to 15% of body weight through water loss. Skin immaturity increases insensible water losses, which may be exacerbated by phototherapy and radiant warmers.

Also, inability of the kidneys to conserve water predisposes the premature neonate to dehydration. Assess the neonate regularly for signs of dehydration, such as depressed fontanels, decreased skin turgor, excessive weight loss, urine output below 1 to 2 ml/hour, urine specific gravity over 1.012, and dry mucous membranes. If the neonate's oral intake is insufficient to maintain fluid balance, administer intravenous (I.V.) fluids, as prescribed.

Fluid loss, decreased electrolyte stores, or inadequate intake may cause electrolyte imbalances, principally calcium and sodium. Also, monitor laboratory serum glucose, calcium, and sodium values. As prescribed, give I.V. electrolyte replacements to manage imbalances, as evidenced by a serum sodium level below 135 mEq/liter, a serum calcium level below 9 mg/dl, or a serum glucose level below 60 mg/dl.

Providing nutrition

Gastrointestinal (GI) motility may be slower in the premature neonate, resulting in infrequent bowel movements, constipation, and abdominal distention. Also, lactose and fat tolerance may be poor.

Be aware that breast milk is preferred for feedings because it is digested more easily than commercial infant formulas and its maternal immunoglobulins help the infant fight infections. If breast milk is not available, give a commercial infant formula.

Coordination of sucking and swallowing does not mature until approximately 34 weeks' gestation. Therefore, the neonate at less than 34 weeks' gestation (and the more mature infant who tires easily) should be fed by gavage. Typically, a tube is passed through the nose or mouth into the stomach. Residual amounts of feeding remaining in the stomach are evaluated periodically to assess how feedings are tolerated. Depending on the infant's feeding tolerance, use an intermittent or continuous-drip gavage method to deliver breast milk or formula. To promote gastric emptying, position the infant on the right side after feeding. There is a risk of aspiration with gavage feedings in infants with no gag reflex. To prevent aspiration, keep the mattress elevated 30 degrees for 30 minutes after intermittent feedings and at all times during continuous feedings. An infant who cannot tolerate oral or enteral feedings may require total parenteral nutrition (TPN).

Preventing skin breakdown

The premature infant's skin is extremely fragile. To help prevent skin breakdown, handle the infant gently, use sheepskin on the mattress, avoid excessive tape, and keep bathing to a minimum. When necessary, clean the infant's skin gently with warm water. Avoid lotions and alkaline soaps because they disrupt normal skin pH, allowing bacteria proliferation and subsequent skin infections. Turn the infant every 2 hours to minimize the development of skin breakdown in pressure-sensitive areas.

Supporting the infant's respiratory effort

The premature infant has less regular respirations than the full-term infant. Weak respiratory muscles and a less rigid thoracic cage may lead to hypoventilation, followed by carbon dioxide retention and acidosis. The premature infant also is at risk for aspiration (caused by weak coughing and gagging reflexes) and respiratory distress syndrome (discussed later in this chapter).

Central nervous system (CNS) immaturity, hypothermia, electrolyte disturbances, sepsis, abdominal distention, and vagal stimulation may result in apnea. Severe or recurrent apneic episodes cause inadequate gas exchange, leading to hypoxemia and bradycardia. Consequently, all premature infants are placed on apnea monitors.

To help prevent apnea, maintain the infant's rectal temperature between 35.5° and 37.5° C (95.9° to 99.5° F). As prescribed, provide sufficient exogenous glucose to maintain a serum glucose level above 60 mg/dl. Minimize abdominal distention by adequate burping and by placing the infant on the right side after feedings. Use care during suctioning and nasogastric (NG) tube insertion to minimize vagal stimulation. To maintain an open airway and help prevent apnea in the infant with weak upper airway muscles, slightly hyperextend the infant's neck.

Avoiding intraventricular hemorrhage

More than half of all premature infants experience intraventricular hemorrhage (IVH), or bleeding into the ventricles of the brain. Fragile cerebral capillaries set the stage for IVH. Sudden changes in arterial or venous pressure, serum osmolarity, or cerebral blood flow may contribute to this problem.

A large hemorrhage may trigger seizures or cause a sudden deterioration in respiratory or cardiac status. A smaller hemorrhage may be hard to detect. Bulging fontanels and increasing head circumference typically develop within 2 weeks of IVH. Hydrocephalus also may follow IVH. Ultrasonography typically confirms hemorrhage. Assess the infant for changes in neurologic status. Measure head circumference daily and assess fontanels for bulging or tenseness. Maintain oxygenation, providing ventilatory support as needed.

Managing jaundice

Liver immaturity predisposes the premature infant to physiologic jaundice, a nonpathologic form of jaundice. Any neonate, not just a premature one, may develop physiologic jaundice. Pathologic jaundice, seen mainly in high-risk neonates, results from blood type or blood group incompatibility, infection, or biliary, hepatic, or metabolic abnormalities.

Physiologic jaundice results from slow or ineffective bilirubin clearance. Unconjugated bilirubin accumulates because of decreased availability of glucuronyl transferase, Y and Z carrier proteins, and albumin. Unconjugated bilirubin can be toxic to the CNS. When the unconjugated bilirubin level reaches 20 mg/dl in the full-term infant (a lower value exists for the premature infant), irreversible brain damage, or kernicterus, occurs.

To manage physiologic jaundice, place the infant in a phototherapy unit, as prescribed. Phototherapy lights break down bilirubin deposited in the skin into compounds that can be excreted. They are available in white or blue ultraviolet light; blue lights are used for infants with more severe jaundice.

Before phototherapy begins, remove the infant's clothes and cover the eyes with patches. Cover the genitals with a mask or diaper to catch urine and stool while leaving the skin surface open to the light. During phototherapy, turn the infant from side to side and from front to back every 2 hours for maximum skin exposure to phototherapy lights. At regular intervals, turn off the phototherapy lights and remove eye patches for several minutes to provide visual stimulation and promote nurse-infant or parent-infant interaction.

Because phototherapy lights serve as an additional heat source, be sure to monitor the infant's temperature closely. Also check for signs of dehydration; bilirubin breakdown increases gastric motility, which can cause loose stools. Monitor fluid intake and output and urine specific gravity.

Managing patent ductus arteriosus

Birth hypoxia may cause patent ductus arteriosus (PDA) in the premature infant. The ductus arteriosus, a connection between the pulmonary artery and aorta in the fetus, typically closes soon after birth when blood oxygenation levels rise. If it fails to close, blood shunts from the aorta to the pulmonary artery, causing increased pulmonary blood flow. Pulmonary circulatory congestion and congenital heart failure may ensue.

Assessment findings in PDA include a continuous, harsh murmur. (For details on PDA, see Chapter 20, Cardiovascular dysfunction). Nursing goals include maintaining adequate cardiopulmonary function. Assess for cyanosis, heart murmurs, arrhythmias, absent or unequal pulses, and respiratory distress. Monitor daily weight and fluid intake and output.

Preventing infection

The premature infant has a reduced capacity to fight infection. Maternal transfer of immunoglobulins does not occur until 28 weeks' gestation; an infant delivered before this time does not receive immunoglobulin A (IgA) transplacentally and therefore has no protection against common bacterial infections, such as diphtheria, measles, and tetanus.

Pathogens may enter through the premature infant's fragile skin, which is susceptible to breakdown. Respiratory infections also may occur, especially in intubated infants who need frequent suctioning. Septicemia also is more common in premature infants.

Because of an immature inflammatory response, signs of infection in neonates are nonspecific and may include temperature instability, feeding intolerance, jaundice, apnea, hypotonia, and lethargy. To detect pulmonary infection, monitor for tachypnea, increased respiratory secretions (especially yellow or green secretions), retractions of the chest wall, hypoxia, and hypercapnia.

To guard against infection, always wash hands thoroughly with bactericidal soap before handling the infant. Be sure to use aseptic technique when performing any invasive procedure. If necessary, restrict visitors to parents only. Isolate any infant with a suspected or confirmed contagious infection. As prescribed, administer I.V. antibiotics to treat infection.

Providing for psychosocial needs

No matter how critical the infant's physiologic needs, be sure to consider the psychosocial needs of both the infant and family. Maintain an appropriate sensory environment and provide opportunities for parent-infant interaction.

The parent's first visit to the nursery may be frightening. For some, this is the first glimpse of their child. Before parents enter the nursery, prepare them for the infant's appearance and briefly mention the medical devices and technological supports near the infant. (These can be explained more fully once the parents are inside the nursery.)

After the parents enter the nursery, sit with them by the infant's side, if possible, so they can be closer to the infant than they would be if standing. Stay with the parents during this initial visit. Encourage them to touch or gently stroke the infant; if necessary, show the parents how to do this. Also, urge parents to talk to the infant quietly. Once the infant is stable and the parents seem comfortable, introduce care-giving tasks, such as diaper changing and bottle- or breast-feeding.

Most infants tolerate visual stimulation well. To provide such stimulation, the nurse may tape simple pictures of human faces to the walls of the Isolette. Encourage the parents to bring their faces close to the infant's when holding the infant. Instruct them to stroke the infant gently, if tolerated, and to bring audiotapes of their voices to soothe the infant. (Audiotaped heart tones may have the same effect.) However, be aware that some premature infants tolerate sensory stimulation poorly. Monitor the infant closely to evaluate the response to touch, sound, and position changes. Avoid multiple stimuli.

Parents of premature infants may experience a grief response similar to that experienced by parents of infants with congenital defects. They may mourn the loss of the perfect full-term infant they anticipated. (For details on parental responses, see Chapter 11, The infant with disturbances in physical development.) Nursing support of the family begins at the time of the initial parent-infant contact and continues throughout the infant's hospitalization and the discharge process.

Not all hospitals provide care for premature infants. Those born at facilities where premature infant care is not available are transported by ambulance or helicopter to the nearest facility providing such services. Long distances may separate these infants from their parents, who may be not able to visit often. Be sure to take extra time to help these parents feel connected to their infant. If possible, telephone them often to keep them informed of their infant's progress. Send them photographs of the infant achieving growth and developmental milestones (such as the first feeding). Also consider keeping a diary of daily events and sharing it with the parents.

Respiratory distress syndrome

Respiratory distress syndrome (RDS, formerly called hyaline membrane disease) is characterized by respiratory distress and impaired gas exchange. Lack of surfactant, a substance that prevents alveoli from collapsing after each breath, puts the premature neonate at risk for RDS. Surfactant deficiency results in progressive atelectasis, hypoxia, and hypercapnia. Prolonged hypoxia leads to metabolic acidosis, while hypercapnia causes respiratory acidosis. Acidosis further compromises the neonate by causing pulmonary vasoconstriction, arrhythmias, cerebral vasodilation, and an even greater surfactant deficiency.

The effects of RDS peak 3 to 5 days after birth. Unless complications occur, however, most neonates improve within 7 to 10 days after birth.

Assessment
Signs and symptoms of RDS, which generally appear within 2 hours of birth, include tachypnea, grunting during expiration, retractions, nasal flaring, decreased breath sounds, fine crackles, and cyanosis.

Medical management
Halting premature labor may prevent RDS or lessen its severity by allowing fetal lungs to develop more fully. To stimulate surfactant production in the fetus, steroids may be administered to a pregnant woman 24 hours to 7 days before the expected delivery date. Surfactant replacement after birth has been attempted with varying results.

Other treatment measures are supportive and include oxygen supplementation. Based on the degree of hypoxia (arterial oxygen deficiency) and hypercapnia (arterial carbon dioxide excess), the neonate may need continuous positive airway pressure (CPAP) or mechanical ventilation. CPAP provides continuous pressure during inspiration and expiration, improving gas exchange by helping to prevent alveolar collapse. However, for CPAP to be effective, the neonate must have spontaneous respirations. CPAP may be delivered through nasal prongs or an endotracheal tube. Mechanical ventilation is reserved for neonates who cannot maintain adequate gas exchange with CPAP.

Positive end-expiratory pressure (PEEP) may be used in conjunction with mechanical ventilation to improve gas exchange. Respiratory acidosis is treated by improving gas exchange — either by raising CPAP or by increasing the mechanical ventilation rate. The physician may order chest physiotherapy to loosen and move bronchial secretions from small airways into large bronchi.

Severe metabolic acidosis warrants I.V. sodium bicarbonate administration. An umbilical arterial catheter is placed to monitor arterial blood gas (ABG) levels. All oral intake is withheld and the neonate receives I.V. fluids.

Nursing management

Monitor the neonate's temperature, heart rate, respiratory rate, blood pressure, skin color, and ABG levels frequently to evaluate the effectiveness of therapy and to detect complications. Be sure to maintain a neutral thermal environment, because hypothermia increases oxygen use in the already compromised neonate.

Monitor fluid balance closely. Document intake and output, and check urine specific gravity. Because overhydration may result in pulmonary edema and congestive heart failure, be sure to assess for edema. If the infant is on nasal CPAP, perform periodic nasopharyngeal and oral suctioning, as prescribed. Take measures to prevent nasal necrosis caused by applying nasal prongs too tightly. If the infant is intubated, perform endotracheal instillation and suctioning, as prescribed.

Complications of respiratory support

Although mandatory for many premature neonates, respiratory therapy may have serious consequences. The use of supplemental oxygen and positive-pressure ventilation — which may cause hyperoxemia — in treating RDS increases the risk of complications in neonates, including retinopathy of prematurity, bronchopulmonary dysplasia, and extraneous air syndromes.

Retinopathy of prematurity

Retinopathy of prematurity (ROP) is a disease of the retinal vasculature related to oxygen therapy in the premature infant. Retinal vasoconstriction leads to ischemia in some retinal vessels. To compensate, new capillaries arise to supply oxygen and nutrients to damaged tissue. However, these vessels rupture and hemorrhage, causing scar tissue formation. Scar tissue becomes rigid and shortened, causing traction that results in retinal detachment.

Most common in neonates weighing less than 1,500 g, ROP results in varying degrees of visual impairment. Some neonates become blind. Immature retinal vasculature and hyperoxemia (increased arterial oxygen content, as from supplemental oxygen) contribute to the development of ROP.

Nursing management includes monitoring the neonate's respiratory status and ABG levels closely and notifying the physician of significant findings. The physician may adjust the percentage of supplemental oxygen to minimize ROP. To prevent ROP, avoid indiscriminate oxygen use.

Bronchopulmonary dysplasia

Bronchopulmonary dysplasia is a chronic lung disorder that may occur in any infant receiving oxygen therapy. Alveolar walls become thickened, and widespread atelectasis and fibrosis develop. Oxygenation and positive-pressure ventilation both seem to play a role in damaging alveolar surfaces. Bronchopulmonary dysplasia is most common in neonates who are intubated and on CPAP or mechanical ventilation.

The infant with bronchopulmonary dysplasia requires long-term respiratory support, and full recovery may take up to 5 years. However, most infants can be discharged on supplemental oxygen delivered via nasal cannula. (Long-term intubation may damage the trachea.)

Be sure to monitor the infant's respiratory status closely. If the infant needs long-term oxygen supplementation, help the parents adjust to caring for an infant with a chronic pulmonary disorder. (For more information on helping families cope with chronic illness, see Chapter 15, Illness concepts.)

Air-leak syndromes of the chest

Air-leak syndromes of the chest, disorders that result from alveolar rupture and the escape of air to tissues in which air is not normally present, may develop in an infant receiving CPAP or mechanical ventilation. Pressure delivered by these systems may cause immature alveoli to overdistend and rupture. Extraneous air syndromes include interstitial emphysema, pneumothorax, and pneumopericardium.

Interstitial emphysema often precedes other air syndromes. When alveoli rupture, air enters the connective tissue between the alveoli, thus impeding gas exchange.

Extraneous air syndromes may not cause obvious effects. Signs of pneumomediastinum (also called mediastinal emphysema), which occurs when leaking air enters the mediastinum, typically are mild. For instance, heart sounds may be distant or muffled and tachypnea may develop.

Pneumothorax occurs when accumulated mediastinal air leaks into the pleural cavity, thereby impairing lung expansion and gas exchange. The infant becomes tachypneic and cyanotic, and breath sounds in the affected lung may decrease. A small pneumothorax may respond to needle aspiration. A large or persistent pneumothorax requires chest tube insertion.

In pneumopericardium, a life-threatening disorder, air passes through the mediastinal wall into the pericardial space, causing cardiac tamponade. The infant becomes severely cyanotic, pulse pressures decline, and heart sounds may become inaudible. To treat the disorder, the physician enters the pericardial space and removes accumulated air. A pericardial catheter may be inserted to remove the air.

Hemolytic disease of the newborn

Hemolytic disease of the newborn is a progressive disorder of the fetal blood and blood-forming organs characterized by hemolytic anemia and hyperbilirubinemia. Rhesus factor (Rh) and ABO incompatibility are the major forms of hemolytic disease of the newborn.

Rh incompatibility

In this isoimmune hemolytic anemia, maternal antibodies cause destruction of fetal red blood cells (RBCs), leading to severe anemia and jaundice in the neonate. The disorder occurs when an Rh-negative woman is exposed to the Rh-positive antigen when carrying an Rh-positive fetus. The woman subsequently develops anti-Rh antibodies, which cross the placenta and attack the RBCs of the fetus, causing hemolysis of fetal RBCs.

An Rh-negative woman most commonly produces anti-Rh antibodies after her first pregnancy with an Rh-positive fetus. Anti-Rh antibodies also are produced after pregnancy termination or accidental transfusion with Rh-positive blood.

Fetal RBC hemolysis leads to profound anemia, which taxes the heart of the fetus and may cause congestive heart failure. Severe jaundice also occurs. Fetal consequences are most severe when hemolysis starts early in pregnancy.

Assessment

After birth, the neonate has severe jaundice and may be edematous. Laboratory findings reveal moderate to high levels of unconjugated serum bilirubin (hyperbilirubinemia) and anemia. A positive Coombs' test indicates the presence of a hemolytic process.

Medical management

Administration of Rh immunoglobulin to an Rh-negative woman within 72 hours of first delivery prevents production of maternal anti-Rh antibodies. This therapy does not destroy anti-Rh antibodies already produced during a previous pregnancy.

Prenatal maternal blood screening detects the presence of circulating anti-Rh antibodies and measures antibody titers. High antibody titers indicate a potential fetal risk, warranting amniocentesis to determine the degree of fetal hemolysis, anemia, and jaundice.

The severely anemic fetus is a candidate for intrauterine transfusion of Type O packed RBCs, transfused via a catheter into the fetal peritoneal cavity or umbilical vein. (Type O blood is not susceptible to hemolysis by anti-Rh maternal antibodies.) Intrauterine transfusions correct fetal anemia, improve tissue oxygenation, and help alleviate fetal heart failure. These transfusions are repeated at 3-week intervals until the fetus reaches 32 to 34 weeks' gestation. The neonate is delivered prematurely, after the last transfusion.

Because the hemolytic process continues after birth, the neonate is placed under phototherapy lights. If bilirubin levels continue to rise, an exchange transfusion is performed, using an umbilical vein catheter to replace approximately 85% of the infant's blood volume with Type O negative blood. This removes circulating anti-Rh antibodies and accumulated bilirubin, thereby slowing hemolysis and reducing the serum bilirubin level. Complications of exchange transfusion include air emboli or thrombus formation, anaphylactic reaction, sepsis, and electrolyte disturbances (such as hyperkalemia and hypocalcemia).

Nursing management

During phototherapy, care for the infant as described in the section on managing jaundice. During an exchange transfusion, assist the physician as appropriate, and record the infant's vital signs every 10 to 15 minutes. On a blood exchange flow sheet, document the amount of blood administered, the amount of blood withdrawn, and medications given.

After the transfusion, monitor the infant closely for 24 to 48 hours. Obtain vital signs and bilirubin levels frequently. Note lethargy, increased irritability, or convulsions, which may indicate neurologic injury. Also check for signs of infection, such as temperature instability, apnea, hypotonia, lethargy, and RDS.

ABO incompatibility

Hemolytic disease also may result from fetal-maternal incompatibility of ABO groups. ABO incompatibility occurs when a woman carries a fetus with a blood type that differs from her own. She develops anti-A and anti-B antibodies after exposure to A and B antigens naturally found in food and gram-negative bacteria. Because these antibodies are present before pregnancy, ABO incompatibility may arise during the first pregnancy.

The most common form of ABO incompatibility occurs in women with blood group O who are pregnant with a fetus whose blood group is A or B. (A fetus with group O blood is never affected because such RBCs lack antigenic sites.) Anti-A and anti-B antibodies cross the placenta, causing hemolysis of fetal RBCs. The hemolysis is less severe than in Rh incompatibility.

Assessment

The infant with ABO incompatibility has moderate to severe hyperbilirubinemia. Rarely, anemia and heart failure occur. A positive Coombs' test indicates a hemolytic process.

Management

Phototherapy typically is effective in reducing circulating serum bilirubin levels.

Infants of insulin-dependent diabetic mothers

Maternal insulin-dependent or gestational diabetes mellitus may cause fetal and neonatal complications. In the fetus, high maternal glucose levels stimulate insulin production. Continued fetal hyperglycemia and hyperinsulinemia lead to excessive fetal growth and fat deposition, resulting in an LGA infant. Fetal pancreatic hyperplasia also occurs.

Infants of diabetic mothers are at greater risk for congenital anomalies, which most often involving the GI tract or heart. This risk may be reduced by closely managing glucose metabolism in the pregnant woman with diabetes.

Assessing for substance withdrawal in the neonate

Maternal use of drugs during pregnancy can have severe consequences for the neonate, including the need to go through substance withdrawal. The withdrawal symptoms are listed below.

Neurologic signs
- Sweating
- Inconsolability
- Sleep disturbances
- Irritability
- Continuous high-pitched crying
- Increased response to auditory stimulation
- Labile motor behaviors (may alternate between hyperactivity and lethargy)
- Tremors
- Seizures
- Hypertonic, hyperactive reflexes

Gastrointestinal signs
- Vomiting
- Diarrhea
- Ineffective sucking
- Extreme urge to suck

Pulmonary signs
- Sneezing
- Tachypnea

Neonates of women with poorly controlled diabetes also are at risk for hypoglycemia after delivery. Although the neonate's pancreas continues to secrete insulin, the maternal glucose supply no longer is available, so hypoglycemia quickly sets in.

Assessment

The infant of a diabetic mother may show characteristics of LGA status, moderate to severe hypoglycemia, hyperbilirubinemia, and lethargy. Also, the infant may have difficulty feeding.

Medical and nursing management

Monitor the neonate's reagent strips immediately after delivery and at least every 2 hours until the neonate is stable. Initially, hypoglycemia may be treated with oral administration of 5% to 10% glucose. If hypoglycemia persists, I.V. glucose may be needed. Glucose regulation generally is established by 48 hours after birth. If the neonate is premature, implement care measures as discussed earlier in this chapter.

Fetal exposure to alcohol or cocaine

Narcotics, alcohol, and cocaine readily cross the placenta and enter the fetal system, possibly causing congenital anomalies. Habitual use of these substances also leads to fetal addiction, which places the infant at risk for complications after birth. The incidence of substance abuse during pregnancy is estimated conservatively at 10%.

Assessment

Passively addicted neonates experience withdrawal signs. Depending on when the mother last used the substance, these signs may appear within 12 hours of birth. (For signs of withdrawal in the neonate, see *Assessing for substance withdrawal in the neonate*.) However, withdraw-

Signs of fetal alcohol syndrome

The infant with fetal alcohol syndrome (FAS) may exhibit characteristic signs involving the central nervous system (CNS) and other body systems.

CNS manifestations of FAS include microcephaly, poor coordination, hypotonicity, irritability, and hyperactivity. Later, the child may be diagnosed with mild to moderate mental retardation. Cardiovascular signs include cardiac anomalies, such as congenital heart disease. Musculoskeletal signs include pectus excavatum (tunnel chest), atypical palmar creases, and limited joint movement. Urogenital findings may include kidney defects and labial hypoplasia.

Other signs of FAS include growth deficiency; failure to thrive; and such facial characteristics as short palpebral fissures, ptosis, strabismus, a short upturned nose, hypoplastic philtrum, a thin upper vermilion (lip border), and retrognathia (underdevelopment of the lower jaw).

---

al signs may not appear for 3 to 4 days, making identification of withdrawal difficult. Many passively addicted infants are small for their gestational age and have related complications.

Neonates born to mothers who ingested alcohol during pregnancy also are at risk for fetal alcohol syndrome (FAS) or alcohol-related birth defects. (For information on assessing FAS, see Signs of fetal alcohol syndrome.) Signs of CNS irritability, such as hyperactivity and a disturbed sleep pattern, may persist for up to 6 months after birth.

Medical and nursing management

Management aims to alleviate the neonate's clinical manifestations. As prescribed, administer decreasing doses of paregoric to the neonate with withdrawal symptoms decreasing doses of paregoric. (Paregoric, a narcotic, eases withdrawal symptoms.) Administer phenobarbital for seizures, as prescribed.

If the neonate experiences vomiting or diarrhea, monitor fluid and electrolyte balance. Provide a quiet environment for the neonate who is easily overstimulated. To limit exposure to overhead lights and to minimize environmental noise, cover the Isolette or crib.

Swaddling in blankets can help calm the passively addicted neonate. Give a pacifier if the neonate needs additional sucking activity. To improve sucking efficiency during feeding, apply pressure under the neonate's chin to pull the lower jaw forward.

Once stable and no longer exhibiting withdrawal signs, the infant may be discharged. Depending on local laws and policies, the infant may be discharged to the mother if she is deemed capable of providing for the infant responsibly. Otherwise, the infant may be discharged to a foster home.

STUDY ACTIVITIES   **Short answer**

1. Jennifer, 10 hours old, was born at 35 weeks' gestation. To address her increased risk for skin breakdown related to her prematurity, the nurse formulates the following nursing diagnosis: High risk for impaired skin integrity related to fragile, immature skin. The expected outcome is that Jennifer's skin will remain intact, clear, and free from signs of irritation and infection. Identify at least four nursing interventions that would help achieve this outcome.

_____

_____

_____

2. Susan, 3 hours old, was born by spontaneous vaginal delivery at 32 weeks' gestation. With a birth weight of 1,725 g, Susan is average for her gestational age. Her main problem at this time is poor thermoregulation. Identify the physiologic and environmental factors that predispose Susan to poor thermoregulation.

_____

_____

_____

3. As a premature infant, Susan is at risk for respiratory distress. What should the nurse watch for when assessing Susan for developing respiratory distress?

_____

_____

_____

Multiple choice

4. Seeley, born at 29 weeks' gestation, develops mild respiratory distress and is given supplemental oxygen. If oxygen supplementation causes hyperoxemia, Seeley will be at risk for which of the following?
   A. Intracranial hemorrhage
   B. Respiratory depression
   C. ROP
   D. Pneumonia

5. How does surfactant affects respiratory function?
   A. It keeps pulmonary capillaries dilated.
   B. It prevents alveoli from collapsing.
   C. It clears mucus from the airway.
   D. It stimulates chest wall muscles to contract.

6. Blue phototherapy lights are prescribed for Steven, 12 hours old. During phototherapy, what should the nurse closely monitor?
 A. Hydration status
 B. Circulatory status
 C. Oxygenation status
 D. Nutritional status

7. Which vein typically is used to administer an exchange transfusion to a neonate?
 A. Jugular vein
 B. Femoral vein
 C. Temporal vein
 D. Umbilical vein

8. What should the nurse expect to administer to a neonate with withdrawal symptoms?
 A. Paregoric
 B. Nalline
 C. Thorazine
 D. Ampicillin

ANSWERS **Short answer**

1. Place sheepskin under Jennifer. Gently turn Jennifer from side to side and from back to front every 2 hours. Avoid excessive use of tape. Minimize bathing.

2. Physiologic factors predisposing Susan to poor thermoregulation include a large body surface area relative to size, minimal subcutaneous tissue, and lack of brown fat (adipose tissue). Environmental factors include heat loss via convection, radiation, evaporation, and conduction.

3. The nurse should watch for such signs of respiratory distress as tachypnea, grunting during expiration, retractions, nasal flaring, decreased breath sounds, fine crackles, and cyanosis.

Multiple choice

4. C. ROP is associated with hyperoxemia in the premature neonate.

5. B. Surfactant keeps alveoli from collapsing after expiration.

6. A. Because phototherapy may increase body temperature and may lead to dehydration, the nurse should monitor the neonate's hydration status closely.

7. D. The umbilical vein is used to administer an exchange transfusion to a neonate.

8. A. The neonate exhibiting withdrawal symptoms typically receives paregoric in decreasing doses.

CHAPTER 13

The child with a developmental disability

OBJECTIVES
After studying this chapter, the reader should be able to:
1. Define developmental disability and mental retardation.
2. Identify etiologic factors associated with developmental disabilities.
3. Name major disorders that cause developmental disabilities.
4. Describe the nurse's multiple roles in working with disabled children and their families.
5. Describe the nurse's role in promoting optimal development of the mentally retarded child.
6. Discuss the etiology, clinical manifestations, and medical and nursing management of Down syndrome and cerebral palsy.

OVERVIEW OF CONCEPTS
The Developmental Disabilities Act of 1984 defines a developmental disability as a severe, chronic condition causing cognitive or physical impairment that manifests before age 22, resulting in significant functional limitations in three or more of the following areas: self-care, receptive and expressive language, learning, mobility, self-direction, capacity for independent living, and economic self-sufficiency.

This chapter focuses on three disorders causing developmental disability: mental retardation, Down syndrome, and cerebral palsy. Mental retardation and Down syndrome result in cognitive impairment (mental deficiency) and thus affect learning. Cerebral palsy results in physical impairment and thus affects mobility. All three disorders may impair language development, self-direction, self-care, the capacity for independent living, and economic self-sufficiency.

Causes of developmental disability
Disorders causing developmental disabilities have been linked to genetic factors, antepartal and perinatal factors, and environmental conditions (see *Factors associated with developmental disability,* page 168).

Nursing care for the child with a developmental disability
Nursing responsibilities include preventing disabling conditions in children, identifying children with existing disabilities, and minimizing

Factors associated with developmental disability

This chart describes possible causes of disorders associated with developmental disability.

FACTOR	DISABILITY-CAUSING DISORDER
Genetic	
Chromosomal disorders	• Down syndrome • Fragile X syndrome • Tay-Sachs disease • Duchenne type muscular dystrophy
Metabolic disorders	• Phenylketonuria • Galactosemia
Antepartal	
Maternal infections	• Toxoplasmosis • Rubella (German measles) • Cytomegalovirus • Herpesvirus
Physical or chemical agents	• Maternal alcohol use • Maternal drug abuse
Perinatal	
Hypoxia	• Birth asphyxia • Respiratory distress • Cerebral palsy • Birth injury
Postnatal	
Accidental injury	• Head injury
Infections	• Meningitis • Encephalitis • Malnutrition
Psychosocial conditions	• Failure to thrive
Poverty	• Malnutrition
Lead exposure	• Lead toxicity

problems associated with disabilities. However, keep in mind that children with developmental disabilities — and their families — require many of the same interventions used with nondisabled children.

To promote primary prevention of developmental disabilities, the nurse conducts lead-screening programs and teaches the public about the importance of abstaining from alcohol, tobacco, and drugs during pregnancy. To identify children with existing disabilities, the nurse and other health care professionals conduct physical, behavioral, and developmental assessments. (For details on assessment, see Chapter 5, Child health assessment.) For example, a nurse working in a community health program may act as the primary case-finder, identifying children with developmental disabilities and those at risk for disability.

To minimize problems associated with disabilities, the nurse provides ongoing family support and education. When parents learn that their child is disabled, they experience feelings similar to those of parents who learn that their child has a chronic illness. Typically, they move through a series of stages while working toward acceptance. (For information on the family's response to disability and chronic illness, see Chapter 15, Illness concepts.)

Other important nursing responsibilities for the disabled child and family include:
• providing anticipatory guidance
• providing well-child care
• assisting with long-term planning
• arranging for services or coordinating care
• assisting parents to carry out the prescribed medical plan.

The nurse also promotes optimal development of the disabled child, such as by providing developmental stimulation or assisting the child and family with use of adaptive devices.

Mental retardation

Mental retardation refers to impaired cognitive functioning, as reflected by an intelligence quotient (IQ) below 70, accompanied by impaired adaptive functioning. Although the cause of mental retardation sometimes can be identified, it often remains unknown.

Classification

Depending on the child's IQ, mental retardation may be classified as mild, moderate, severe, or profound.

Mild mental retardation

Indicated by an IQ of 50 to 70, mild mental retardation may be hard to detect during infancy. The child is slow to acquire motor, language, and self-help skills. Generally, the child achieves academic skills up to approximately the sixth-grade level and acquires the social and vocational skills needed for independent living.

Mildly retarded persons typically cannot provide the intellectual and social stimulation necessary for successful child-rearing. Therefore, they are discouraged from bearing children (although some eventually marry). For those who do become parents, support services are available to help them develop parenting skills.

Moderate mental retardation

Children with moderate mental retardation, indicated by an IQ of 35 to 49, have delayed motor and language development. However, most eventually acquire basic communication skills. These children usually achieve bowel and bladder control and some are able to acquire self-care skills, including simple health and safety skills.

The older child or adolescent may be able to travel independently to school or work, perform simple counting skills, and recognize names and letters. Older adolescents and young adults typically can function in a sheltered workshop setting, performing simple manual tasks. However, most do not progress to independent living and must live with relatives or in supervised group homes.

Severe mental retardation

Indicated by an IQ of 20 to 34, severe mental retardation causes marked delays in motor and language development. Expressive language skills are affected more significantly than receptive language skills. Most severely retarded children eventually learn how to walk and acquire minimal communication skills, such as a basic vocabulary. They may be hard to understand because of articulation problems.

Most severely retarded children can follow simple directions and learn self-care skills, such as feeding and basic grooming. However, they have difficulty with bowel and bladder training. These children require constant direction and supervision. In the past, many were institutionalized. Today, most live at home or in supervised group homes.

Profound mental retardation

This condition, characterized by an IQ below 20, necessitates complete custodial care. Some profoundly retarded children show emotional and physical responses to environmental stimulation. Their communication skills may consist of simple grunting. With support, many families choose to care for the child at home. Otherwise, the profoundly retarded child typically lives in a supervised group home.

Medical management

Health supervision and illness management of the mentally retarded child resemble those provided for any child. Most mentally retarded children benefit from early intervention programs, which provide physical, cognitive, and social stimulation and aim to maximize developmental potential in all areas. Preferably, the child is enrolled in the program early in infancy and parents participate in the program. The physician often initiates referral to an infant stimulation or special education program.

Nursing management

Mentally retarded children have the same basic physical and emotional needs as children of normal intellect. Although they learn more slowly than others, they learn in the same way — through manipulating the environment, interacting socially, playing, exploring, and undergoing systematic training.

If the child is enrolled in a special program, promote follow-through at home by teaching the family stimulation activities appropriate for the child's mental age. (For developmental stimulation activities appropriate for infants, see Chapter 6, The infant and family.)

Encourage parents to expose the child to children of normal intellect. Such exposure benefits all involved: the retarded child learns appropriate social behavior by being with and observing other children play; the other children learn to accept those who are different. Including mentally retarded children in typical child-socialization experiences (called normalization) helps the child to become a participating member of the family and community. For older children, socialization commonly is accomplished through school and group activities.

Encourage the family to provide typical socialization experiences, such as taking the child for walks, on shopping trips, and to the zoo. To avoid frustration in the child, teach parents to modify play activities to match the child's mental age rather than chronological age.

Be aware that mentally disabled adolescents have the same sexual feelings as other adolescents, and many are sexually active. Because the adolescent's sexual development may frighten or confuse the child and worry the parents, offer parents information appropriate for the child's developmental level. Give the adolescent simple explanations about anatomy and physical development as well as instruction on how to avoid pregnancy and sexually transmitted diseases. Also provide information on personal safety. For example, caution the child not to go alone with any unfamiliar person. Encourage appropriate activities to provide social experiences.

The mentally retarded child may have trouble developing a positive self-concept. Frustration, ridicule from others, and lack of appropriate socialization experiences may erode the child's self-esteem. Therefore, encourage parents to help the child gain a sense of accomplishment — even from completing minor tasks — by praising appropriate behavior, for example.

Down syndrome   Down syndrome is a congenital condition characterized by some degree of mental retardation and multiple physical defects. The most common chromosomal disorder of a generalized syndrome, it occurs in 1 of 800 to 1,000 live births. It is slightly more common in Caucasians than Blacks.

Down syndrome may be accompanied by other defects. Approximately one-third of children with Down syndrome have congenital heart disease — most commonly ventricular septal or endocardial cushion defects. Gastrointestinal (GI) defects may include tracheoesophageal fistula and duodenal atresia. Ocular disorders associated with Down syndrome include strabismus, myopia, and cataracts.

Children with Down syndrome have a high incidence of chronic myelogenous leukemia and hypothyroidism and are at increased risk for Alzheimer's disease. Many have frequent respiratory infections, resulting from inadequate lung expansion secondary to hypotonia or from upper respiratory congestion secondary to an underdeveloped nasal bridge. Some have atlantoaxial instability (instability of the first and second vertebrae), which puts them at risk for cervical injury. Also, Down syndrome predisposes the child to otitis media, which may lead to conductive hearing loss. Many children with Down syndrome have communication disorders, partly because a large, protruding tongue makes articulation difficult.

Most children with Down syndrome are overweight and shorter than normal. Sexual development varies. Males are infertile and may have underdeveloped genitalia and decreased facial hair. Females develop more typically, menstruating between ages 10 to 14; some can reproduce. Breasts are small to moderate in size.

Down syndrome confers a shorter-than-normal life expectancy. Most affected persons reach adulthood, but mortality increases after age 44.

Etiology and classification

Down syndrome has three forms, each resulting from a distinct pattern of chromosomal abnormality. About 92% to 95% of affected persons have trisomy 21, characterized by the presence of an extra chromosome. Why this occurs is unclear; however, the risk of trisomy 21 is significantly higher in children of mothers over age 35 or fathers over age 55. Trisomy 21 has a relatively low recurrence rate in families.

The translocation form of Down syndrome, seen in about 4% to 6% of cases, involves translocation (transfer) of chromosomes 15 and 21, or 15 and 22. This form commonly is hereditary and is not linked to advanced parental age.

Roughly 1% to 3% of cases of Down syndrome involve the mosaic form, in which some cells have the normal 46 chromosomes and others have an extra chromosome 21. The degree of impairment with the mosaic form depends on the percentage of cells with the abnormal chromosomal makeup.

Assessment

Amniocentesis or chorionic villi sampling can detect all forms of Down syndrome prenatally.

Clinical assessment of children with Down syndrome reveals characteristic physical features, including:
• a relatively flattened face
• eyes that slant upward and outward, with inner epicanthal folds
• small, low-set ears
• a small nose with a depressed nasal bridge
• a short neck with extra skin folds
• a large, protruding tongue
• short, stubby fingers and simian palmar creases
• widely spaced first and second toes, with a plantar crease between them.

Other findings include decreased muscle tone and lax, hyperextensible joints. Intellectual functioning ranges from low-normal to severely retarded; most children with Down syndrome show an intellect within the moderate range. Social skills seem advanced in relation to the child's mental age. Typically, the child enjoys being around people and behaves well.

Medical management

The child with Down syndrome requires supportive treatment. Physical anomalies, such as cardiac and GI defects, may be corrected surgically. Hearing function is evaluated and referrals are made to an ear, nose, and throat specialist, as needed. Otitis media is treated promptly to prevent hearing loss. Thyroid function also is evaluated.

Children who wish to engage in sports that cause neck stress, such as diving, soccer, football, and gymnastics, should be evaluated for atlantoaxial instability. If this skeletal deformity is found, such activities are contraindicated.

Many children with Down syndrome require referrals for speech therapy. If appropriate, they should be taught alternate forms of communication, such as sign language, until they develop verbal skills.

Nursing management

Primary nursing goals for children with Down syndrome and their families include promoting optimal development; preventing and managing such complications as frequent respiratory infections, feeding difficulties during infancy, constipation, and obesity; and supporting the family.

Begin parent teaching early in the child's development. To reduce the risk for respiratory infection, instruct parents to change the infant's position frequently and to use an infant seat to hold the child upright to improve respiratory expansion. Also teach them how to use a bulb syringe for nasal suctioning. Encourage them to use a cool-mist vaporizer and to ensure an adequate fluid intake to help loosen nasal secretions and keep the child's respiratory passages moist. Advise them to supplement feedings with additional water or juices, if needed.

The infant may have difficulty feeding because of hypotonia, nasal congestion, and a large, protruding tongue. Advise parents to suction the infant's nose if congestion occurs, and show them how to support the infant in an upright position for feeding. Demonstrate techniques to encourage the infant to take the entire nipple in the mouth.

Recommend that parents introduce solid foods with a spoon. To encourage the child to swallow, instruct them to place solid foods toward the back and side of the infant's mouth. Reassure them that tongue thrusting does not mean the child is refusing food. Because the infant with Down syndrome may become frustrated easily during feeding, suggest shorter, more frequent feedings.

Decreased gastric motility secondary to hypotonia may lead to constipation. To prevent constipation, instruct parents to provide sufficient fluids. For an infant, giving supplemental water and fruit juices may be appropriate. If the child can ingest solid foods, advise parents to provide dietary fiber, such as fresh fruits (pureed for the infant) and prune juice. Instruct parents to encourage the older child to drink at least 8 glasses of fluid daily, to eat bran cereal, and to exercise.

Closely monitor the child's weight. For the overweight child, implement nutritional counseling, restrict foods high in fat and sugar, and encourage exercise — preferably in an organized sports program.

Cerebral palsy

Cerebral palsy is a nonprogressive disorder characterized by varying degrees of impaired motor function and, in some cases, impaired cognitive function. Cerebral palsy is the most common permanent disability in children.

Etiology

Cerebral palsy is caused by brain damage or by a brain lesion present at or shortly after birth. Common causes include birth asphyxia (as from a difficult delivery) and hypoxic brain damage associated with respiratory distress syndrome. Less commonly, cerebral palsy results from neurologic injury secondary to metabolic disturbances, congenital infections, and central nervous system infections. The premature neonate is most vulnerable to cerebral palsy.

Classification

Cerebral palsy is classified according to the type of motor dysfunction. The three main forms are described below.

Spastic cerebral palsy, the most common form, is characterized by general hypotonia (reduced skeletal muscle tone) during infancy, possibly persisting for up to 1 year. Later, the child develops increased muscle tone accompanied by muscle weakness and toe-walking. Asymmetric crawling is an early sign of spastic cerebral palsy. Unilateral hand preference before age 3 also may suggest this form. Some children have impairment of all four extremities (quadriplegia), of only one extremity (monoplegia), of one side of the body (hemiplegia), or of both arms or both legs (diplegia).

Athetoid or dyskinetic cerebral palsy is characterized by abnormal involuntary movements (which increase with stress and are absent during sleep), athetosis (slow, involuntary, writhing movements of the tongue and extremities, including the fingers and toes, sometimes accompanied by facial grimacing), drooling, and dysarthria (poorly articulated speech). This form of cerebral palsy may affect expressive language skills severely.

Ataxic cerebral palsy is characterized by a widely spaced gait and coordination problems, especially in the upper extremities. Coordination tends to improve with age.

Some children have mixed cerebral palsy, exhibiting characteristics of both the spastic and athetoid (dyskinetic) forms. Typically, they have severe delays in motor and speech development.

Assessment

Cerebral palsy is diagnosed from neurologic findings and the patient's history. Because early signs and symptoms (such as feeding difficulty, hypotonicity or hypertonicity, and seizures) are nonspecific, diagnosis is hard to establish at birth. Older children show delayed gross motor development as well as abnormalities in motor performance, muscle tone, posture, and reflexes.

Persistence of the nonobligatory tonic neck reflex is an early sign of cerebral palsy. Normally, this reflex disappears by age 6 months; persistence beyond this age is considered abnormal. To elicit the reflex, position the infant supine, then turn the infant's head to one side and note the position of the extremities. The nonobligatory tonic neck reflex is present if extremities on the side toward which the head is turned extend and the opposite extremities flex.

Medical management

Goals of medical management include promoting locomotion, communication, and self-care skills. Braces may be prescribed to prevent or reduce deformity and to aid ambulation. However, young children may comply poorly with braces and may fare better by using mobility devices, such as scooters, to propel themselves along. Infant walkers are avoided because they delay motor development and may cause abnormal motor patterns.

The child with cerebral palsy may require surgery to improve muscle function, physical therapy to improve musculoskeletal functioning, and occupational therapy to aid adaptive functioning. Speech therapy may be beneficial for the child with poor articulation. Microcomputers with voice synthesizers may aid communication.

Medications have little effect on the spasticity associated with cerebral palsy. The child with seizures may receive anticonvulsant drugs.

Nursing management

Nursing goals for the child with cerebral palsy include:
• promoting a positive self-image in the child
• preventing injury
• providing rest and nutritional needs
• supporting the family.

To promote a positive self-image, encourage the child to maintain an attractive physical appearance, praise independent actions, and maximize the child's strengths. To prevent injuries, teach parents to modify the environment as appropriate. Suggest a helmet if the child frequently falls or bumps into walls.

Because of involuntary movements and the increased effort needed to carry out daily activities, the child with cerebral palsy expends tremendous amounts of energy. Therefore, encourage the child to rest frequently and to consume more calories.

STUDY ACTIVITIES   **Fill in the blank**

1. Mental retardation is associated with an IQ below _____.

2. Some children with Down syndrome must avoid activities that cause neck stress because they have _____.

3. The speech of a child with cerebral palsy may be hard to understand because of _____.

Short answer

4. What abnormal reflex may be found in a child with cerebral palsy?

_____

_____

5. How can locomotion be improved in a child with cerebral palsy?

_____

_____

_____

6. Why does the child with cerebral palsy have increased rest and nutritional requirements?

_____

_____

_____

Multiple choice

7. Which history finding suggests cerebral palsy?
   A. Perinatal history of a difficult delivery
   B. Maternal aunt who is mentally retarded
   C. Milk allergy
   D. Frequent respiratory infections

8. What is a major physical characteristic of the child with Down syndrome?
   A. Hypotonic musculature
   B. Tall stature
   C. Inflexible joints
   D. A prominent nasal bridge

9. Genetic counseling is most critical for parents of children with which form of Down syndrome?
   A. Trisomy 21
   B. Translocation
   C. Mosaic
   D. Mixed type

ANSWERS

Fill in the blank

1. 70

2. Atlantoaxial instability

3. Dysarthria

Short answer

4. A child with cerebral palsy may exhibit a persistent nonobligatory tonic neck reflex.

5. The child with cerebral palsy can use braces or a scooter to aid locomotion.

6. The child with cerebral palsy has increased rest and nutritional requirements because of the increased energy expended in carrying out activities of daily living and expended during involuntary movements.

Multiple choice

7. A. A difficult delivery is associated with birth asphyxia — a common cause of cerebral palsy. Hereditary factors, allergies, and respiratory infections are not linked with cerebral palsy.

8. A. Children with Down syndrome exhibit hypotonic musculature, short stature, hyperextensible joints, and an underdeveloped or depressed nasal bridge.

9. B. Most types of the translocation form of Down syndrome are inherited. The Trisomy 21 and mosaic forms are not inherited. Classification of Down syndrome does not include a mixed type.

CHAPTER 14

Child abuse and maltreatment

OBJECTIVES

After studying this chapter, the reader should be able to:

1. Discuss theories of child abuse and maltreatment.

2. Differentiate among the forms of child abuse and maltreatment: physical abuse, physical neglect, sexual abuse, emotional neglect, and psychological abuse.

3. Describe characteristics of physically abusive parents.

4. Identify physical and behavioral signs in victims of each form of child abuse and maltreatment.

5. Describe nursing documentation and reporting of suspected cases of child abuse and maltreatment.

6. Discuss the nurse's role in preventing child abuse and maltreatment.

7. Describe the causes, clinical manifestations, and management of nonorganic failure to thrive.

OVERVIEW OF CONCEPTS

Child abuse and maltreatment occur in all socioeconomic groups. The effects of these problems may appear not only in the child and family but also in society at large. Nurses play a crucial part in preventing and detecting child abuse as well as in managing the victim and the abuser.

This chapter begins by presenting a theoretical perspective on child abuse and maltreatment. It defines the various forms of child abuse and maltreatment. Then, the chapter explores the nurse's role in preventing, detecting, and managing these problems. The chapter concludes by discussing nonorganic failure to thrive.

Theoretical perspective

The Human Ecologic Model, developed by Garbarino in 1977, helps the nurse understand the complex problem of child abuse and maltreatment. The model also can be used to guide assessment and intervention strategies.

Garbarino's model proposes that child abuse results from an interaction of factors involving society, the family, the parent, the child, and stress. For example, in American society, violence is pervasive on television and in the movies; in these media, the violent person rarely is punished, and sometimes is rewarded, for violent behavior. To many, this conveys the impression that violence is an acceptable way to gain power over another person.

The family historically has been allowed to carry out its functions without interference. The parents are viewed as experts on rearing and controlling children, and punishment is considered appropriate in shaping a child's behavior — even when it injures the child physically.

Parental factors, such as immaturity, poor impulse control, and unrealistic expectations of children's behavior, contribute to the potential for child abuse and maltreatment. A child whom the parent perceives as difficult, different, or unwanted may provoke abusive parental behavior.

Taken in isolation, none of these factors alone is thought to cause child abuse or maltreatment. However, multiple factors may interact to result in abusive behavior by some parents and other caregivers during periods of environmental, family, or parental stress.

Defining child abuse

Although the judicial system determines the actual definitions of child abuse and neglect, American culture generally accepts the following definitions:
- Physical abuse — physical injury of a child under age 18 by a parent, legal guardian, or other adult
- Sexual abuse — sexual activity with a child under age 18 engaged in by a parent, legal guardian, or other adult
- Psychological abuse — emotional harassment of a child under age 18 by a parent, legal guardian, or other adult; emotional harassment includes belittling or degrading comments, frequent criticism, and name-calling
- Physical neglect — failure of the parent or legal guardian to provide adequate food, clothing, shelter, or education for a child under age 18, resulting in harm or the danger of harm to the child's physical condition
- Emotional neglect — failure of the parent or legal guardian to provide adequate nurturance, support, and love to a child under age 18, resulting in harm or the danger of harm to the child's emotional health.

Assessment

The nurse who can recognize risk factors for child abuse and maltreatment and detect characteristic signs in abusers and their victims can identify high-risk families and promptly initiate preventive and supportive care. After performing a thorough assessment to identify such families, the nurse makes the necessary referrals to agencies that provide preventive and supportive services. *Remember* — nurses are legally obligated to report all suspected cases of child abuse. Most often, nurses working in emergency departments, ambulatory care settings, and schools are involved in case-finding and reporting.

Regardless of the form of suspected child abuse or maltreatment, first assess the child for evidence of physical injury and note any behavioral signs of abuse. If findings suggest abuse, interview the child in a quiet, nonthreatening manner. To help accustom the child to the nurse, start with a casual discussion and play with the child, if appropriate. This helps to establish trust — a prerequisite to making the child feel safe enough to disclose abuse.

As appropriate, use play and art activities during the interview. For instance, the nurse may ask the child to act out what has happened. If trained in art therapy, the nurse may evaluate the child's drawings, which may reveal such problems as low self-esteem, dysfunctional family relationships, and sexual abuse.

Carefully document the nature of any physical injuries, behavioral characteristics, and the child's description of the alleged abuse.

Next, interview the parents. If the child sustained a physical injury, ask them to explain how the child was hurt. Note whether the explanation is consistent with the child's injury; a parent's inability to explain the injury, or inconsistency between the injury and the parent's explanation or the child's developmental age, is the strongest indicator of physical abuse. If the nurse suspects the parents harmed the child physically, assess their discipline practices. In all cases of abuse, assess the parent-child interaction style. Note parental characteristics that suggest an abusive nature (see below).

Physical abuse

Evaluate the parents or other caregivers for risk factors of and characteristics of abusive behaviors and traits. Also assess the child for physical and behavioral signs of abuse.

Characteristics of physically abusive parents

If the nurse suspects actual or potential physical abuse, evaluate the parents or other caregivers for the following:
• history of abuse or neglect as a child
• lack of support from friends, relatives, neighbors, or the community
• low self-esteem
• marital problems, including spouse abuse
• alcohol or substance abuse
• becoming a parent during adolescence
• lack of child-rearing skills
• irrational behavior
• poor impulse control
• use of corporal punishment
• unrealistic expectations of the child's needs and behavior, including the expectation that the child should fulfill the parent's emotional needs
• belief that the child is bad, evil, or different

• history of violent behavior directed at others or the environment (such as hitting walls or throwing furniture).

Also suspect abuse in families who change health care providers frequently, who delay or fail to seek health care for a child's injuries, or who seek treatment in various emergency department settings (commonly at night). Stress also predisposes a family to abuse. Assess for family stressors, such as unemployment, debt, and housing problems.

Physical signs of physical abuse
Suspect physical abuse if the parent cannot explain the child's physical injuries or if the injuries are inconsistent with the parent's explanation or the child's developmental age. (For types of injuries that may indicate child abuse, see *When to suspect physical abuse,* page 182.)

Behavioral signs of physical abuse
The child who has been abused physically may exhibit the following behavioral signs:
• wariness of parents and other adults
• aggression
• withdrawal
• reluctance to go home
• low self-esteem
• wearing clothing that hides injuries
• self-injurious behaviors, such as head-banging in a younger child or substance abuse in an older child
• history of running away from home
• history of suicide attempts.

Physical neglect
Physical neglect of a child can be just as damaging as physical abuse. The physically neglected child commonly appears listless, tired, unkempt, and dirty and is dressed inappropriately for the weather. The hair may be matted and the teeth discolored and stained. The child may be hungry frequently and may resort to stealing and hoarding food. When fed, the child eats quickly and may overeat to the point of becoming sick.

Physically neglected children may be unsupervised and left to fend for themselves for prolonged periods of time. They may be absent from school chronically, or may arrive for school early and leave late. Some exhibit developmental delays.

Some physically neglected children show such behavioral disturbances as destructive behavior. Others may be overly compliant and eager to please adults.

Sexual abuse
Identifying the victim of sexual abuse may be difficult because physical signs may be absent. Most victims are extremely reluctant to tell an adult about the abuse. Also, most sexual abusers are family members or close friends of the child's family. Shame, guilt, and fear of losing

When to suspect physical abuse

Suspect physical abuse if the child has any of the following injuries:
- Bruises or welts on the face, lips, mouth, neck, wrist, ankles, torso, back, buttocks, or thighs. (In contrast, accidental injuries usually occur over bony or prominent body parts, such as the forehead, nose, elbows, and knees.) The bruises or welts may be clustered over one part of the body. Welts may be shaped like the article used to inflict the injury, such as a belt buckle or an electrical cord.
- Injuries to both eyes or both cheeks. (Accidental injuries, in contrast, generally affect just one side of the face.)
- "Grab marks" on the arms or wrists
- Human bite marks, as evidenced by the characteristic tooth pattern on the skin
- Injuries in various stages of healing
- Lacerations or abrasions of the mouth, lips, gums, eyes, external genitalia, backs of arms, legs, or torso
- Cigarette burns on the soles of feet, palms, back, or buttocks
- Immersion burns caused by scalding water, suggested by doughnut-shaped burns on the buttocks and perineal area
- Rope burns on the arms, legs, neck, or torso
- Fractures of the skull, nose, or facial bones (may be multiple or spiral fractures)
- Dislocation of the shoulder or hip
- Patches of missing hair, caused by hair pulling
- Subdural hematoma caused by head injury
- Retinal hemorrhages caused by head injury
- Eye injuries

the family member or friend contribute to the child's difficulty in reporting the abuse. To compound the problem, the abuser may threaten to abandon, injure, or even kill the child if the abuse is reported.

Physical signs of sexual abuse

Suspect sexual abuse if the child has the following signs or symptoms:
- difficulty walking or sitting
- genital pain or itching
- bloody underclothes
- bruising or bleeding in the external genitalia, vagina, or rectum
- bruises in the soft and hard palate
- sexually transmitted diseases (vaginal or oral, especially in prepubescent girls)
- pain on urination
- frequent urinary tract infections
- foreign bodies in the vagina or rectum.

Behavioral signs of sexual abuse

The following behavioral signs may indicate sexual abuse in a child:
- social withdrawal
- lack of friends

- provocative sexual behavior, such as overly friendly behavior or rubbing up against people
- dislike of being touched, even in a casual manner
- inappropriate knowledge of sexual activities
- acting out of sexual activities with other children or dolls
- low self-esteem
- fearfulness
- history of suicide attempts
- history of running away from home.

Emotional neglect and psychological abuse
Assess both the parents and child for characteristic behaviors and traits.

Characteristics of the abuser
Certain characteristics in parents or other caregivers may suggest they are neglecting a child emotionally or abusing the child psychologically. For instance, the emotionally neglectful parent may seem indifferent to the child, not engaging in play or social activities with the child and showing no warmth toward or emotional investment in the child. The psychologically abusive parent may belittle or degrade the child (for example, calling the child lazy or stupid), criticize the child frequently, or state that the child is inadequate in some way.

Behavioral signs in the victim
The victim of emotional neglect or psychological abuse typically has low self-esteem and has trouble establishing emotional relationships with others. An emotionally neglected infant seems wary of adults, does not establish eye contact, and may not seek adults for comfort. Other signs of emotional neglect in infants include developmental delays and failure to thrive.

An older child who has been emotionally neglected or psychologically abused may engage in disruptive behavior, such as acting out in school. Such a child shows little empathy in play or social situations and does not seem attached to dolls or stuffed animals. The child does not seek out others when hurt or frustrated and may have frequent psychosomatic complaints.

Reaching a conclusion
After the child and family assessment and interview are completed, the nurse, physician, and, possibly, the social worker collaborate to determine the likelihood that abuse or maltreatment has taken place. If the assessment indicates a possibility of abuse or maltreatment, inform the parents that child protective services are being notified of the problem. Explain that the purpose of such notification is to strengthen the family and prevent further harm or injury to the child. *Important:* Always maintain a nonjudgmental attitude toward the parents.

Medical and nursing management

Dealing effectively with child abuse and maltreatment requires a multi-disciplinary effort. The nurse collaborates with physicians, social workers, psychologists, and teachers in preventing and managing the problem.

The child who has sustained significant physical injury may require hospitalization. Be sure to explain to the child the reason for the hospital admission, which may seem like punishment to the child or may make the child feel guilty for disrupting the family.

A child who does not require hospitalization but who may be in continued danger of abuse or maltreatment may be placed in temporary foster care until the family is evaluated fully. This child may feel at blame for removal from the family. To help the child understand the situation, explain in a nonjudgmental way that the child cannot go home with the parents because they cannot take care of the child right now.

A child who is considered at low risk for further abuse or maltreatment may be discharged to the home. Child protective services then conducts a complete child and family assessment.

All confirmed cases of child abuse must be referred to the judiciary system. Depending on the circumstances, the court may decide to terminate parental rights, place the child in temporary foster care while the family receives therapy, or allow the child to remain in the home with supportive services (such as home therapy aides, parental teaching, or therapeutic day care) in place.

Failure to thrive

Failure to thrive refers to abnormal slowing of growth and development in a child, resulting from conditions that interfere with normal metabolism, appetite, and activity.

Classification and etiology

Failure to thrive may be organic or nonorganic. Organic failure to thrive is caused by a pathologic condition, such as congenital heart disease. Nonorganic failure to thrive stems from psychosocial factors, such as a maladaptive parent-child interaction. For instance, the parents of a child with nonorganic failure to thrive may lack effective communication skills and be unable to support each other. Typically, the family is isolated, receiving little support from relatives or friends, and may be experiencing stress, such as from unemployment or work-related demands. The parents appear overwhelmed with the demands of child care. Although they may attempt to provide for the child's physical needs, they may do so in an unemotional way. Commonly, they cannot interpret infant behavior correctly and thus respond to the infant inappropriately. For instance, they may attempt to play with the infant when the infant is fussy and trying to sleep. Some parents seem overly anxious or depressed. The mother may report that the pregnancy and delivery were particularly difficult.

A poor match between infant and parent temperament contributes to nonorganic failure to thrive. For instance, an irritable, fussy infant and a tense, anxious parent will reinforce each other's behavior. The parent initially may be unable to calm the irritable infant; continuing to try without success, the parent becomes increasingly tense. The infant senses parental anxiety and responds with yet more crying. On the other hand, a parent who is depressed may pay too little attention to an easygoing, nondemanding infant.

Assessment

When assessing a child for failure to thrive regardless of its classification, stay alert for both physical and behavioral indicators.

Physical signs of failure to thrive

With an infant, use a growth chart to document growth patterns. Most infants grow consistently from month to month. For example, an infant whose birth weight was in the 50th percentile should continue to grow within close range of that percentile; plotting the infant's growth should yield a gentle, convex curve without sudden dips.

In an infant with failure to thrive, the growth pattern is inconsistent. Suspect failure to thrive in any infant whose weight is below the 5th percentile or whose growth slows suddenly. The infant with nonorganic failure to thrive also exhibits developmental delays, poor muscle tone, and decreased muscle mass. Poor abdominal muscle tone makes the abdomen appear distended.

Behavioral signs of failure to thrive

The behavior of the infant with nonorganic failure to thrive resembles that of an emotionally neglected infant. Assess for avoidance of eye contact, wariness of adults, and lack of discrimination between parents and other adults. In an older infant, note lack of stranger anxiety or separation anxiety, self-stimulating behavior (such as head-banging or rocking), and atypical affect (such as continual fussing or apathy).

Admission interview

If the child is admitted to the hospital, obtain information about the prenatal, perinatal, and postnatal history during the admission interview. Be sure to elicit specific information about the parents' perceptions about the child during the prenatal and postnatal periods.

Conduct a complete infant feeding and nutritional assessment. Observe the infant and parent (or other primary caregiver) during a feeding situation and a play situation. Note the infant's position during feeding, the parent's manner when feeding the infant, and any parent-infant interaction during feeding. During play, note the parent-infant interaction style, the parent's verbal interaction with the infant, the parent's responses to the infant's behavior, and the infant's responses to the parent's behavior. Also, perform a thorough developmental assessment of the child.

Medical management

The infant with failure to thrive may be hospitalized for observation and definitive diagnosis. Nonorganic failure to thrive may be diagnosed from weight gain in response to nurturing, an age-appropriate diet, and provision of adequate calories.

The infant may be discharged once weight gain patterns are established and signs of appropriate infant-parent interaction appear. Follow-up care is essential and includes close monitoring of weight gain patterns and achievement of developmental milestones.

Nursing management

Nursing goals for the child with failure to thrive include:
• providing an age-appropriate diet, with sufficient calories for growth
• promoting a nurturing environment
• supplying developmentally appropriate stimulation
• serving as a role model for adult-infant interactions
• providing parent support and teaching.

Initially, increase the child's caloric intake to promote weight gain, as prescribed. Feed the child in a quiet environment, without distractions. Hold the infant during a feeding and make eye contact. After the feeding, take the time to cuddle the infant. Document the amount of food ingested, urine and stool output, and the infant's behavioral responses during feeding. Weigh the infant daily and plot the results on a growth chart.

Provide developmentally appropriate activities. For visual stimulation, place brightly colored mobiles in the crib; for auditory stimulation, use a music box. Talk to the infant when providing physical care. Take the infant for walks in the hallway or to the playroom. If appropriate, schedule developmental stimulation sessions with the child life specialist or occupational therapist.

Most importantly, act as a role model for the parents. Remember that these parents must overcome problems in their relationship with the infant. By observing the nurse feeding and playing with the infant, the parents learn how to interact with their infant effectively. Point out infant cues, such as the need to burp or to sleep, to the parents. Be sure to use positive reinforcement, such as praise, for all appropriate parenting behavior. Document parenting behaviors and indicators of parent-infant attachment, such as eye contact, mutual smiling, and the infant searching for the parent.

A single nurse should be responsible for planning the infant's care. To promote consistency of care, the number of nurses providing care should be limited. Ideally, the infant should receive care from only one nurse per shift, and the same nurse should provide care on consecutive days. Nursing care activities should be consistent, with all nurses following the same routines each day.

After the child is discharged, provide the family with ongoing support and teaching, as appropriate, to help them maintain the gains made during hospitalization and provide a nurturing environment for the infant's physical and emotional development.

STUDY ACTIVITIES

Short answer

1. Define psychological abuse and emotional neglect.

_____

_____

_____

2. Explain why sexual abuse may be hard to confirm.

_____

_____

_____

3. Dale and Jeanne Santello bring Timmy, their 2-year-old son, to the emergency room at 10:00 p.m. They report that he "fell off the couch and hurt his head." The nurse suspects Timmy has been abused. How should the nurse proceed when assessing Timmy?

_____

_____

_____

Multiple choice

4. The nurse suspects that Jimmy, age 4, is being physically neglected. To best assess his nutritional status, the nurse should ask his parents which of the following questions?

A. "Has Jimmy always been so thin?"
B. "Is Jimmy a picky eater?"
C. "What did Jimmy eat for breakfast today?"
D. "Do you think Jimmy eats enough?"

5. Most adults who sexually abuse children are:

A. Strangers
B. Relatives or family friends
C. Homosexual
D. Psychotic

6. When caring for the hospitalized infant with nonorganic failure to thrive, the nursing staff should:

A. Maintain a consistent, structured environment.
B. Encourage the child to hold a bottle.
C. Keep the child on bed rest to preserve energy.
D. Rotate caregivers to provide stimulation.

ANSWERS **Short answer**

1. Psychological abuse is emotional harassment of a child under age 18 by a parent or other person legally responsible for the child's care. Emotional harassment includes belittling or degrading comments, frequent criticism, and name-calling. Emotional neglect refers to failure of the parent or legal guardian to provide adequate nurturance, support, and love to a child under age 18, resulting in harm or the danger of harm to the child's emotional health.

2. Sexual abuse may be hard to confirm because physical signs may be absent and the sexually abused child typically is extremely reluctant to report the abuse.

3. The nurse should observe Timmy and his parents, noting parent-child interaction styles and checking for behavioral signs of physical abuse in Timmy. Next, the nurse conducts a physical examination, focusing on Timmy's physical injuries, followed by a private interview with Timmy to elicit his account of the incident. Then, the nurse interviews Timmy's parents, noting whether their explanation is consistent with his injuries; assesses them for characteristics of abusiveness; and asks them about family stressors.

Multiple choice

4. C. The nurse should determine objectively the child's nutritional intake for the day. The other responses are subjective and thus are open to varying interpretations.

5. B. Most sexual abusers are relatives or friends of the child's family. Strangers, homosexuals, and psychotics rarely commit child sexual abuse.

6. A. Nurses caring for the infant with nonorganic failure to thrive should strive to maintain a consistent, structured environment. The infant should never be encouraged to hold the bottle, which reinforces a negative, uncaring feeding environment. The infant with failure to thrive should be exposed to social stimulation and need not conserve calories; therefore, bed rest is unnecessary. The number of caregivers should be minimized to ensure consistency in care.

CHAPTER 15

Illness concepts

OBJECTIVES
After studying this chapter, the reader should be able to:
  1. Describe the impact of acute illness and hospitalization on the child and family.
  2. Discuss the effects of chronic illness on the child and family.
  3. Identify coping strategies used by children and families to adapt to illness and hospitalization.
  4. Describe the reactions of family members to a child's life-threatening illness and impending death.
  5. Discuss the nurse's role in helping children and families cope with illness and hospitalization.

OVERVIEW OF CONCEPTS
This chapter explores the responses of the child and family to a child's illness, hospitalization, and impending death. It investigates such problems as separation anxiety, fear of an unfamiliar environment, uncertainty about expectations, and loss of control in the acutely ill child. Then, the chapter discusses the effects of chronic illness on the child and family. Next, it explores life-threatening illness in a child. It explains how a child's perception of death varies with age, and discusses the reactions of all family members to a child's impending death. The chapter highlights nursing strategies to help family members cope with a child's illness and death.

Responses to acute illness
An acutely ill child may need to be hospitalized, placing additional stress on the child and family. Common stressors in the hospitalized child include separation from family and friends, fear of harm or injury, fear of an unfamiliar environment, uncertainty about expectations, and loss of control. Children age 8 to 9 months also have stranger anxiety, which creates further stress for the child, parents, and nurse (the stranger). How these stressors manifest depends on the child's developmental age. Also, the child's adaptation to hospitalization depends on child's developmental stage.

Separation anxiety

In children age 8 months to 4 years, separation from the family is the primary stressor. Children in this age group do not understand the need for hospitalization or why they must be separated ("taken away") from their families. Consequently, they are most vulnerable to the negative effects of hospitalization. In younger infants, the disruption in routine caused by hospitalization seems to cause more stress than actual separation from the family. Between birth and age 5 months, the infant has not yet attached strongly to the primary caregiver. Stress resulting from a change in the caregiver or the number of caregivers and a change in the environment can be seen in altered sleeping, feeding, and elimination patterns. Infants age 5 to 7 months experience stranger anxiety, which is evidenced by the infant clinging to the parents and crying when approached by health care workers. Infants age 7 to 9 months experience separation anxiety, which is demonstrated as the infant cries when the parents leave and refuses to be comforted by others.

Nursing strategies

To help the child cope with separation, it is important that the health care facility and staff to adapt to the family's needs and the family adapt to the facility's rules and policies. Liberal visiting and rooming-in policies as well as shorter hospital stays can alleviate many of the long-term consequences of separation. Because continuity of care helps to relieve the infant's stress, the nursing staff should arrange for the same nurse to care for the infant during a single shift.

To relieve anxiety caused by disruption in routine, ask the parents about the child's feeding, sleeping, napping, and play routines; if possible, incorporate these routines into the plan of care.

Inform the parents (and child, if appropriate) of visiting and rooming-in policies at the time of admission. Encourage the parents to stay with an infant during hospitalization and to participate in the infant's feeding and play experiences. For an older child, encourage at least one family member to stay with the child, if possible. Urge parents to bring familiar objects from home.

However, be aware that even if a parent can stay with the child, separation anxiety is likely to arise when the parent leaves the unit for short periods. An infant or young child typically cries and clings to the parent when trying to leave; during the first separation, the child may cry loudly to try to bring the parent back. Explain to parents that this behavior is normal and indicates a healthy attachment to the parents. Mention that short separations will not harm the child.

Advise parents to tell the child in advance when they are leaving and to mention when they will return. Counsel them to be truthful with the child about the circumstances of separation; sneaking out of the room when the child is distracted or telling the child they are going to the gift shop when they actually are going home can have harmful effects. After parents leave, the nurse should stay with the child until the child calms down.

With prolonged separations from the family, a child may respond by withdrawing from the environment. The child who has experienced prolonged separations seems uninterested in the hospital environment and staff, may show no interest in food, and may spend more time sleeping. Crying diminishes, although it may begin anew when parents visit. Explain to parents that the child's crying during their visits indicates the desire to be with them. Help the family find ways to arrange for more regular visits. In the parents' absence, provide emotional support and spend extra time with the child. Diversional activities also may be helpful.

Children who require lengthy hospitalizations and experience prolonged separation from their families also may repress their need for their families. These children may seem happy, engaging in play (which may be superficial) and seeking attention from any adult present. Although they acknowledge their parents during visits, they do not seem distressed when the parents leave. Take care not to mistake this behavior as adaptive. These children still need their family's love and support but cannot express this need. If parents are distressed that the child seems disinterested, reassure them that with continued regular visits, the child will resume a normal relationship with them.

School-age children and particularly adolescents experience distress over separation from friends. Help the child find ways to stay connected with peers, such as through telephone calls, letters, and even videotapes. Depending on visiting policies, older school-age children and adolescents may visit their hospitalized friend.

Fear of harm or injury
Starting with the toddler period, children develop an increased awareness of their bodies. Injuries, however slight, cause marked anxiety. Young children fear irreparable harm from loss of body integrity. They may believe all their blood will run out after an injection or that their insides will fall out after an abdominal incision. Preschool-age children may have castration anxiety, fearing their genitals will be mutilated for some perceived wrongdoing. Toddlers and preschool-age children may believe that illness and treatment procedures are punishment for past misbehavior or "bad" thoughts. Adolescents fear mutilation, especially if undergoing surgery. Fear of death is common in older school-age children and adolescents.

Nursing strategies
To help the child cope with fear of harm or injury, explain the reason for all procedures. Encourage the child to ask questions and express feelings. Provide bandages, even for such minor "wounds" as needle sticks and injections. Inform the child that all incisions will be closed

tightly by the physician and will not open. (For more information on fear related to surgery, see Chapter 16, Management principles.)

Fear of an unfamiliar environment

Like many patients, the child perceives the hospital as a place filled with unfamiliar and potentially frightening people and equipment.

Nursing strategies

To help the child deal with related fears, encourage parents to arrange a preadmission orientation visit to the nursing unit and playroom. After admission, explain all equipment in simple terms. Let the child handle equipment used in procedures (except sharp objects, such as needles and scissors). Encourage parents to stay with the child as much as possible. As appropriate, use therapeutic play to help the child to express fears.

Uncertainty about expectations

Illness and hospitalization may necessitate restrictions on a child's behavior and activity. Young children are particularly threatened by activity restrictions. Older children, including adolescents, may be frustrated by restrictions on television watching or radio playing.

Nursing strategies

Avoid using restraints unless absolutely necessary for the child's safety. Explain any activity restriction, including the reason for the restriction. Because inconsistencies in expectations increase with multiple caregivers, limit the number of caregivers. If possible, provide the child with same-age roommates.

Reward behavior consistent with expectations. Avoid punishment for "breaking the rules". If the child misbehaves, review the expectations again. Help an older child identify strategies to make behavior less disruptive to others—for instance, by providing earphones for the television and radio.

Loss of control

Starting in later infancy and increasing during the toddler and preschool-age years, the child becomes capable of performing self-care, and gains self-esteem by doing so.

However, illness and hospitalization may make the child feel a loss of control. The sick child may become dependent on others for assistance in dressing, feeding, and ambulating. Such dependency and loss of control may cause anxiety and frustration. Intrusive procedures over which the child has little control also cause anxiety.

Nursing strategies

Anticipate that dependency and intrusive procedures will threaten the child's sense of well-being and control. To counter these effects, let the child participate as fully as possible in self-care activities. Give the child a sense of control by offering realistic choices.

Stress in family members

The families of children hospitalized with acute illness also experience stress. Common family responses include anxiety and guilt. Parents may feel anxious if they do not understand the child's diagnosis or treatment plan. Some may have fear regarding the child's prognosis; others may fear the child will experience harm or pain. Many parents feel they somehow are responsible for their child's illness, and suffer feelings of guilt.

Parents of an acutely ill, hospitalized child also may feel they have lost control of their parenting role and no longer are solely responsible for their child's well-being. Some become overprotective and try to do everything for their child.

Like parents, young siblings may feel responsible for the sick child's illness. They also may resent the attention the sick child receives, as well as the need to take on additional responsibilities because of changes in family routines and roles brought on by the hospitalization. For example, if a parent rooms-in with the sick child, other family members may have extra responsibilities at home. Siblings also may react with anger or jealousy. They may have behavioral problems, difficulty concentrating in school, or the desire to be alone.

Nursing strategies

To help the family cope, explain to the parents and siblings the reason for the child's hospitalization, the implications of the child's diagnosis, and the rationale for the treatment plan. Spend time with the family, and encourage them to discuss their feelings about the child's illness and hospitalization.

Also discuss changes in family routines brought on by the child's hospitalization, and explore family members' feelings about these changes. Identify family support systems, and enlist the aid of support personnel to help the family manage stress and changes related to the child's illness and hospitalization.

Encourage the parents to spend additional time with well siblings. If facility policy permits, encourage siblings to visit the sick child.

Urge parents to take part in the child's care and to participate in decisions about treatment options. Advise them to let the ill child participate in medical and nursing care as much as possible.

Nursing diagnoses

Depending on assessment data, nursing diagnoses for the hospitalized child and family may include those listed below.

For the child:
- *Anxiety related to separation from parents and an unfamiliar environment*
- *Fear related to medical procedures, the diagnosis, or the possibility of harm*
- *Anxiety related to uncertainty about expectations*

- *Anxiety related to loss of control*
- *Social isolation related to separation from peers*
- *Altered growth and development related to the disease process, hospitalization, and separation from peers.*

For the family:
- *Altered family processes related to role changes*
- *Ineffective family coping, compromised, related to anxiety and fear about the hospitalized child*
- *Powerlessness related to loss of control*
- *Altered parenting related to the perceived need to protect the child and feelings of guilt*

Responses to chronic illness

A chronic illness has one or more of the following characteristics:
- It endures over time.
- It is progressive.
- It leads to impaired physical or mental functioning.
- It requires long-term health-care supervision.

Some chronic illnesses, such as sickle cell anemia, are characterized by stable periods during which the child is managed as an outpatient, interrupted by exacerbations or crises necessitating acute-care intervention. Other chronic illnesses, such as bronchopulmonary dysplasia, require such extensive medical and nursing support that long-term hospitalization is necessary.

Children's responses

The response of a sick child to chronic illness depends on:
- the degree of disability involved
- amount of medical support required
- number of hospitalizations required
- effect on the child's activities and ability to perform self-care
- effect on the child's socialization, including school and outside activities
- the degree to which the illness impedes mastery of developmental tasks
- long-term implications of illness, including the possibility of death.

Parents' responses

Parents of a chronically ill child may experience considerable stress. Sources of stress include the potentially overwhelming medical expenses, role strain related to caring for the child, and decreased socialization opportunities related to the physical demands of caring for the sick child or inability to obtain satisfactory child care. They also may suffer marital strain from the overwhelming nature of caring for the child and decreased time spent with each other, as well as anxiety and fear about the possibility that the acute illness could become worse or their child's possible death.

To cope with the stress involved in caring for a chronically ill family member, the parents may need assistance in performing family developmental tasks. (For a complete discussion of family developmental tasks, see Chapter 2, Pediatric nursing concepts).

Siblings' responses

As with siblings of an acutely ill child, siblings of a chronically ill child may resent the sick child for taking more of the parents' time and attention or because they must become more independent and self-sufficient. Such resentment may lead to anger toward the sick child. Also, some siblings of disabled or disfigured children are ashamed of their sibling and may be reluctant to bring friends home or be seen in public with the sibling.

Nursing management

The nurse can use various strategies to help the child and family cope with chronic illness.

Strategies for the child

To help the sick child maintain as much independence as possible, teach the child to manage his or her own care. Expect the child to perform age-appropriate self-care tasks. Explore opportunities for the child to socialize with well peers. Encourage an older school-age child or adolescent to join a support group.

Help and encourage the child to discuss feelings about the illness. With an older child, discuss both short-term and long-term implications of the illness.

Strategies for parents

Discuss the short-term and long-term implications of the child's illness. Teach parents how to help the child master age-appropriate developmental tasks. (For details, see *How chronic illness affects a child's growth and development,* pages 196 and 197.)

If the parents need a respite from caring for the child, help them find and train qualified alternate caregivers. Encourage them to spend time alone together, to join a parents' support group, and to express their feelings about their child's illness.

Strategies for siblings

Explain the implications of the child's illness to the siblings. Encourage them to express their feelings about the illness and the family situation. Urge them to engage in social activities or sports outside the home.

Respect a sibling's reluctance to bring friends home. If a sibling is ashamed of the sick child, encourage the sibling to join a sibling support group to deal with these feelings.

To help siblings cope with their family situation, advise parents to keep family routines as consistent as possible. Explore realistic ways to include siblings in the care of the sick child—but urge parents to avoid making inappropriate demands on siblings. Help parents arrange for

How chronic illness affects a child's growth and development

Chronic illness in a child may hinder mastery of developmental tasks. This chart describes the effects of illness on the developmental tasks for each age group, and presents nursing interventions to help the sick child master these tasks.

AGE-GROUP AND DEVELOPMENTAL TASK	EFFECT OF ILLNESS ON DEVELOPMENTAL TASK	NURSING INTERVENTIONS
Infant (birth to 12 months): Trust vs. mistrust	• Frequent separations from parents, inconsistent care, and pain resulting from illness or procedures may interfere with establishment of trust. • For neurologically impaired infants, parents may have trouble interpreting infant cues and thus fail to meet infant's needs.	• Provide consistency of care during hospitalization. • Help parents interpret infant cues. • Encourage parents to room-in with infant. • Use appropriate pain relief measures during procedures.
Toddler (ages 12 to 36 months): Autonomy vs. shame	• Early in this period, the child gains independence and autonomy by exploring the environment. Illness or hospitalization may interfere with exploration and motor play. Overprotective parents may restrict child's exploration. Overindulgent parents may not set appropriate behavioral limits; without such limits, the child who oversteps boundaries may experience shame.	• Allow child to make simple choices when possible. • Help parents find ways for child to play independently. • Advise parents of importance of setting limits. Suggest appropriate disciplinary strategies.
Preschool child (ages 3 to 6 years): Initiative vs. self-doubt	• Child needs exposure to larger environment to try out new ideas and skills. Parental overprotection and lack of exposure (caused by frequent hospitalization, limitations on motor activity, or isolation) hinders this process. Consequently, child does not learn how to cope with larger environment, resulting in self-doubt.	• Encourage child to try new methods to overcome obstacles. • Let child perform as many self-care tasks as possible. • Help parents find ways to expose child to outside environment, such as in preschool or play group. • Discuss appropriate disciplinary strategies with parents.
School-age child (ages 7 to 12 years): Industry vs. inferiority	• Illness, frequent hospitalization, and school absences may jeopardize child's sense of industry. • Decreased opportunities to socialize with peers or sense of being different may cause feelings of inferiority.	• Let child perform as many self-care tasks as possible. • Help parents find ways to increase child's opportunities to socialize with peers, such as clubs, sports, or church groups. • Explain importance of normalization in school and home life. • Discuss age-appropriate disciplinary strategies with parents. • Help parents identify household tasks for which child can be responsible. • Urge parents to let child help make decisions about hairstyle and clothing.

How chronic illness affects a child's growth and development (continued)

AGE-GROUP AND DEVELOPMENTAL TASK	EFFECT OF ILLNESS ON DEVELOPMENTAL TASK	NURSING INTERVENTIONS
Adolescent (ages 13 to 18 years): Identity vs. role confusion	• Feelings of being "different" and decreased access to peer group may hinder child's identification with peer group. • Decreased social opportunities or disability may prevent child from developing peer relationships with members of the opposite sex. • Stress caused by illness may impede child's search for a vocation. • Illness may make child dependent on others.	• Allow child to be as independent as possible. • Explain to parents that child has same feelings and needs as healthy adolescents. • Explore with child and parents the child's choices after high school (such as college, vocational school, or independent living options). • To help parents "let the child go," urge them to establish a social life outside immediate family. • Explore with child and parents activities in which child can initiate friendships.

help with household tasks, if necessary, so that siblings' responsibilities are reasonable. To help parents meet siblings' emotional and developmental needs, encourage them to spend extra time with siblings.

Nursing diagnoses
Depending on assessment data, nursing diagnoses for the chronically ill child and family may include those listed below.
For the child:
• *Social isolation related to overprotective parents and decreased exposure to the community*
• *Altered growth and development related to overprotective parents and lack of exposure to the larger environment*
• *Altered growth and development related to the disease process, hospitalization, and separation from peers*
• *Body image disturbance related to feelings of being different*
• *Anxiety related to the uncertain prognosis*
• *Fear related to the uncertain prognosis*
For the family:
• *Social isolation related to the time spent caring for the sick child*
• *Altered family processes related to role changes*
• *Ineffective family coping, compromised, related to anxiety, fear, and uncertainty regarding the child's illness*
• *Altered parenting related to perceived helplessness of the sick child and feelings of guilt*
• *Impaired home maintenance management related to parental knowledge deficit regarding care of the child.*

Responses to life-threatening illness

Traumatic injury, cancer, and cardiovascular disease account for the majority of deaths from disease in American children. The meaning of death and dying to children and their families depends on several factors.

How children view death

A child's understanding of death depends on the level of cognitive development. Obviously, assessing the meaning of death for an infant is extremely difficult because of language limitations. Based on their cognitive abilities, it is possible that infants have no concept of death. Toddlers also do not have a concept of death; they can only think about events in terms of their own frame of reference—living. They do, however, react to loss and separation. Toddlers and preschool-age children do not view death as permanent, seeing it instead as a temporary separation or as "going to sleep." When told that someone has died, a toddler or preschool-age child may ask when the dead person is coming back, and may express the desire to see the person as if nothing has happened. The child also may refuse to remove the dead person's belongings. Young children who equate death with going to sleep may fear being alone or going to bed after a loved one dies. Also, toddlers and preschool-age children may believe they somehow caused the dead person to "go away."

School-age children begin to view death as permanent but may fantasize about the dead person returning to life. Young school-age children may believe that only older people die and that they themselves somehow are protected from death. Because of a limited coping ability, the school-age child may respond to death by making light of the situation—behavior that should not be confused with lack of feeling. The school-age child also takes great interest in post-death rituals and services and may ask questions about what happens to the body after death.

Older school-age children and adolescents, who have acquired formal operations skills, understand that death is permanent and can occur at any age. They also begin to associate internal disease processes with death. Adolescent responses to the death of a loved one vary greatly. Extreme sadness, anger, withdrawal, and apparent unconcern are the most common ones.

Stages of dying

According to Kübler-Ross (1965), older school-age children, adolescents, and adults who are confronted with their anticipated death progress through a series of stages—denial, anger, bargaining, depression, and acceptance. The nurse can use Kübler-Ross's framework to help assess the responses of an older child or adult to impending death. However, be aware that not all people progress through all the stages.

Denial

This stage commonly begins at the time the patient is told the diagnosis. A patient's typical response to a grim diagnosis is "This couldn't possibly be happening to me. There must be some mistake." A person using denial as a coping mechanism may not really hear what the health care professional is saying, and may ask the same questions over and over.

Complete denial may be maladaptive because it may delay treatment. However, partial denial—accepting the fact that the person is ill but denying that the illness is serious—may be adaptive, because it permits the ill person to maintain hope. The length of time spent in denial varies from person to person.

Nursing strategies. During this stage, provide clear, simple explanations of the diagnosis and treatment plan. Respond to questions with simple, factual information. Listen actively to the patient, and support the patient by remaining with the patient. Do not try to force the patient out of denial. Instead, recognize this response as a temporary stage during which the patient needs support and understanding.

Anger

During this stage, the patient realizes the seriousness of the diagnosis. Attempting to make sense of the situation, the patient wonders, "Why me?" Trying to assign blame for the illness, the patient may become angry with self or others. The patient also may be angry about major lifestyle changes brought on by the illness, such as activity restrictions or frequent visits to the physician. A family member may feel anger because of the need to take on responsibilities the patient can no longer carry out. Many dying patients direct anger at health care professionals.

Nursing strategies. Accept the patient's anger as a normal response, and do not take it personally. Acknowledge the patient's anger without assigning blame or causing guilt.

Try to devise acceptable alternatives to the lifestyle changes caused by the illness. Listen actively to the patient, and support the patient and family by spending time with them.

Bargaining

During this stage, the patient tries to "make a deal" with God or another being perceived to have power. The patient may promise to "be a better person" in return for a special favor, such as a visit home, the ability to return to school or work, or a cure from the illness. When such agreements between the patient and God fail, the patient's religious beliefs may be threatened seriously.

Nursing strategies. Use active listening to determine if the patient is bargaining. Ask the patient "If you could do one more thing, what would it be?" The answer often will reveal a hidden desire. Also, attempt to understand the patient's symbols, for example, the wish for another trip home, drawings, dreams.

Depression

A patient who realizes that bargaining has little or no effect on the illness may become depressed and feel sad about losses brought on by the illness, such as the accustomed lifestyle, school or work routine, social contacts, or self-care ability. The patient also may feel profound sadness about the anticipated loss of everything and everyone of importance. Some patients also respond by withdrawing.

Nursing strategies. Work with the patient to find substitutes for losses. For example, arrange for school work to be brought to the hospital or the patient's home, or suggest the parents negotiate with the school to have the patient attend classes for several hours a day.

The depressed or withdrawn patient needs support to work through feelings of loss. Most patients receive support from close family members. Recognize this need, and arrange opportunities for extended family contact. Also, provide emotional support to the child and family by spending time with them.

Acceptance

During this stage, the patient comes to terms with anticipated death and seems to be at peace with the self and the world. Some patients talk freely about happier times in the past; such reminiscing may help them put their lives in perspective. Other patients simply say they are ready to die.

Nursing strategies. During this stage, listen actively and support the patient by spending time with him or her.

Parents' responses

Parental responses to the impending death of a child resemble those of the dying child. After hearing the diagnosis, parents initially may respond with shock and denial. Once they accept the reality of the diagnosis, they may feel anxious, hostile, angry, and guilty. They also may go through a bargaining stage before finally accepting their child's death as inevitable.

Guilt feelings are particularly common. Many parents feel they are responsible somehow for their child's illness. They wonder if they missed early signs of illness, which may have been treatable if reported sooner. Guilt may contribute to parental overindulgence toward the sick child. Guilty, overindulgent parents have trouble setting behavioral limits for the child or following through with disciplinary strategies.

Siblings' responses

Some of the responses seen in parents may occur in older siblings of a terminally ill child. However, siblings also may react with crying, hyperactivity, excessive talking, or withdrawal. Some have nightmares, enuresis, somatic complaints (such as stomachache and headache), and problems in school. Some fear that they themselves may die. These responses seem to be linked to the stressors associated with a sibling's illness— separation from parents (including loss of parents' attention), disruptions in family routines, and role changes.

Nursing management

Pay attention to the language children use to convey their thoughts and emotions. Assist the child in expressing how he or she feels. Offer support and guidance to the child and family.

Anticipate shock and denial when parents first hear the child's diagnosis. Take the parents to a private place to recover from the news. Provide emotional support, and answer any questions they have about the diagnosis or treatment plan.

If parents feel guilty and have trouble disciplining the child, recognize and acknowledge their feelings and behavior as normal. If they need help understanding their behavior, explain that nothing they did, or failed to do, contributed to the seriousness of their child's illness. Also explain the importance of maintaining a sense of normality in the child's life, including continuing with pre-illness behavioral expectations.

Help parents and siblings understand the source of their feelings. Explain to parents that healthy siblings continue to need their presence and support. Help parents find ways to spend time with healthy siblings.

Determine if the family needs assistance with housekeeping or child care so that older siblings need not assume these burdens. Encourage parents to inform siblings of the child's prognosis and to let siblings visit the child in the hospital.

During the child's final days, parents may need help in finding ways to comfort their dying child. Advise them that their simple presence is most important to the child and that conversation is not necessary.

Grief responses

According to Lindemann (1944), after the death of a loved one, a person may have the following responses:

• physical sensations—tightness in the throat, muscle weakness, shortness of breath, or an "empty" feeling
• preoccupation with the deceased—the perception that the dead person is present (such as reports of hearing or seeing the dead person or imagining the person is near), feelings of isolation, or a fear of "losing my mind"
• guilt—a belief that the person is responsible for the loved one's death
• hostile feelings—anger, irritability, inability to show warmth or love toward others, or withdrawal
• loss of usual behavior patterns—restlessness, purposeless movement, or inability to concentrate or to start or complete the task at hand
• adopting the behavior of the dead person.

Lindemann believed these grief responses last 4 to 6 weeks. However, more recent research suggests that the grieving process takes much longer. Glick, Weiss, and Parkes (1974) described three phases of grief. These phases may not occur in sequence and may recur at any time. *Phase one* starts at the time of death and lasts for several weeks after burial. Common feelings during this phase include numbness, emptiness, disbelief, and profound sadness.

Phase two begins several weeks after the funeral and lasts approximately 1 year. During the early part of this phase, family members may be preoccupied with reviewing the cause of the loved one's illness, the appropriateness of the treatment plan, and the cause of death. They may experience intense yearning for the dead person. After a few months, family members start to reorganize and adjust to life without the loved one. New family goals and responsibilities are negotiated and established.

Phase three begins during the second year after the death. Family members start to resume typical social and work functions. They may feel sad and lonely occasionally, but these feelings are not incapacitating.

Nursing strategies

The nurse who works with grieving families must recognize that although most people experience some of the grief responses described above, grief is a highly individualized process. To help family members cope with the death of a child, use the following interventions:

- Encourage all family members to participate in burial or cremation rituals.
- Listen actively.
- Help the family understand the source of any guilt, hostility, or anger they feel.
- Assure the family that their distress will subside gradually, but advise them that full recovery takes time.
- Identify the family's physical and emotional support systems, such as relatives and clergy. Physical support, such as food preparation and cleaning, is most critical during the first few weeks after the death. For emotional support, suggest parents and siblings join formal support groups, as appropriate.
- Assist in the reminiscing process. For example, talk about what the child liked to do.

STUDY ACTIVITIES   **Short answer**

1. Identify at least three stressors that hospitalized children experience.

_____

_____

_____

2. List at least four stressors that parents of a chronically ill child experience.

_____

_____

_____

3. How does a typical 3-year-old child view death?

_____

_____

_____

4. Explain why denial may be an adaptive coping response for a person with a life-threatening illness.

_____

_____

_____

5. David, age 7, has a chronic illness. To help his siblings cope with their feelings about his illness, the nurse formulates the following nursing diagnosis: _Ineffective family coping, compromised, related to anger and resentment toward the sick brother._ The expected outcomes are that David's siblings will express anger in an acceptable way; will discuss their feelings of anger and resentment; will verbalize an understanding of their anger and resentment; and will exhibit a decrease in anger and resentment over time. Identify four nursing interventions that would help achieve these outcomes.

_____

_____

_____

Multiple choice
6. Which response by the parents of a chronically ill child may indicate feelings of guilt about the child's illness?
- **A.** Sadness
- **B.** Anger
- **C.** Overindulgence
- **D.** Shock

7. Which child is most likely to believe that illness is a punishment for past misdeeds?

    A. Infant
    B. Preschool-age child
    C. School-age child
    D. Adolescent

8. A chronically ill school-age child is especially vulnerable to which stressor?

    A. Mutilation anxiety
    B. Anticipatory grief
    C. Anxiety over school absences
    D. Fear of hospital procedures

9. Susan, age 12, is near death from respiratory failure secondary to cystic fibrosis. Her parents ask the nurse what they can do to help Susan at this time. What would be the nurse's best response?

    A. "Sit quietly with Susan."
    B. "Bring Susan's favorite toy."
    C. "Read to Susan."
    D. "Ask Susan if she would like her friends to visit."

10. Which nursing intervention is most important for a hospitalized 3-month-old infant?

    A. Ask the parents about special routines at home.
    B. Encourage the infant's siblings to visit.
    C. Assign another infant as a roommate.
    D. Encourage the parents to leave when the infant cries.

11. For the hospitalized adolescent, which of the following is a major stressor?

    A. Anxiety related to separation from parents
    B. Fear of the unknown
    C. Fear of an altered body image
    D. Anger related to activity restrictions

ANSWERS **Short answer**

1. Stressors in hospitalized children include separation from family and friends, fear of harm or injury, fear of an unfamiliar environment, uncertainty about expectations, and loss of control.

2. Stressors in such parents include potentially overwhelming medical expenses, role strain related to caring for the child, decreased socialization opportunities related to the physical demands of caring for the sick child or inability to obtain satisfactory child care, marital strain from the overwhelming nature of caring for the sick child and decreased time spent with each other, and anxiety and fear about the possibility that acute illness becomes worse or their child's possible death.

3. A toddler typically views death as a temporary separation or as "going to sleep", and may feel responsible for causing the dead person to "go away."

4. Denial may be adaptive because it allows the sick person to maintain hope.

5. Encourage David's siblings to express their feelings about his illness. Encourage David's parents to keep family routines as consistent as possible. Encourage the siblings to participate in a support group. Help David's parents meet the sibling's emotional and developmental needs and advise them to spend additional time with siblings.

Multiple choice

6. C. Parents who feel guilty about a child's illness may overindulge the child. Sadness, anger, and shock are common in parents of chronically ill children, but are not linked specifically to feelings of guilt.

7. B. Preschool-age children are most likely to view illness as punishment for past misdeeds.

8. C. The developmental task of the school-age child is to become industrious, such as by mastering school-related activities. Therefore, school absences are particularly stressful for this child. Mutilation anxiety is more common in adolescents. Anticipatory grief is rare in a school-age child. Fear of hospital procedures is most common in preschool-age children.

9. A. The parents' presence shows their support for the child (being available to the child, such as by sitting quietly); this is most important to the dying child.

10. A. A young infant is particularly affected by the disruption in routines caused by separation from family. Therefore, the nurse should ask about special routines at home.

11. C. Fear of an altered body image is a major stressor for adolescents, who are concerned about their physical appearance and may fear disfigurement resulting from procedures and treatments. Separation anxiety rarely is a major stressor in this age group. Adolescents may fear the unknown, but will ask questions if they want information. Activity restrictions are most stressful for toddlers.

CHAPTER 16

Management principles

OBJECTIVES After studying this chapter, the reader should be able to:
1. Discuss the transport of fluid and electrolytes in the body.
2. Describe the mechanisms that regulate the body's fluid, electrolyte, and acid-base balances.
3. Identify signs and symptoms of fluid, electrolyte, and acid-base disturbances.
4. Discuss nursing management for the child with a fluid, electrolyte, or acid-base imbalance.
5. Describe the nurse's role in assessing pain in children.
6. Identify general guidelines for managing pain in children.
7. Discuss pharmacologic and nonpharmacologic pain management methods for children.
8. Describe preoperative and postoperative nursing care for a child and family.

OVERVIEW OF CONCEPTS This chapter explores management principles for children with fluid, electrolyte, and acid-base disturbances; children who are in pain; and children who undergo surgery. For each of these broad topics, it presents general principles and details clinical assessment and management. The chapter highlights the nurse's role in caring for children with fluid, electrolyte, and acid-base imbalances; relieving pain; and providing preoperative and postoperative care.

Fluid, electrolyte, and acid-base imbalances Many pediatric illnesses place a child at risk for fluid, electrolyte, and acid-base imbalances. Children under age 2 are more susceptible than older children to such imbalances.

Fluids
The body needs fluid to excrete solutes produced by cellular metabolism, to maintain homeostasis, and to dispel the heat produced by metabolic activity. Body fluids are replenished through oral or intravenous (I.V.) intake. The body regulates fluid balance so that imbalances do not occur under normal conditions—despite fluctuations in dietary intake and metabolism.

Body fluids exist both within cells (intracellular fluid [ICF]) and outside cells (extracellular fluid [ECF]). ECF fall into three major categories:
• intravascular fluids—fluids in the plasma
• extravascular or interstitial fluids—fluids in spaces between cells
• other fluids—cerebrospinal fluid, ocular fluid, gastrointestinal (GI) fluid, and lymphatic fluid.
Normally, fluid is lost through the kidneys (0.5 to 2 ml/kg/hour), through the skin via sweat and evaporation (which yield losses of variable amounts), through the lungs (300 to 400 ml/24 hour), and through the GI tract (100 to 200 ml/24 hour).

Fluid transport

Within the body, water moves by osmosis. In osmosis, a passive transport process, a solvent (in the body, this is water), moves through a semipermeable membrane from an area of lower solute concentration to one of higher solute concentration. Water movement and distribution depend on the concentration of solute within the compartment. Obeying the same principles, water moves from the intravascular to the intracellular spaces.

Water and solute movement occur continuously between the vascular and interstitial fluid compartments. Movement of water depends on hydrostatic and colloid osmotic pressures in the capillaries. The active pumping of the heart creates a pressure gradient (hydrostatic pressure) between the arterial bed and venous bed that favors water movement out of the arterial side of the capillary and into the tissues. Once the fluid moves into the tissues, another pressure gradient is established to move fluid back into the venous bed. The colloid osmotic pressure (also called oncotic pressure) is determined by the concentration of protein molecules in the blood. This pressure causes water to move from the interstitial spaces into the venous bed.

Oncotic pressure, determined by serum osmolarity, exerts a force within vascular spaces that counteracts osmosis. Plasma proteins, such as albumin, primarily are responsible for oncotic pressure. (Sodium, an extracellular electrolyte, also plays a role in serum osmolarity; I.V. fluids that have a high osmolarity—such as Ringer's lactated solution and dextrose 10% in water—increase oncotic pressure within the vascular space.) Under normal conditions (when the serum protein level is normal), oncotic pressure keeps water within the vascular spaces. However, if the serum protein level falls (such as in nephrotic syndrome or severe malnutrition), decreased oncotic pressure causes water to move from the intravascular to the extravascular spaces.

Water also moves from an area of higher hydrostatic pressure (fluid pressure within the vascular spaces) to an area of lower hydrostatic pressure. Therefore, hypervolemia (characterized by high hydrostatic pressure) causes water to shift from the vascular to the extravascular spaces.

Fluid regulation

Various natural mechanisms maintain the body's fluid balance:

- Thirst stimulates fluid ingestion.
- The kidneys regulate ECF volume by selectively retaining and excreting body fluids.
- The hypothalamus produces antidiuretic hormone (ADH), which is stored in the posterior pituitary gland. ADH maintains the osmotic pressure of the cells by controlling renal retention and excretion of water. When osmotic pressure is high—that is, when the osmotic pressure of ECF exceeds that of ICF (as in hypernatremia)—ADH is secreted, and the kidneys respond by retaining water. When osmotic pressure is low—that is, when the osmotic pressure of ICF exceeds that of ECF (as in hyponatremia)—ADH is *not* secreted, and the kidneys respond by excreting water.
- Aldosterone, a hormone produced by the adrenal cortex, causes the kidneys to retain sodium and water. Sodium retention, in turn, induces potassium excretion. Both aldosterone and ADH play a role in controlling blood volume. In hypovolemia (fluid volume deficit), ADH and aldosterone are secreted. In response to ADH secretion, the kidneys retain water; in response to aldosterone secretion, the kidneys retain sodium and water and excrete potassium. In hypervolemia (fluid volume excess), ADH and aldosterone secretion is inhibited. Responding to the lack of ADH, the kidneys excrete water; responding to the lack of aldosterone, the kidneys excrete sodium and water.

Electrolytes

Electrolytes exist within the ICF and ECF compartments. The major intracellular electrolytes are potassium, phosphorus, and magnesium. The major extracellular electrolytes are sodium, chloride, and calcium. Hydrogen and bicarbonate also are extracellular electrolytes.

Electrolytes typically are replenished by oral intake of food high in the particular electrolyte. The body regulates electrolytes to avoid imbalances under normal conditions. (For more information on electrolytes and their functions, see *Major electrolytes.*)

Electrolyte transport

Electrolytes move from the intracellular spaces to the extracellular spaces by means of diffusion and active transport. Their size and electrical charge prevent them from moving as readily as water.

Some electrolytes, such as sodium and potassium, are transported by means of the concentration gradient, moving from an area of higher concentration to one of lower concentration. However, sodium, potassium, calcium, iron, hydrogen, and chloride also move by active transport. During active transport, physiologic pumps actively move substances *against* the gradient; that is, from lower- to higher-concentration areas. For example, the sodium-potassium pump moves sodium out of cells and into the intravascular spaces, and moves potassium out of the intravascular spaces into cells.

Major electrolytes

This chart describes the primary functions and normal serum ranges for the body's major electrolytes.

ELECTROLYTE	PRIMARY FUNCTIONS	NORMAL SERUM RANGE
Sodium (an extracellular cation)	• Acid-base regulation • Maintenance of serum osmolality • Muscle and nerve irritability	135 to 145 mEq/liter
Chloride (an extracellular anion)	• Acid-base regulation	98 to 106 mEq/liter
Bicarbonate (an extracellular anion)	• Acid-base regulation	22 to 28 mEq/liter
Hydrogen (an extracellular cation)	• Acid-base regulation	Cannot be measured directly; indirectly measured by pH (normal value ranges from 7.35 to 7.45)
Calcium (an extracellular cation)	• Bone and tooth development • Muscle contraction and relaxation • Acid-base regulation • Cardiac function • Assistance in blood clotting	8.8 to 10.8 mg/dl
Potassium (an intracellular cation)	• Cellular metabolism • Nerve impulse conduction • Muscle contraction • Acid-base regulation	3.5 to 5.5 mEq/liter
Phosphorus (an intracellular anion)	• Bone and tooth development • Acid-base regulation • Cell division	3.0 to 4.5 mg/dl in children ages 5 and over; 3.5 to 6.8 mg/dl in children under age 5
Magnesium (an intracellular cation)	• Neurologic function • Muscle contraction	1.5 to 2.0 mEq/liter

Electrolyte regulation

Various mechanisms regulate the body's electrolyte balance:
• The kidneys regulate chloride, sodium, potassium, and magnesium levels in ECF by selectively retaining needed electrolytes and excreting others.
• The kidneys also regulate the pH of ECF by retaining or excreting hydrogen.
• Parathyroid hormone (PTH), secreted by the parathyroid gland, regulates calcium and phosphorus balance. PTH influences bone resorp-

tion of calcium, calcium absorption from the intestines, and calcium reabsorption and phosphorus excretion from the renal tubules.

Acid-base balance

The chemical reactions of the body rely on a delicate balance between acids and bases. Even a slight imbalance can threaten a person's well-being.

The lungs, under control of the brain's medulla oblongata, help regulate acid-base balance. For example, they govern hydrogen ion concentration (pH) by controlling carbon dioxide (CO_2) levels within ECF. In metabolic alkalosis, the lungs respond by initiating hypoventilation, which increases CO_2 retention. In metabolic acidosis, the lungs respond by initiating hyperventilation, which reduces CO_2 retention. Blood-buffering systems, which involve chemical buffers in the blood, also play a role in acid-base balance. These buffer systems act quickly to temporarily take up or release extra hydrogen ions, thereby preventing rapid, drastic changes in pH. The three major buffer systems in the body are the carbonic-bicarbonate system, the phosphate system, and the protein buffer system.

Medical and nursing management

For information on medical and nursing measures for pediatric patients with selected fluid, electrolyte, and acid-base imbalances, see *Managing fluid, electrolyte, and acid-base imbalances,* pages 211 to 214.

Pain management

Regardless of the medical diagnosis, all hospitalized children are likely to experience some pain. Needle sticks, I.V. line insertion, dressing changes, and transfer techniques are examples of procedures that cause at least transient discomfort. Children undergoing surgery may experience acute pain of longer duration. Those with certain chronic diseases, such as cancer and juvenile rheumatoid arthritis, typically have chronic pain.

Assessing pain in children

Components of the pediatric pain assessment include a pain experience history, subjective data on pain characteristics, and objective data on behavioral indicators of pain. Knowledge about previous pain that the child has experienced and the strategies that relieved the pain successfully are important factors to consider when assessing a child's pain.

Preferably, obtain a pain experience history during the admission interview, when the child is more likely to be free of pain. Be sure to obtain both subjective and objective data when planning nursing care. Evaluate the child's pain level and the effectiveness of management strategies at regular intervals. Self-reporting methods for pain assessment have been designed for children as young as age 3 and have proven accurate in measuring pain intensity.

(Text continues on page 214.)

Managing fluid, electrolyte, and acid-base imbalances

This chart presents the causes, assessment findings, medical management, and nursing interventions for major fluid, electrolyte, and acid-base imbalances.

IMBALANCE	CAUSE	SIGNS AND SYMPTOMS	LABORATORY FINDINGS	TREATMENT	NURSING INTERVENTIONS
FLUID IMBALANCES					
Fluid volume deficit (hypovolemia, dehydration)	Excessive fluid loss (burns, fever, vomiting, diarrhea, nasogastric [NG] tube suctioning, diabetes insipidus, fistulas, inappropriate antidiuretic hormone secretion, or hemorrhage)	• Thirst • Dry skin and mucous membranes • Poor skin turgor • Poor perfusion (as indicated by a weak pulse and slow capillary refill) • Tachycardia • Decreased blood pressure • Weight loss • Decreased urine output	• Urine specific gravity above 1.025 • Hematocrit above 45% • Serum osmolality above 290 mOsm/kg	• Fluid replacement.	• Carefully measure and record patient's fluid intake and output. • Continuously assess the patient's hydration status.
Intravascular fluid volume excess	• Excessive fluid intake (hypertonic fluid overload) • Inadequate fluid output (renal disease or renal failure)	• Bounding pulses • Tachycardia • Weight gain • Elevated blood pressure	• Urine specific gravity below 1.005 • Hematocrit below 35% • Serum osmolality below 270 mOsm/kg	• Fluid restriction. • Diuretic therapy.	• Carefully measure and record patient's fluid intake and output. • Continuously assess the patient's hydration status.
Extravascular fluid volume excess	• Increased capillary hydrostatic pressure (congestive heart failure) • Decreased plasma oncotic pressure (nephrotic syndrome) • Reduced oncotic pressure (severe malnutrition)	• Edema • Weight gain	• Urine specific gravity from 1.015 to 1.022 • Hematocrit from 42% to 45% • Serum osmolality from 270 to 290 mOsm/kg	• Fluid restriction. • Diuretic therapy. • For nephrotic syndrome in children with persistent edema: administration of hyperosmolar fluids (such as albumin) to move water from extravascular to intravascular spaces, followed by diuretic therapy.	• Carefully measure and record patient's fluid intake and output. • Continuously assess the patient for edema. • Monitor the patient's weight daily.
ELECTROLYTE IMBALANCES					
Sodium depletion (hyponatremia)	• Increased sodium loss (sweating associated with cystic fibrosis; vomiting;	• Thirst • Same as for fluid volume deficit because sodium loss	• Serum sodium level below 135 mEq/liter • Serum sodi-	• For severe hyponatremia: rapid I.V. fluid and sodium replacement to raise	• Carefully measure and record patient's fluid intake and output.

(continued)

Managing fluid, electrolyte, and acid-base imbalances *(continued)*

IMBALANCE	CAUSE	SIGNS AND SYMPTOMS	LABORATORY FINDINGS	TREATMENT	NURSING INTERVENTIONS
ELECTROLYTE IMBALANCES *(continued)*					
Sodium depletion (hyponatremia) *(continued)*	diarrhea; NG tube drainage; or fistulas)	accompanies fluid loss • Lethargy • Apathy • Seizures (in severe hyponatremia)	um level below 120 mEq/liter in severe hypo-natremia	serum sodium level to 120 mEq/liter, followed by slower replacement (over 24 to 36 hours) to raise level to 135 mEq/liter.	• For a patient with severe hyponatremia, institute these seizure precautions: raise side rails of the bed and keep oxygen and suctioning equipment nearby.
Sodium excess (hypernatremia)	• Increased sodium intake (inappropriate dietary salt intake) • Decreased sodium loss (diarrhea in which water losses exceed sodium losses)	• Thirst • Dry, sticky mucous membranes • Decreased urine output • Disorientation or confusion • Seizures (in severe hypernatremia or sudden serum sodium decrease)	• Serum sodium level above 145 mEq/liter	• Slow fluid replacement (over 24 to 36 hours) with isotonic fluid, such as dextrose 5% in water, 0.9% sodium chloride (normal saline) solution, or Ringer's lactated solution.	• Carefully measure and record patient's fluid intake and output. • Continuously assess the patient's hydration status. • Institute seizure precautions.
Potassium excess (hyperkalemia)	• Increased potassium intake (inappropriate I.V. potassium administration) • Inadequate potassium excretion (renal disease or renal failure) • Cellular damage causing potassium to move from intracellular to extracellular spaces (crushing injury or burns) • High potassium concentration relative to water within intravascular spaces (severe dehydration) • Movement of potassium from intracellular to extracellular spaces in exchange for hydrogen (acidosis)	• Nausea • Muscle weakness • Hyperreflexia • Abdominal cramping • Diarrhea • Arrhythmias	• Serum potassium level above 5.5 mEq/liter	• Removal of excess potassium; for example, via dialysis or Kayexalate enema. • Sodium bicarbonate or glucose administration (with or without insulin) to promote movement of potassium into intracellular spaces.	• Monitor the patient's vital signs. • Monitor the patient's electrocardiogram (ECG).

Managing fluid, electrolyte, and acid-base imbalances *(continued)*

IMBALANCE	CAUSE	SIGNS AND SYMPTOMS	LABORATORY FINDINGS	TREATMENT	NURSING INTERVENTIONS
ELECTROLYTE IMBALANCES *(continued)*					
Potassium depletion (hypokalemia)	• Inadequate potassium intake (starvation or malabsorption) • Excess potassium loss (diarrhea, vomiting, draining fistulas, NG tube suctioning, or excess urine output [diuretic use]) • Movement of potassium from extracellular to intracellular spaces in exchange for hydrogen (alkalosis)	• Drowsiness • Apathy • Muscle weakness • Hyporeflexia • Arrhythmias	• Serum potassium level below 3.5 mEq/liter	• Oral or I.V. potassium replacement.	• Carefully measure and record patient's fluid intake and output. • Monitor the patient's vital signs. • Monitor the patient's ECG.
ACID-BASE IMBALANCES					
Metabolic acidosis	• Hydrogen increase secondary to excess ketone acids produced by fat metabolism (starvation or diabetes mellitus) • Bicarbonate loss (diarrhea or fistulas) • Hydrogen increase secondary to inadequate hydrogen excretion (renal disease or renal failure) • Dehydration	• Deep, rapid respirations (compensatory mechanism)	*Uncompensated metabolic acidosis:* • Arterial pH below 7.35 • Plasma bicarbonate below 22 mEq/liter • Partial pressure of carbon dioxide in arterial blood ($Paco_2$) from 35 to 45 mm Hg	• Treatment of underlying cause. • For severe acidosis, sodium bicarbonate administration.	• Monitor the patient's fluid intake and output. • Administer I.V. sodium bicarbonate replacement, as prescribed.
Respiratory acidosis	• Impaired respiratory function leading to hypoventilation and CO_2 retention (head injury or barbiturate overdose) • Pulmonary disease accompanied by hypoventilation and CO_2 retention	• Shallow respirations • Respiratory distress • Headache • Blurred vision • Restlessness • Anxiety • Somnolence	*Uncompensated respiratory acidosis:* • Arterial pH below 7.35 • Plasma bicarbonate from 22 to 26 mEq/liter • $Paco_2$ above 45 mm Hg	• Treatment of underlying cause. • Measures to improve gas exchange, such as manual or mechanical ventilation.	• Monitor the patient's respiratory status. • Monitor arterial blood gas (ABG) values.

(continued)

Managing fluid, electrolyte, and acid-base imbalances *(continued)*

IMBALANCE	CAUSE	SIGNS AND SYMPTOMS	LABORATORY FINDINGS	TREATMENT	NURSING INTERVENTIONS
ACID-BASE IMBALANCES *(continued)*					
Metabolic alkalosis	• Hydrogen losses (vomiting or NG tube suctioning) • Bicarbonate increase (bicarbonate ingestion [baking soda used as antacid]) • Movement of hydrogen into intracellular spaces (hypokalemia) • Hydrogen losses (misuse of diuretics)	• Patient may be asymptomatic • Deep, slow respirations (compensatory mechanism) • Mental confusion	*Uncompensated metabolic alkalosis:* • Arterial pH above 7.45 • Plasma bicarbonate above 26 mEq/liter • $PaCO_2$ from 35 to 45 mm Hg	• Treatment of underlying cause. • Administration of I.V. fluids with sodium chloride, which causes kidneys to excrete bicarbonate.	• Monitor the patient's fluid intake and output. • Monitor ABG values.
Respiratory alkalosis	• Hyperventilation leading to excessive CO_2 loss (acute anxiety, tachypnea, or early salicylate poisoning)	• Light-headedness • Tingling of extremities • Altered consciousness • Muscle cramps	*Uncompensated respiratory alkalosis:* • Arterial pH above 7.45 • Plasma bicarbonate from 22 to 26 mEq/liter • $PaCO_2$ below 35 mm Hg	• Treatment of underlying cause. • Use of rebreather mask to slow respirations and increase CO_2 retention.	• Monitor ABG values.

Older children who understand numbers may use simple numerical scales to report pain. Although such scales have been used with children as young as age 5, they are most reliable with children age 8 and over. (For an example of a simple numerical scale, see *Rating pain on a numerical scale,* on the next page.)

Also observe the child for behavioral and physiologic indicators of pain. Behavioral indicators of pain include:
• motor activity—thrashing, jaw and fist clenching, tensing of muscles, rigidity, grinding of teeth, and lack of movement
• facial expressions—grimacing, frowning, closing the eyes tightly, lowering and drawing together the brows, and wrinkling the forehead
• verbal expressions—crying, screaming, and reporting pain or discomfort
• behavioral changes—irritability, restlessness, refusal to eat, altered sleep patterns, decreased ability to concentrate, and disinterest in playing or watching television.

Rating pain on a numerical scale

A child age 8 or over may use a numerical scale, such as the one shown here, to report pain severity. The scale may be oriented in a horizontal or vertical plane; younger children find a vertical scale easier to understand.

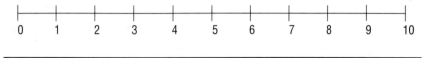

Physiologic indicators of pain are highly variable. In patients with acute pain, the sympathetic nervous system initially responds by increasing the heart and respiratory rates, raising the body temperature and blood pressure, and dilating the pupils. Typically, the child becomes restless and diaphoretic. These responses may last up to 1 hour. Then, the parasympathetic nervous system triggers a decrease in the respiratory and heart rates and a drop in blood pressure. If pain persists, however, the body adapts and these responses stabilize.

Also, these physiologic indicators are not specific to pain; they also occur in response to such stressors as fear and anxiety. Because of the variable, nonspecific nature of physiologic indicators, do not rely solely on these when assessing pain in children.

General pain management principles

When implementing pain management measures in children, keep the following principles in mind:

- Children of all ages, including infants, experience pain.
- Children may be unable to report pain because of developmental considerations, unwillingness to share their feelings, cognitive impairment, or language differences.
- Unrelieved pain has negative physical and psychological effects.
- Preventing pain is easier than treating pain that already exists.
- Encourage the child and family to be actively involved in pain assessment and management.
- Administering narcotics for acute pain does not lead to addiction or physical dependence and rarely causes respiratory depression.

Specific pain management strategies depend on the type and duration of pain (such as acute, transient, or long-term) as well as the underlying cause. Most hospitalized children undergo diagnostic or treatment procedures that cause temporary pain. Management of procedure-related pain may differ from management of postoperative pain. Regardless of the type, duration, or cause of pain, the nurse should act as the patient advocate, making sure that adequate pain control is achieved.

To manage pain associated with procedures, prepare the child and family adequately for the procedure. Reducing fear and anxiety may change the child's perception of the pain and help the child cope with the experience. Also, allow the parents to be present during the procedure and prepare them for their role, which is to comfort the child.

Coping with postoperative pain

Prepare the child and family for the likelihood of postoperative pain. Be sure to tell the child to inform the parents, nurse, and physician if pain occurs. Also inform the child and parents of pain treatment options, such as patient-controlled analgesia or intermittent I.V. analgesia for major surgery and oral analgesia for minor surgery.

Pharmacologic pain control

For mild pain, the physician may order nonsteroidal anti-inflammatory drugs (NSAIDS), such as ibuprofen. For moderate pain, NSAIDS may be combined with oral opiates, such as acetaminophen with codeine. Moderate to severe pain may call for such opiates as morphine, meperidine, or hydromorphone. Meperidine should be given only for brief periods of time because normeperidine, a toxic by-product, accumulates in the body and causes adverse central nervous system effects ranging from mood changes to seizures.

Administration guidelines

Titrate dosages, as prescribed, depending on the severity of the child's pain. Be aware that recommended starting doses may be inadequate to relieve pain. As prescribed, give opiates around the clock (at set intervals) (rather than as needed) or by continuous infusion because a drug must reach steady-state blood level to be effective continuously. For breakthrough pain, administer "rescue" doses, as prescribed.

Consider giving analgesics before procedures known to cause severe pain, such as bone marrow aspiration. Administer local anesthetics as prescribed and as needed, such as for I.V. line insertion or lumbar puncture. Be aware that sedatives and antianxiety agents decrease behavioral responses to pain but do not reduce pain.

When administering opiates, be sure to monitor for adverse effects, such as respiratory depression (relatively rare), constipation, urine retention, nausea and vomiting, pruritus, orthostatic hypotension, and sleepiness. If respiratory depression occurs, an opiate antagonist, such as naloxone, may be used to reverse the effects of the opiate. To prevent constipation, administer stool softeners and laxatives. To promote urination, help the child to an upright or standing position when voiding. As prescribed, administer oral antihistamines to ease pruritus, and antiemetics (rectally or intramuscularly) to relieve nausea and vomiting.
Administration routes. I.V. administration of analgesics is preferred during the immediate postoperative period. When the child can tolerate oral fluids, switch to oral administration, as prescribed. For children over age 7, consider patient-controlled analgesia.

Intramuscular (I.M.) injections cause additional pain and anxiety; the child may not report pain as readily when this route is used. Thus, use the I.M. route only when I.V. or oral administration is not possible.

Nonpharmacologic pain control

Nonpharmacologic methods may be used alone to relieve mild pain, or in conjunction with drugs to relieve more severe pain.

Distraction

Distraction—taking the child's mind off the pain—works best for pain of short duration, such as the transient pain caused by procedures. It generally is ineffective in relieving longer-lasting pain.

To use distraction, ask the parents (and child, if appropriate) to identify effective distractors. Examples of distractors include use of a pacifier, music box, or mobile for infants; singing or listening to music for toddlers and preschoolers; and listening to music or rhythmic breathing for school-age children and adolescents. Jokes and humor also may be used to distract the child.

Relaxation

This method changes the child's response to pain by altering the activity of the autonomic nervous system. Choose a relaxation technique appropriate for the child's age. For instance, swaddle and hold an infant in a comfortable position, rock the infant rhythmically, and speak to the infant softly.

With an older child, use deep-breathing or muscle-relaxing exercises. Deep breathing is easy to teach a child and can be effective in relieving acute pain of short duration. Although a child can learn muscle relaxation, doing so takes more time. Therefore, this method is a better choice for a child with pain of longer duration or chronic pain.

Guided imagery

In this method, ask the child to use the imagination to create pleasant, distracting images or to review pleasurable memories. Then have the child describe the image or memory, focusing on the most pleasurable parts.

Guided imagery has been used with children as young as ages 6 and 7. It is most effective at relieving pain of short duration.

Positive self-talk

To use this method, teach the child to talk to himself or herself when pain occurs, repeating such phrases as "It'll be over soon," "I can handle it," and "It's not so bad." Positive self-talk works best with pain of short duration.

Thought-stopping

With this method, the child interrupts thoughts about pain. Instruct the child to memorize phrases, such as "I love ice cream," and then repeat these over and over when pain occurs. Like guided imagery and positive self-talk, thought-stopping works best with pain of short duration.

Cutaneous stimulation

Massage, heat or cold application, or transcutaneous electrical nerve stimulator (TENS) may help manage pain of either short or long duration. For example, TENS sends low-voltage electricity to the painful area. Used with children as young as age 4, TENS is most effective against chronic pain.

Evaluating the effectiveness of pain management

Routinely evaluate the child's response to pain management by checking for a change in the child's self-report of pain and assessing for behavioral and verbal indicators of pain. Be sure to document initial pain assessment findings, methods of pain relief used, and the effectiveness of these methods. If the methods do not relieve pain adequately or if they cause undesirable effects, choose alternative techniques.

The child who requires surgery

All children require similar preoperative and postoperative care, regardless of the type of surgery.

Preoperative nursing care

To minimize anxiety regarding surgery—the primary preoperative nursing goal—be sure to prepare both the child and parents for the procedure. (For details on preparing the child, see *Preparing a child for surgery.*)

Parental concerns related to surgery include separation (especially with an infant or young child), fear of the surgical outcome (including the possibility of the child's death), and concern for the child's postoperative comfort.

Begin preparing the parents as soon as they are informed that the child needs surgery. Explain the reason for surgery and the type of procedure the child will undergo. Advise parents how they can assist in their child's care. Also prepare them for the child's postoperative appearance, and explain how the child's pain will be managed. Orient the parents to the nursing unit, and explain visiting policies. Reinforce verbal information with written material.

Postoperative nursing care

When the child returns to the unit after surgery, formulate appropriate nursing diagnoses and implement nursing interventions. Nursing diagnoses for the child recovering from surgery may include:
- *High risk for infection related to the surgical procedure*
- *Pain related to the surgical incision and invasive procedures*
- *Ineffective airway clearance related to ineffective coughing and immobility*
- *High risk for fluid volume deficit related to nausea, loss of appetite, vomiting, or nasogastric tube (NG) drainage*
- *Anxiety related to an unfamiliar environment*
- *Fear related to an unfamiliar environment*
- *Urine retention related to the effects of anesthesia, narcotics, and immobility*
- *Constipation related to lack of oral intake, narcotics, and immobility.*

Preparing a child for surgery

When preparing a child for surgery, the nurse should formulate interventions that are appropriate for the child's age. This chart present concerns of children in each pediatric age group, along with strategies the nurse can use to ease these concerns.

AGE-GROUP	CONCERNS OF CHILD	PREPARATION STRATEGIES
Infant (birth to age 12 months)	• Separation from parents • Unfamiliar environment	• Be aware that the level of cognitive development prevents infants from understanding explanations of surgery and hospitalization. • Encourage parents to bring transitional objects (such as blankets and toys) to the hospital to help ease separation anxiety. • Use measures to reduce parents' anxiety because this has a calming effect on the infant as well as the parents.
Toddler and pre-school-age child (ages 1 to 6)	• Separation from parents • Unfamiliar environment • Mutilation anxiety (in preschool-age children)	Prepare this child 1 to 3 days before admission by: • using simple verbal explanations of surgery • showing the child the body part that will be affected • using dolls to explain procedures, dressings, and intravenous lines • letting the child manipulate medical equipment, if appropriate • explaining that parents will visit the child in the hospital • arranging for the child to visit the playroom • urging the child to bring a favorite blanket, book, or toy to the hospital • explaining activity limitations imposed by surgery.
Young school-ages child (ages 6 to 9)	• Fear of surgery • Fear of mutilation • Loss of control	Prepare this child 5 to 7 days before admission by: • using the strategies described above for the toddler and preschool-age child • using books and pictures to aid explanations • informing the child of the anticipated length of hospital stay • showing the child films of children recovering from similar surgery • teaching the child how to assist in self-care • arranging for the child to visit the nursing unit in advance • explaining visiting policies.
Older school-age child (ages 10 to 12)	• Separation from friends • Loss of control • Fear of pain	Prepare this child 1 to 2 weeks before admission by: • explaining the reason for surgery, using simple written material and verbal explanations (with correct medical terms) • reviewing the types of procedures and treatments expected • explaining what the child will hear, see, and feel before, during, and after surgery • showing the child a film of children recovering from similar surgery • explaining pain-management strategies in simple terms • teaching the child how to assist in self-care • informing the child of the anticipated length of the hospital stay • arranging for the child to visit the nursing unit • reviewing visiting policies • explaining policies on telephone use • informing the child of activity limitations imposed by surgery • using pictures to review the child's expected postoperative appearance.
Adolescent (ages 13 to 18)	• Loss of control • Fear of the surgical outcome (including the possibility of death) • Fear of disfigurement • Separation from friends	Prepare adolescent as soon as the need for surgery is established by: • using strategies described above for the older school-age child, but providing more detail • providing written materials for the child to review independently • using detailed books and diagrams.

Goals of postoperative nursing care include preventing infection, promoting comfort, managing pain, maintaining a patent airway, promoting hydration, monitoring electrolyte status, promoting urination and bowel evacuation, and relieving anxiety.

Preventing infection

Monitor the child's temperature. Stay alert for signs of infection, such as fever and yellow or green wound drainage. Maintain aseptic technique during dressing changes. Keep the wound clean and the dressings intact. As prescribed, administer wound care and give antibiotics.

Promoting comfort and managing pain

Administer pain medications, as prescribed, and use nonpharmacologic pain management strategies as needed. Monitor the child's pain status and response to pain-management methods.

If the child cannot take foods or fluids by mouth, provide mouth care. Lubricate the child's nostrils with a water-soluble lubricant to decrease irritation from a NG tube.

Medicate the child for pain before performing wound care. Help the child find a comfortable position. Splint the wound during coughing and deep-breathing exercises.

Maintaining a patent airway

Monitor the child's breath sounds. Encourage the child to change position at least every 2 hours. Teach coughing and deep-breathing exercises, and assist the child with incentive spirometry. Perform percussion and postural drainage and suction airway secretions, as prescribed.

Promoting hydration

Administer I.V. fluids, as prescribed. Encourage oral fluid intake, unless contraindicated. Closely monitor the child's hydration status. When recording fluid intake and output, be sure to include emesis and output from drainage tubes.

Monitoring electrolyte status

Monitor serum electrolyte laboratory values. Record potential sources of electrolyte loss, such as drainage tube output and emesis.

Promoting urination and bowel evacuation

Monitor the child's urinary status, checking for bladder distention. Help the child to an upright position to use a bedpan or urinal, or help the child to the bathroom, if allowed. To stimulate voiding, turn the faucet on and run warm water over the child's pubic area. Assist with ambulation, if allowed.

To promote bowel evacuation, administer stool softeners, as prescribed. Again, assist the child to an upright position when using the bedpan, or help the child to the bathroom, if allowed. Assist with ambulation, and increase the child's dietary fiber intake. Provide adequate fluids, as prescribed.

Relieving anxiety

Maintain a calm, reassuring manner. Explain all procedures in advance. Encourage the child to discuss any fears and concerns. Stay with the child during times of stress and anxiety; also encourage parents to stay at the child's side.

STUDY ACTIVITIES

Short answer

1. How does ADH help regulate the body's fluid balance?

_____

_____

2. Explain why the nurse should not rely solely on physiologic indicators when assessing a child's pain.

_____

_____

_____

3. Eric, age 7, is recovering from an appendectomy. His NG tube is suctioned intermittently and an abdominal dressing is in place. Placed on NPO status, he is receiving I.V. fluids. The physician orders I.V. meperidine for pain. Why is Eric at risk for dehydration?

_____

_____

True or false

4. Immediately after surgery, the I.M. route is preferred for administering pain medications to a child.
☐ True   ☐ False

5. Children who receive narcotics for pain may have difficulty voiding.
☐ True   ☐ False

6. Nausea and vomiting are adverse effects of codeine.
☐ True   ☐ False

7. Infants are less likely than older children to experience pain.
☐ True   ☐ False

Multiple choice

8. Which condition predisposes a child to dehydration?
  A. Fever
  B. Renal failure
  C. Congestive heart failure
  D. Cystic fibrosis

9. Which assessment finding in a child may indicate hypokalemia?
  A. Edema
  B. Arrhythmias
  C. Hypertension
  D. Mental confusion

10. Which of the following actions should the nurse implement for a child whose serum sodium level is 118 mEq/liter?
  A. Monitor arterial blood gas values.
  B. Raise the side rails of the bed.
  C. Encourage oral fluid intake.
  D. Administer diuretics, as prescribed.

ANSWERS

Short answer

1. When hypovolemia or high osmotic pressure occurs, ADH is secreted, and the kidneys respond by retaining water. When hypervolemia or low osmotic pressure occurs, ADH is *not* secreted, and the kidneys respond by excreting water.

2. Physiologic indicators of pain are highly variable; if pain persists, the body's responses to pain stabilize and these indicators no longer appear. Also, physiologic indicators are not specific to pain; they also occur in response to such stressors as fear and anxiety.

3. Eric is at risk for dehydration because of fluid losses associated with the NG tube suctioning and lack of oral intake associated with his NPO status.

True or false

4. False. The I.V. route is preferred.

5. True.

6. True.

7. False. Children of all ages experience pain.

Multiple choice

8. A. Fever increases fluid losses. Renal failure and congestive heart failure are associated with fluid volume excess, not fluid volume deficit. Cystic fibrosis does not predispose a child to fluid volume deficit.

9. B. A potassium imbalance, such as hypokalemia, can cause arrhythmias. Edema occurs with extravascular fluid volume excess; hypertension, with intravascular fluid volume excess. Mental confusion is associated with sodium imbalance and acid-base disturbances.

10. B. A severe sodium imbalance may cause seizures. The nurse should raise the side rails of the bed to protect the child from injury during a seizure.

CHAPTER 17

Neurologic disorders

OBJECTIVES   After studying this chapter, the reader should be able to:

1. Describe the nursing assessment of a child with a neurologic disorder.

2. Identify the causes, pathophysiology, and signs and symptoms of increased intracranial pressure and acute intracranial infection.

3. Describe medical and nursing management of the child with increased intracranial pressure or acute intracranial infection.

4. Identify the causes, pathophysiology, and signs and symptoms of seizure disorders.

5. Discuss medical and nursing management of the child experiencing seizures.

6. Describe nursing management of the unconscious child.

OVERVIEW OF CONCEPTS   The nurse caring for a child with a neurologic disorder must know how to conduct an acute neurologic assessment, understand the pathophysiology of neurologic disorders, and be familiar with medical and nursing management of the specific disorder.

This chapter describes the acute neurologic assessment, including evaluation of level of consciousness (LOC). It discusses the causes and pathophysiology of selected neurologic disorders—increased intracranial pressure (ICP), acute intracranial infections, and seizure disorders—and delineates assessment and management of children with these disorders. Finally, the chapter outlines the nursing management of an unconscious child.

Acute neurologic assessment   The nurse conducts an acute neurologic assessment to monitor the hospitalized child with a neurologic disorder. (For information about a complete neurologic assessment of children, see Chapter 5, Child health assessment.) The acute neurologic assessment includes evaluation of these elements:

• LOC
• pupillary response and eye movement
• motor function and responses
• reflexes

- respiratory pattern
- vital signs.

Level of consciousness

The child's LOC reflects the degree of neurologic dysfunction. To evaluate LOC, the nurse may use the Glasgow Coma Scale. Most reliable for children over age 12 months, the Glasgow Coma Scale assesses three neurologic responses: eye response, motor response, and verbal response. Because of these limited response categories, do not base evaluation of a patient's LOC function solely on the basis of the Glasgow Coma Scale score. (For details, see *Glasgow Coma Scale.*)

To further assess the child's LOC, the nurse evaluates the level of arousal and notes which of the following categories applies to the child:

- Alert—the child is awake, oriented to person and place, and responsive to developmentally appropriate stimuli.
- Lethargic—the child is drowsy but easily aroused (awakened) with minimal stimulation.
- Stuporous—the child is difficult to arouse, appears confused (does not know where he or she is), and may be irritable.
- Unconscious—the child responds to painful stimulation with motor activity, may be restless, and may sit or lie with eyes open but does not follow objects or light, turn the head toward sound, or speak.
- Comatose—the child does not respond to painful stimuli.

Pupillary response and eye movement

Next, assess the child's pupil size, pupil reactivity to light, and eye movements. Normally, both pupils are equal in size (2 to 6 mm in diameter) and react to light, constricting when a bright light is directed at them. A bilateral increase in pupil size (dilation of both pupils) may signal hypoxic injury, drug effects, or increased ICP. Unilateral dilation with fixation (no response to light) may indicate intracranial hemorrhage. A bilateral decrease in pupil size (constriction of both pupils) suggests brain stem injury. A slow response or no response to light indicates a disturbance on the same side of the brain as the abnormal pupil.

Assess eye movements by asking the child to follow an object up, down, sideways, and obliquely. Normally, both eyes move together (conjugate movement). Disconjugate eye movement indicates dysfunction of cranial nerve III, IV, or VI.

The nurse may attempt to elicit the "doll's eyes" reflex by swiftly moving the child's head from side to side with the child's eyes open. (*Important:* Do not perform this test if the child has a cervical spinal injury.) Normally, both eyes move in the direction opposite the side to which the head moves. A negative response—failure of one or both eyes to move in the opposite direction—may signal midbrain or brain stem dysfunction.

Glasgow Coma Scale

For a child over age 1, the nurse may use the Glasgow Coma Scale to evaluate the level of consciousness. First, score the child's response in all three categories—eye response, motor response, and verbal response. Then, add the scores to determine the patient's total score. The total score may range from 3 to 15. A total score below 7 indicates coma; approximately half of those children with a score of 8 also are comatose.

TEST	SCORE
Eye response	
• Opens spontaneously	4
• Opens to verbal command	3
• Opens to painful stimuli	2
• No response	1
Motor response	
• Reacts to verbal commands	6
• Reacts to painful stimuli	
—Identifies local pain	5
—Exhibits abnormal flexor response*	3
—Exhibits abnormal extensor response**	2
• No response	1
Verbal response	
• Is oriented and uses age-appropriate language	5
• Makes confused conversation	4
• Uses inappropriate words	3
• Makes incomprehensible sounds (cries, screams, moans, or grunts)	2
• No response	1

* Decorticate positioning: Patient's arms are adducted and flexed, with wrists and fingers flexed on the chest; legs extended stiffly and rotated internally; and feet plantarflexed.
** Decerebrate positioning: Patient's head is retracted; arms are adducted and extended, with wrists pronated and fingers flexed; legs are extended stiffly; and feet are plantarflexed.

Motor function and responses

Observe the child for spontaneous movement in all extremities. Then check for purposeful movement, using an age-appropriate activity. For instance, hold a brightly colored toy in front of an infant and watch for reaching behavior; ask an older child to raise the right arm. Also observe for symmetry of movement.

To assess muscle strength, ask the child to grasp the nurse's index and middle fingers and squeeze as hard as possible. Normally, the child squeezes equally hard with both hands.

Test flexor muscle strength by asking the child to pull the nurse's hands toward the child while the nurse resists the child's pulling. Test extensor muscle strength by asking the child to push the nurse's hands away from the child while the nurse resists the pushing. Normally, flexor and extensor muscle strength are bilaterally equal.

The nurse also may test muscle strength by performing the pronator drift test. Ask the child to extend the arms, palms up, and then close the eyes. Normally, both arms stay in the same position. If the muscles of one arm are weak, that arm will drift slightly downward and pronate (rotate so that the palm faces downward and backward).

If the child cannot respond to verbal commands, assess motor responses by using painful stimuli. However, be sure to use the least amount of stimulation needed to provoke a motor response. In a normal response, the child pushes away or withdraws from the stimuli. Decerebrate or decorticate positioning in response to painful stimuli is abnormal and indicates brain stem dysfunction. (For details on these positions, see *Glasgow Coma Scale,* page 225.)

Reflexes

The corneal and gag reflexes are normal protective reflexes in children with intact neurologic functions. To elicit the corneal reflex, gently touch the outer cornea with a wisp of cotton. The normal response is prompt bilateral blinking; however, an infant may respond with prompt, asymmetrical blinking. Lack of response may indicate trigeminal nerve or pons dysfunction.

To elicit the gag reflex, press firmly on the child's tongue with a tongue depressor and then observe for symmetry of palatal movements. Persistence of the tonic neck reflex in an infant over age 6 months or the Babinski reflex in an infant over age 12 months indicates neurologic dysfunction. (For details on the tonic neck reflex, see Chapter 13, The child with a developmental disability.)

Respiratory pattern

Changes in the child's respiratory pattern indicate injury deep within the central hemispheres of the brain or the brain stem. Check for the following respiratory patterns:

- Cheyne-Stokes respirations—gradually increasing and decreasing respiratory rate and depth, with episodes of apnea; associated with disturbances in the cerebral hemispheres and basal ganglia
- Cluster breathing—periods of irregular breathing with episodes of apnea at variable intervals; may signal a disturbance in the upper portion of the medulla oblongata

- Ataxia or Biot's respirations—irregular respirations characterized by periods of hyperpnea followed by episodes of apnea, with deep or shallow breathing; suggests medullary dysfunction
- Apneusis—prolonged inspiratory phase, followed by an expiratory pause, then expiration; may indicate pons or brain stem damage
- Hyperventilation—increased respiratory rate and depth; central neurogenic hyperventilation may result from a disturbance in the lower region of the midbrain or pons.

Vital signs

Monitor the child's vital signs regularly. Watch for increases in the respiratory rate and blood pressure accompanied by a decrease in the heart rate—this cluster of changes suggests increased ICP. With persistently elevated ICP, blood pressure falls and the pulse becomes irregular and thready.

Hyperthermia (a higher than normal body temperature) may accompany increased ICP or an intracranial infection. Hypothermia (a body temperature below 95° F [35° C]) may accompany hypothalamic dysfunction.

Increased intracranial pressure

An increase in any of the three cranial components—brain mass, cerebral blood volume, or cerebrospinal fluid (CSF)—may cause ICP to rise. Increased ICP is a life-threatening condition.

During infancy, when the fontanels and suture lines are open, the skull can expand somewhat to prevent increased ICP. However, when maximum expansion is reached, ICP increases. Even with skull expansion, increases in CSF may cause compression of brain tissue.

After the fontanels and sutures close, the skull becomes an unyielding, bony structure with a fixed volume capacity. Under normal circumstances, brain mass, cerebral blood volume, and CSF volume are balanced and ICP remains constant. If any of these components increases, the other two components must decrease in order for ICP to remain constant. For example, in a head injury, the body initially attempts to compensate for cerebral edema by increasing the rate of CSF absorption and reducing cerebral blood volume. With continued edema, however, these compensatory mechanisms cannot maintain constant ICP, and ICP rises.

Unless treated, increased ICP may cause cerebral ischemia and, eventually, brain cell death. Brain tissue may herniate or become displaced into other brain structures. With continuous, severe ICP (above 20 mm Hg), the brain stem may herniate through the foramen magnum, causing damage to brain stem structures.

Etiology and pathophysiology

An increase in brain mass may result from cerebral edema secondary to a head injury, cerebral inflammation secondary to intracranial infection, a brain tumor or cyst, or cerebral hemorrhage. Causes of in-

Assessing for increased ICP

Signs and symptoms of increased intracranial pressure (ICP) vary with the duration of the ICP increase and with the child's age.

Early signs generally include irritability, restlessness, and lethargy. In infants, also expect poor feeding, a high-pitched cry, full scalp veins, and tense fontanels. In children over age 18 months, also expect headache and an unsteady gait.

Intermediate signs generally include a slow heart rate, increased blood pressure, seizures, slow and unequal pupillary responses, papilledema, strabismus, and vomiting. In infants, also expect a shrill cry, a bulging fontanel, and increased head circumference. Children over age 18 months typically also have vision problems, such as blurring and diplopia (double vision).

Late signs generally include a decreased level of consciousness, reduced reflex responses, respiratory pattern changes, elevated body temperature, fixed and dilated pupils, and decorticate or decerebrate posturing. In infants, also expect "sunset" eyes.

---

creased cerebral blood volume include systemic hypertension and cerebral vasodilation secondary to hypercapnia (excess carbon dioxide in the blood). An increase in CSF volume may stem from increased CSF production secondary to a choroid plexus tumor, decreased CSF absorption related to arachnoid villi malfunction, or obstructed CSF flow resulting from an infratentorial tumor or Arnold-Chiari deformity.

Assessment

Signs and symptoms of ICP vary with the child's age, and may be classified as early, intermediate, or late assessment findings. (For early, intermediate, and late assessment findings and age-related differences, see *Assessing for increased ICP*.)

A diagnosis of increased ICP typically is based on clinical findings. However, ICP can be measured noninvasively or invasively. For example, a transducer placed over the fontanel indirectly measures ICP by measuring the fullness of the fontanel. Invasive ICP monitoring devices include the subarachnoid bolt, intraventricular catheter, and epidural probe. Normally, ICP ranges from 0 to 15 mm Hg.

Medical management

Medical therapy for the child with increased ICP depends on the underlying pathophysiology. Surgery may be required to evacuate large volumes of blood resulting from an intracranial hemorrhage, to remove a brain tumor or cyst, or to insert a shunt to drain CSF accumulation caused by a CSF obstruction.

Nonsurgical methods also may be attempted. Induced hyperventilation decreases arterial oxygen (PaO_2) tension, causing hypocapnia; the resulting cerebral vasoconstriction leads to reductions in cerebral blood volume and ICP.

CSF removal, via such devices as an intraventricular catheter or subarachnoid screw, reduces ICP by decreasing overall CSF volume.

Fluid restriction—for example, one-half or two-thirds the child's maintenance level—decreases ICP by preventing excess cerebral blood volume. The child receives only isotonic fluid to prevent fluid shifts into or out of the cerebrovascular spaces.

I.V. osmotic diuretics, such as mannitol, cause fluid to shift from brain tissue into the cerebrovascular space, thus reducing ICP by decreasing brain mass. The kidneys excrete the excess fluid. Loop diuretics, such as furosemide (Lasix), decrease total body water, thereby reducing ICP.

I.V. corticosteroids reduce ICP by relieving cerebral edema; this, in turn, decreases brain mass. I.V. barbiturates may be given in high doses to decrease cerebral blood flow and metabolism, which, in turn, reduces ICP.

Blood pressure maintenance—keeping systolic pressure between 100 and 160 mm Hg—may decrease cerebral perfusion and relieve brain ischemia. (Hypertension, in contrast, may cause ICP to increase.)

Nursing management

Nursing goals for the child with ICP include monitoring neurologic status, reducing ICP, maintaining adequate cerebral perfusion, preventing injury, and providing parental support.

Monitoring the child's neurologic status is critical. Assess LOC regularly, check for signs of increased ICP, and record ICP hourly. Also, document vital signs and hourly fluid intake and output, and evaluate for signs and symptoms of fluid volume excess or deficit.

To help reduce ICP, maintain adequate cerebral perfusion, such as by elevating the head of the bed 30 degrees. By promoting venous return, this action reduces cerebral blood volume and decreases ICP. Keep the child's head in a neutral position; this also promotes venous return. Do not allow the child to flex or extend the neck—actions that may increase ICP. If necessary, use sandbags to keep the neck in a neutral position.

Minimize nursing care activities, such as turning and suctioning, because these can cause transient ICP increases. Also, reduce stimulation, which may increase ICP, and alternate nursing care activities with frequent rest periods.

Check the child's vital signs regularly. Hyperthermia speeds cerebral metabolism and may raise ICP. If the child has a fever, administer antipyretics, as prescribed, and use cooling devices to reduce body temperature. Be sure to maintain a patent airway because airway obstruction causes hypercapnia and cerebrovascular dilation, which raise ICP. Administer diuretics to reduce increased ICP and fluids to maintain fluid balance, as prescribed.

To minimize crying and agitation, which may increase ICP, explain all procedures to the child. The presence of a family member also may reduce agitation. If the child is in pain, administer analgesics, as prescribed.

Limit coughing and straining, which cause transient increases in ICP. As needed, administer stool softeners to prevent constipation.

The child with increased ICP may be prone to injuries because of an altered LOC. To prevent injury, keep the side rails of the bed up. If the child is agitated or confused, make sure someone stays with the child at all times to prevent self-injury.

Parents may have difficulty understanding the rationale for invasive ICP monitoring and other aspects of the child's care. Some parents may find the intensive care environment frightening. To reduce their anxiety and fear, explain all procedures, medical treatments, and nursing care. Allow time to answer their questions directly and honestly.

Acute intracranial infection

Bacterial and viral meningitis and encephalitis are the most common acute intracranial infections in children. Meningitis is characterized by inflammation of the meninges; encephalitis is an inflammation of the brain.

Bacterial meningitis is a life-threatening disease. Viral meningitis, caused by a variety of organisms such as measles, mumps, or herpesvirus, is less serious; most children recover fully. Bacterial meningitis is most common in children under age 5. *Haemophilus influenzae* Type B, *Neisseria meningitidis,* and *Streptococcus pneumoniae* are the bacteria most frequently implicated in meningitis. The meninges can become infected by vascular dissemination of an infection that initially originated elsewhere in the body. For example, organisms from the nasopharynx may enter the nasal blood supply and travel to the meninges. Bacteria also may infect the meninges directly after a skull fracture or penetrating head wound. Encephalitis may be caused by a variety of organisms, including bacteria, spirochetes, protozoa, helminths, and viruses. Most infections are associated with viruses, such as measles, mumps, varicella, and rubella.

This section focuses on bacterial meningitis. Assessment and management of viral meningitis and encephalitis are similar.

Pathophysiology

In bacterial meningitis, the inflamed meninges become covered with exudate. Brain edema occurs, and ICP rises. Complications of bacterial meningitis may include:
- obstructive hydrocephaly secondary to infection of the ventricles and occlusion of the ventricular passages by exudate or fibrinous material
- deafness or blindness resulting from cranial nerve damage
- behavioral and intellectual changes.

Assessment

Clinical findings vary with the child's age. (See *Assessment findings in meningitis.*)

Assessment findings in meningitis

Signs and symptoms of meningitis vary with the child's age. In children up to age 2, expect fever; disinterest in feeding; seizures; and signs and symptoms of increased intracranial pressure (ICP), such as irritability, a high-pitched cry, vomiting, and a bulging fontanel.

In children over age 2, symptoms typically arise suddenly. (However, some children have a slower onset of symptoms, which is preceded by several days of mild respiratory or gastrointestinal symptoms.) The nurse should stay alert for the abrupt onset of:

- fever
- chills
- seizures
- nuchal rigidity (resistance to neck flexion)
- purpuric rash (with meningococcal infection)
- behavior changes, such as agitation, delirium, aggression, drowsiness, or stupor
- signs and symptoms indicating increased ICP, such as headache, vomiting, and irritability.

Also check for Kernig's and Brudzinski's signs, which are positive when the child has meningitis. To test for Kernig's sign, place the child supine, with the leg flexed at the hip and knee. Then, ask the child to extend the knee. Resistance or pain upon leg extension is abnormal and indicates a positive Kernig's sign.

To test for Brudzinski's sign, place the child supine and have the child flex the neck. Pain or involuntary flexion of the knees and hips is abnormal and indicates a positive Brudzinski's sign.

For a definitive diagnosis, the child undergoes lumbar puncture to draw a sample of CSF. In bacterial meningitis, CSF analysis reveals an elevated white blood cell count, a glucose level lower than the serum glucose level, and an elevated protein level. CSF culture determines the causative bacteria.

Medical management

The child with an acute intracranial infection usually requires the following therapy:

- I.V. antibiotic therapy, intrathecal antibiotic therapy, or both
- measures to reduce ICP (as described earlier)
- measures to control seizures (as described in the section on "Seizures" below)
- fluid management, such as restriction to two-thirds the maintenance level, to prevent fluid overload and cerebral edema
- pain management, typically with acetaminophen.

Nursing management

Nursing goals for the child with an intracranial infection include:

- maintaining adequate cerebral perfusion
- reducing ICP
- preventing spread of the infection
- controlling the infectious process
- managing irritability and pain

• preventing injury
• providing parental support.
For nursing measures that help maintain adequate cerebral perfusion and reduce ICP, see the section on "Increased intracranial pressure" above.

Preventing spread of the infection
Place the child on respiratory isolation precautions for at least 24 hours after antibiotic therapy begins.

Controlling the infectious process
Administer I.V. medications, as prescribed. Always give medications on time to ensure a therapeutic blood drug level. Because the antibiotics used to control bacterial meningitis are highly potent, be sure to monitor the child's blood urea nitrogen and serum creatinine levels. As prescribed, obtain peak and trough blood samples. Draw the trough sample immediately before administering the antibiotic. Draw the peak sample 30 minutes after the antibiotic infusion ends.

Managing irritability and pain
The child with meningitis is extremely irritable. Give acetaminophen, as prescribed, to help manage fussiness and irritability. Because meningitis causes extreme sensitivity to noise, lights, and sudden position changes, be sure to keep the child's room quiet, minimize environmental stimulation, and reposition the child slowly.

Preventing injury
Be sure to implement seizure precautions (discussed in the section on "Seizures" below.)

Seizures

A seizure is a sudden, violent, involuntary contraction of a group of muscles. It may be paroxysmal and episodic, or acute and transient. Epilepsy is characterized by recurrent seizures; its cause generally is unknown.

Some seizures are idiopathic (associated with no known cause). Others result from one of a wide range of conditions, including the following:
• asphyxia during birth or following head trauma
• intracranial hemorrhage
• an electrolyte disturbance (such as hypoglycemia, hypocalcemia, hypomagnesemia, hyponatremia, or hypernatremia)
• intracranial infection
• drug withdrawal
• acute cerebral edema
• brain cyst or tumor
• high fever.
In some patients, seizures do not recur once the underlying cause is controlled. In others, seizures recur chronically, even after the primary cause is controlled.

Seizures are classified as partial or generalized. (For descriptions of these classifications, see *Seizures: Classifications and clinical manifestations,* pages 234 and 235.)

Pathophysiology

Regardless of the underlying cause, a seizure occurs when the seizure threshold of nerve cells in the brain is low, allowing excess discharge of electrical impulses. The excess discharge disrupts normal brain function, thus provoking a seizure.

Assessment

Clinical manifestations of a seizure depend on the origin of the excess electrical discharge. (See *Seizures: Classifications and clinical manifestations,* pages 234 and 235.)

Diagnosis of a seizure disorder begins with a detailed patient history. The physician tries to identify the underlying cause of the condition. To help classify the child's seizures, the physician asks the parents to describe the body parts involved in the seizure, the length and duration of the seizure, whether the child loses consciousness, and the child's behavior before and after the seizure.

Electroencephalography (EEG) is the most important diagnostic tool for evaluating the child with seizures. Although an EEG cannot determine the cause of a seizure, it can reveal its brain origin and help classify the seizure.

Blood studies may be done to determine if the seizure results from an electrolyte disturbance or a toxic substance (such as lead or drugs). Typically, the child also undergoes lumbar puncture to rule out intracranial infection or increased ICP as the cause of seizures. Computed tomography may be done to detect such possible causes as an intracranial tumor or intraventricular obstruction.

Medical management

Medical goals include correcting the underlying cause of seizures (when known) and reducing the incidence of seizures. Certain factors that precipitate seizures—for example, electrolyte imbalances, intracranial infection, acute cerebral edema, drug withdrawal, and high fever—can be treated successfully, thus ending seizures permanently.

For the patient whose seizures continue even after the underlying cause has been treated, or for whom the cause of seizures cannot be determined, medical therapy aims to reduce the incidence of seizures. Typically, the physician prescribes anticonvulsant drugs, which raise the seizure threshold or prevent abnormal electrical discharges. The choice of anticonvulsant drug depends on the type of seizure. In most cases, the child receives a single anticonvulsant agent; the dosage is increased slowly until a therapeutic blood drug level is reached. If seizures continue, a second anticonvulsant is added to the drug regimen. (For details, see *Anticonvulsant therapy,* pages 236 and 237.)

Seizures: Classifications and clinical manifestations

Seizures fall into two major classifications—partial and generalized. Each classification has various subdivisions. Partial seizures originate in a localized brain area; generalized seizures involve both hemispheres of the brain.

This chart describes typical behavior and activity before, during, and after the various types of seizures. Before a seizure, for example, the patient may experience an aura—a sensation of light or warmth. After a seizure ends, the patient may have such postictal (postseizure) signs as weakness or drowsiness.

TYPE	AURA	MOTOR BEHAVIOR	SENSORY EFFECTS	IMPAIRMENT OF CONSCIOUSNESS	POSTICTAL FINDINGS
Partial seizures					
Simple partial seizure	Common; may be the only obvious sign of seizure	May include clenching fists, averting eyes, turning head to one side, or tonic-clonic movement; typically restricted to one side of the body.	Common	No	Weakness
Complex partial seizure	Common	Includes automatisms (such purposeless activity as lip smacking), staring, cessation of activity, limpness, or stiffness.	Common	Yes	Drowsiness, followed by sleep
Generalized seizures					
Tonic-clonic seizure	No	Initially, eyes roll upward. Patient then falls to ground and stiffens in generalized *tonic* contraction lasting 1 to 20 seconds. During this phase, patient stops breathing and may become cyanotic. Next, the *clonic* phase is marked by rapidly alternating muscle contraction and relaxation. This phase lasts 30 seconds or more. Patient may experience bowel or bladder incontinence.	Rare	Yes	Patient relaxes, and appears drowsy and confused; may sleep for several hours
Absence seizure	No	Includes minimal change in muscle tone; automatisms; staring; and sudden cessation of activity.	Rare	Yes (may be brief)	Resumption of preseizure activity and behavior, with no drowsiness or weakness
Atonic and akinetic seizures	Rare	Patient experiences sudden loss of muscle tone and falls to ground.	Rare	Yes (may be brief)	Resumption of preseizure activity and behavior, with no drowsiness or weakness

Seizures: Classifications and clinical manifestations (continued)

TYPE	AURA	MOTOR BEHAVIOR	SENSORY EFFECTS	IMPAIRMENT OF CONSCIOUSNESS	POSTICTAL FINDINGS
Myoclonic seizure	Rare	Exhibits sudden, brief, rhythmic contractions of a muscle or a muscle group.	Rare	No	Resumption of preseizure activity and behavior, with no drowsiness or weakness
Infantile spasm	Rare	May start with a sharp cry, followed by sudden dropping forward of patient's head. Rhythmic muscle contractions also may occur.	Rare	Sometimes	Resumption of preseizure activity, with no drowsiness or weakness

Adapted with permission from the Commission on Classification and Terminology of the International League Against Epilepsy. "Proposal for Revised Clinical and Electroencephalographic Classification of Epileptic Seizures." *Epilepsia* 22:489-501. New York: Ravin Press, Ltd., 1981.

Nursing management

Nursing goals for the child with seizures include:
- documenting seizure activity
- preventing or controlling seizures
- protecting the child from injury during a seizure
- supporting the child and family.

Documenting seizure activity

Carefully observe all activity during a seizure, and document observations in the patient's record. Nursing observations during a seizure may help identify precipitating factors, determine the seizure type, and reveal the effectiveness of anticonvulsant therapy. Be sure to document the following information:
- time of seizure onset
- the child's activity, behavior, and sensations before seizure onset
- the child's activity and behavior during the seizure (including body, facial, and eye movements) and any loss of consciousness
- related activity and behavior during the seizure, such as changes in skin color, diaphoresis, respiratory pattern changes (including apnea), and involuntary urination or defecation
- duration of the seizure
- postictal (postseizure) activity, including the child's state of consciousness; orientation to person, place, and time; drowsiness or motor weakness; and speech.

For details on seizure observations, see *Observing the child who has seizures,* page 238.

Anticonvulsant therapy

The choice of anticonvulsant agent is based on the type of seizure the patient has experienced. This chart provides information on drugs used to treat the various types of seizures.

TYPE	ANTICONVULSANT AGENT	NURSING CONSIDERATIONS
Partial seizures, generalized tonic-clonic seizures	*Primary drugs* Carbamazepine (Tegretol)	• Monitor patient for blurred vision, diplopia, and drowsiness. • Monitor patient's blood studies; aplastic anemia is a rare toxic effect.
	Phenytoin (Dilantin)	• Monitor patient for gastric irritation, diplopia, nystagmus, nervousness, ataxia, acne, hirsutism, gingival hyperplasia, and folate deficiency. • Monitor patient's blood studies; thrombocytopenia or folate deficiency may occur. • Drug may increase incidence of absence and myoclonic seizures. • Drug may cause behavioral disturbances in some children. • Teach parents that drug colors urine brown or dark red. Urge preventive tooth and gum care, such as twice-daily cleaning with a soft-bristled toothbrush.
	Secondary drugs • Primidone (Mysoline)	• Monitor patient for drowsiness, nausea, ataxia, and nystagmus. • Monitor patient's blood studies; anemia may be a toxic effect.
	Phenobarbital (Luminal)	• Monitor patient for fever, drowsiness, hyperactivity, irritability, ataxia, decreased cognitive performance, reduced concentration and motor speed, and depression. • Drug may cause vitamin D and folic acid deficiencies. • Use caution when administering with valproic acid; phenobarbital increases both the therapeutic and toxic effects of this drug.
	Ethosuximide (Zarontin)	• Monitor patient for nausea, gastric irritation, anorexia, headache, and drowsiness. • Monitor patient's blood studies; leukopenia is a toxic effect. • Monitor liver function tests; drug may cause liver toxicity. • Teach parents to administer drug with food to reduce gastric irritation. • Drug may increase incidence of generalized seizures.
	Valproic acid (Depakene)	• Monitor patient for nausea, drowsiness, and anorexia. • Check for diarrhea and stomach cramps, which are toxic effects. • Monitor patient's blood studies; altered bleeding times indicate toxicity. • Monitor liver function tests; drug may cause liver toxicity. • Use caution when administering drug with phenobarbital or phenytoin; valproic acid increases both the therapeutic and toxic effects of these drugs.
Absence seizures	*Primary drugs* Clonazepam (Klonopin)	• Monitor patient for lethargy, ataxia, hyperactivity, nystagmus, behavioral disturbances, slurred speech, and rhinorrhea. • Monitor patient's blood studies; thrombocytopenia is a toxic effect. • This drug commonly is given as an adjunct to other anticonvulsant agents.
	Ethosuximide (Zarontin)	• This agent is a drug of choice for absence seizures. • See previous listing.
	Phenobarbital (Luminal)	• This agent is a drug of choice for absence seizures. • See previous listing.

Anticonvulsant therapy *(continued)*

TYPE	ANTICONVULSANT AGENT	NURSING CONSIDERATIONS
Absence seizures *(continued)*	*Primary drugs (continued)* Trimethadione (Tridione)	• Monitor patient for nausea, irritability, drowsiness, rash, and photophobia. • Monitor patient's blood studies; leukopenia and agranulocytosis are toxic effects. • Monitor urinalysis; nephrosis is a toxic effect.
	Valproic acid	• Same as for trimethadione.
Atonic, akinetic, and myoclonic seizures	Combinations of the above drugs, such as phenobarbital and clonazepam	• See individual entries for these drugs.

Preventing or controlling seizures

To prevent or control seizures, administer anticonvulsant drugs, as prescribed. Teach the family about the importance of complying with the therapeutic regimen. Advise them to have the child avoid known precipitating factors, such as bright, blinking lights and emotional stress.

Preventing injury

To prevent injury during a seizure, pad the side rails of the bed. Once the seizure begins, do not restrain the child. If the child was sitting or standing when the seizure began, ease the child onto the floor. Loosen tight clothing, place a blanket under the child, and push furniture away from the child. Do not put anything in the child's mouth. Allow the seizure to end.

After the seizure ends, obtain the child's vital signs. Check for physical injury, such as bruising and tongue or lip bites. If the child is cyanotic, administer oxygen by face mask, as prescribed. If the child is drowsy, make the child comfortable and let the child rest or sleep. If the child urinated or defecated during the seizure, change the child's clothing.

Supporting the child and family

Because epilepsy is a chronic disorder, the nurse should provide support for the child and family as for any child with a chronic illness (see Chapter 15, Illness concepts). Encourage the family to allow the child to participate in age-appropriate activities. If seizures are well-controlled, the child may be allowed to engage in competitive sports, swimming, and bicycle riding. However, advise parents to make sure the child is accompanied during these activities and wears a helmet when riding a bicycle. Discourage climbing because the child would fall if a

Observing the child who has seizures

Before, during, and after a seizure, observe the child closely. After the seizure ends, document observations carefully.

Before the seizure
The child may have an *aura*—a visual, auditory, gustatory, or olfactory sensation that warns of an impending seizure. Immediately before the seizure, a sense of fear or dread may arise.

During the seizure
Note *motor activity,* which may range from minimal to severe. For example, check for cessation of activity, random eye movements or eye movements to one side, automatisms (such purposeless activity as lip smacking or chewing), staring, or muscle contractions. Tonic contractions cause muscle rigidity; clonic contractions cause opposing muscles to contract and relax, resulting in a rhythmic jerking.

Observe for autonomic nervous system activity, such as pallor, sweating, and flushing. Also, check for *sensory effects,* such as tingling, prickling, hallucinations, light flashes, tastes, smells, or sounds. To obtain information about sensory effects, the nurse may have to question the patient after the seizure ends.

In some children, a seizure may induce partial or complete loss of consciousness. The child who loses consciousness is unresponsive to the environment and does not remember the seizure.

After the seizure
Postictal (postseizure) findings may include weakness, confusion, or drowsiness. Some children sleep for several hours after a seizure.

---

seizure occurred during these activities. Motor vehicle restrictions vary from state to state. In some states, an adolescent with well-controlled seizures may be allowed to drive.

The unconscious child

A child with a head injury, increased ICP, or intracranial infection may become unconscious.

Management
The physician typically treats the underlying cause (if known). Nursing goals for the unconscious child include:
• reducing or preventing increased ICP (when indicated)
• maintaining an open airway
• promoting skin integrity
• aiding bowel elimination
• preventing injury
• promoting musculoskeletal functioning
• providing adequate nutrition
• providing sensory stimulation.
For nursing measures that help reduce or prevent increased ICP and prevent injury, see the section on "Increased intracranial pressure."

Maintaining an open airway

If the unconscious child cannot swallow oral secretions, these secretions pool in the oropharynx and may be aspirated. To help prevent aspiration, place the child in a side-lying or semi-prone position to promote drainage of oral secretions. Suction the oropharynx to remove accumulated secretions. Raise the head of the bed to prevent reflux and possible aspiration of gastric contents. If the child's airway is compromised, insert an oral airway, as prescribed.

Airway clearance is jeopardized by impaired coughing, pooling of pulmonary secretions, and decreased lung expansion secondary to immobility. The unconscious child also is predisposed to pneumonia because of the retention of pulmonary secretions and secondary bacterial colonization of such secretions. To promote airway clearance, reposition the child every 2 to 4 hours (unless contraindicated by increased ICP). Administer chest physiotherapy, as prescribed. Monitor the child closely for adventitious breath sounds and atelectasis.

Promoting skin integrity

Immobility places the child at risk for skin breakdown and pressure sores (decubitus ulcers). To prevent pressure on bony prominences, place the child on a low-air-loss mattress. Place sheepskin under the child to prevent friction between the skin and bedsheets. Unless contraindicated, change the child's position every 2 hours.

Inspect the child's skin for redness and other signs of irritation every 4 hours. To promote circulation, gently rub bony prominences with lotion. Bathe the child daily to remove irritating body secretions.

Aiding bowel elimination

Immobility, inactivity, and low dietary fiber intake contribute to constipation in the unconscious child. To stimulate bowel evacuation, administer stool softeners, such as Colace, and glycerine suppositories, as prescribed. Provide adequate fluids.

Promoting musculoskeletal function

Immobility and inactivity contribute to muscle wasting in the unconscious child. Poor positioning may contribute to contractures.

To promote musculoskeletal function, obtain a referral for physical therapy. Perform passive range-of-motion (ROM) exercises, and keep the child in proper body alignment. Place a small, rolled towel in the child's palm to maintain proper finger position. To prevent footdrop, place a footboard at the foot of the bed or use high-top sneakers (on for 2 hours, off for 2 hours).

Providing adequate nutrition

Initially, the unconscious child receives I.V. fluids and caloric intake. Monitor the child's hydration status to detect signs of dehydration or overhydration. Once the child is stable, provide nutrition enterally, by nasogastric (NG) or gastrostomy tube. If the child can have nothing by mouth (NPO), perform oral hygiene.

If the child has an NG tube, gently clean the nares twice a day with sterile water to remove crusted nasal secretions. If the child has a gastrostomy tube, clean the skin around the insertion site twice daily with half-strength hydrogen peroxide. Then dry the skin with a clean, dry, cotton-tipped applicator or gauze.

To prevent accidental removal of an NG tube, tape the tube securely to prevent dislodgment. If the child tries to pull at the tube, place mitts on the hands. Tape a gastrostomy tube securely to prevent tension on the tube if it is pulled.

Before starting a feeding through the NG tube, verify that the distal end of the tube is in the stomach. To do this, release the clamp on the tube. Then apply gentle negative pressure to the tube, using a 20-ml syringe. The tube is placed correctly if this procedure yields gastric contents. Another way to determine proper NG tube placement is to inject 5 ml of air into the NG tube, then auscultate the fundus of the stomach. With correct tube placement, the nurse should hear the rush of air entering the stomach. To determine if unabsorbed formula remains in the stomach, apply gentle negative pressure to the NG tube.

Before starting a feeding through a gastrostomy tube, measure the length of the tube and compare it to length measured immediately after insertion. To mark the length of the tube immediately after insertion, use an indelible pen to draw a line at the appropriate place.

When preparing the enteral feeding formula, make sure the formula is at room temperature to aid absorption. Measure the correct amount of formula prescribed.

The timing of feedings varies with the amount of formula administered. To administer the formula, raise the head of the child's bed to 30 degrees. Next, attach the 20-ml syringe to the feeding tube, keeping the tube at the level of the child's abdomen. Slowly pour the formula into the syringe. Then raise the syringe and tube until a slow flow of formula is established. To ensure a slow, steady flow, adjust the roller clamp. Refill the syringe, as needed. When using a larger enteric feeding bag, fill the bag with the entire volume of formula. Prime the tubing and connect the distal end to the gastrostomy or NG tube. (A Kangaroo pump may be used to administer enteral fluids.)

After the feeding, flush the tube with 20 to 30 ml of sterile water to clear it of formula. Then clamp the tube shut. To minimize regurgitation and promote gastric emptying, place the child in a prone position or on the right side for at least 1 hour. Record the amount of residual formula (the formula obtained when aspirating for tube placement) and the type and amount of formula administered.

Providing sensory stimulation

Providing sensory stimulation—especially auditory—is an important care measure for the unconscious child. Experts believe most unconscious children can hear. Greet the child by name when entering the room, and speak in a normal conservational tone, as if the child were conscious. As appropriate, play a radio softly. Explain procedures, such as feeding and drug administration, to the child in advance.

Tactile stimulation, such as gentle stroking, is soothing to some unconscious children but may agitate others. Carefully observe the child's response to tactile stimulation before using this calming method. Provide age-appropriate visual stimulation, such as mobiles or television.

STUDY ACTIVITIES

Matching related elements

Match the breathing pattern on the left with the description on the right.

1. ___ Cheyne-Stokes respirations   **A.** Hyperpnea followed by episodes of apnea, with deep or shallow breathing

2. ___ Cluster breathing   **B.** Increased respiratory rate and depth

3. ___ Ataxia or Biot's respirations   **C.** Gradually increasing respiratory rate and depth, with episodes of apnea

4. ___ Apneusis   **D.** Periods of irregular breathing followed by episodes of apnea

5. ___ Hyperventilation   **E.** Prolonged inspiratory phase, followed by an expiratory pause, then expiration

Short answer

6. List the three types of neurologic responses assessed by the Glasgow Coma Scale.

_____

7. Compare and contrast decorticate and decerebrate positioning.

_____

_____

_____

8. Describe how to perform the pronator drift test.

_____

_____

9. Rennie, age 7, is unconscious. To address related respiratory problems, the nurse formulates the following nursing diagnosis: *Ineffective airway clearance related to poor cough and stasis of pulmonary secretions.* The expected outcomes are that Rennie will exhibit an effective cough and clear, equal breath sounds. List two nursing interventions that would help achieve these outcomes.

_____

_____

Multiple choice

10. In a 5-year-old child with increased ICP, the nurse would expect to find all of the following signs and symptoms *except*:

    A. Headache

    B. Blurred vision

    C. Increased head circumference

    D. Decreased level of consciousness

11. When assessing a child with bacterial meningitis, the nurse would expect to find:

    A. Dilated pupils

    B. Resistance to neck flexion

    C. An absent gag reflex

    D. Persistence of the Babinski reflex

ANSWERS **Matching related elements**

    1. C

    2. D

    3. A

    4. E

    5. B

Short answer

6. The Glasgow Coma Scale assesses eye, motor, and verbal responses.

7. In decorticate positioning, the patient's arms are adducted and flexed, with the wrists and fingers flexed on the chest; the legs are extended stiffly and rotated internally; and the feet are plantarflexed. In decerebrate positioning, the patient's head is retracted; the arms are adducted and extended, with the wrists pronated and fingers flexed; the legs are extended stiffly; and the feet are plantarflexed.

8. In the pronator drift test, the child extends the arms, with palms up, and then closes the eyes. Normally, both arms stay in the same position. If the muscles of one arm are weak, that arm will drift slightly downward and rotate so that the palm faces downward and backward.

9. Reposition Rennie every 2 to 4 hours. Administer chest physiotherapy, as prescribed. Monitor Rennie closely for crackles or atelectasis.

Multiple choice

10. C. After infancy, the skull cannot expand in response to increased ICP. Therefore, the nurse would not expect increased head circumference in a 5-year-old with increased ICP.

11. B. The child with meningitis exhibits nuchal rigidity. The other responses are uncommon in children with meningitis.

CHAPTER 18

Respiratory disorders

OBJECTIVES

After studying this chapter, the reader should be able to:

1. Describe how the nurse assesses the child with an acute or chronic respiratory disorder.

2. Discuss the causes, pathophysiology, and clinical manifestations of the following acute respiratory disorders: bronchiolitis, bronchitis, pneumonia, acute laryngotracheobronchitis, and acute epiglottitis.

3. Identify medical and nursing management of children with acute respiratory disorders.

4. Discuss the pathophysiology of asthma and cystic fibrosis.

5. Describe medical and nursing management of children with asthma and cystic fibrosis.

OVERVIEW OF CONCEPTS

Respiratory dysfunction is the most common health problem in children. The nurse who cares for the child with a respiratory disorder must be familiar with the underlying pathophysiology as well as medical and nursing management. If the disorder is chronic, the nurse also must recognize—and be prepared to deal with—the impact of the disorder on the child's physical and psychosocial development.

This chapter focuses on acute and chronic respiratory disorders in children. After reviewing the elements of the baseline respiratory assessment, it discusses certain acute disorders—bronchiolitis, bronchitis, pneumonia, acute laryngotracheobronchitis (LTB), and acute epiglottitis. The chapter also explores two chronic disorders—asthma and cystic fibrosis. (For a discussion of the psychosocial effects of chronic illness on children, see Chapter 15, Illness concepts).

Respiratory assessment

A baseline respiratory assessment is essential to ensure effective monitoring of a child with a respiratory disorder. To begin the assessment, obtain a complete health history (described in Chapter 5, Child health assessment). Next, perform a physical examination. Be sure to observe the rate, depth, and quality of respirations; auscultate lung fields; and note the child's skin color. Check for a productive or nonproductive cough, and observe characteristics of sputum or nasal secretions. Also evaluate the ease of the child's breathing.

During the physical examination, stay alert for the following abnormal findings:

- hypopnea—shallow respirations, indicating exchange of small volumes of air
- hyperpnea—deep respirations, indicating exchange of large volumes of air
- green- or yellow-tinged nasal secretions or sputum, which may signal an infection
- dyspnea—shortness of breath or difficulty breathing
- chest retractions—use of accessory chest muscles to assist the breathing effort, which may indicate airway obstruction
- grunting sounds during respiration, indicating respiratory distress
- tachypnea—an increased respiratory rate, which may indicate respiratory compromise or hypoxia
- adventitious breath sounds, such as wheezing, crackles, or rhonchi, which may indicate airway obstruction or increased secretions
- diminished or absent breath sounds, which may signal atelectasis (alveolar collapse) or bronchial obstruction
- cyanosis—bluish tinge to the skin, mucous membranes, and, possibly, nail beds, which may indicate an oxygen deficit
- circumoral cyanosis (bluish ring around the mouth), which may reflect respiratory difficulty
- restlessness, irritability, or anxiety, which may indicate hypoxia
- pain upon inspiration, which may indicate pulmonary or cardiac disease.

Bronchiolitis

Bronchiolitis is an acute respiratory viral infection characterized by inflammation of the bronchiole, one of the finer subdivisions of the bronchial tree. Common in children under age 2, bronchiolitis is rare after this age.

Respiratory syncytial virus (RSV) is the most common underlying cause of bronchiolitis. Normally occurring in the winter and spring, RSV affects more boys than girls.

Pathophysiology

The inflamed bronchioles become edematous and respiratory secretions accumulate, thereby occluding the bronchiolar lumen. The narrowing of the small airways compromises expiration, and causes air to be trapped in the alveoli. The trapped air, in turn, induces lung hyperinflation and may lead to atelectasis. Inadequate ventilation results in hypoxemia and hypercapnia.

Assessment

Initially, the child may have signs and symptoms of an upper airway infection—nasal drainage, sneezing, coughing, poor appetite, and a low-grade fever. As these mild symptoms worsen, expect signs of respiratory distress—tachypnea, shallow respirations, inspiratory crackles, expiratory wheezing, tachycardia, chest retractions, dyspnea, and a productive or congested cough. In infants who are still breast- or bottle-feeding, an inability to suck may cause feeding difficulties from increased respiratory effort.

Diagnosis commonly rests on clinical findings and such defining characteristics as the child's age and the season. Nasal washings revealing RSV provide a definitive diagnosis.

Medical management

A child with mild respiratory symptoms and adequate oxygenation may receive care at home. A child with hypoxia must be hospitalized.

Medical treatment involves oxygen therapy, rest, and fluids. Sufficient oxygen is given by nasal cannula or mist tent to keep arterial oxygen saturation above 95%. Chest physiotherapy, which includes postural drainage, percussion, and vibration, may be prescribed to help rid the lungs of mucus.

The child receives intravenous (I.V.) fluids to thin secretions and prevent dehydration from increased respiratory effort. Bronchodilators, such as albuterol or metaproterenol, may be administered by nebulizer. Ribavirin, an antiviral drug that speeds recovery, may be given via aerosol generator.

Nursing management

Nursing goals for the child with bronchiolitis include:
- preventing spread of the infection
- promoting airway clearance and effective gas exchange
- maintaining an adequate fluid volume
- easing the work of breathing.

RSV can be transmitted by respiratory droplet for up to 9 days. To prevent the spread of RSV, the nurse should wash hands carefully and institute respiratory isolation precautions, as appropriate.

To promote airway clearance and effective gas exchange, perform chest physiotherapy, as prescribed. Reposition the child at least every 2 hours to promote lung expansion and prevent stasis of pulmonary secretions. As prescribed, administer bronchodilators and ribavirin, and give fluids to thin pulmonary secretions. Provide humidified air or oxygen, as prescribed.

To maintain an adequate fluid volume, monitor the child's hydration status by carefully documenting fluid intake and output, urine specific gravity, moistness of mucous membranes, and skin turgor. Administer I.V. fluid therapy, as prescribed.

To ease the work of breathing, position the child comfortably for breathing. A younger infant typically breathes easiest when seated upright in an infant seat; an older infant may prefer lying prone, with the head of the bed raised. Also, provide sufficient rest periods to help conserve the child's energy for breathing.

Bronchitis An inflammation of the mucous membranes of the tracheobronchial tree, bronchitis occurs when an upper respiratory viral infection spreads to the bronchi. Most common in boys under age 4, bronchitis typically occurs during the winter.

Assessment
Initially, the child has a runny nose but no fever. Within 3 to 4 days of becoming infected, the child exhibits a dry, hacking cough, which becomes loose and congested within a few days. The child may have a low-grade fever and may be fatigued. A productive cough, which may persist for up to 10 days, is especially pronounced at night when the child is supine. Lung auscultation may reveal wheezing or fine crackles.

Medical management
A child with bronchitis typically does not require hospitalization. Cough suppressants may be prescribed if the child has trouble sleeping; analgesics are given to reduce fever. A cool-mist humidifier may help loosen bronchial secretions.

Nursing management
Direct interventions are aimed at relieving the child's symptoms. Encourage the parents to provide plenty of fluids and rest periods for the child. Teach them how to use a cool-mist humidifier.

Pneumonia Pneumonia is an acute inflammation of the lungs, including the smallest alveoli.

Etiology
The cause of pneumonia commonly is a viral or bacterial infection. The specific causative agent varies with the patient's age and, to some extent, the season. The following agents can cause pneumonia:
- *Escherichia coli, Klebsiella pneumoniae, Staphylococcus pneumoniae,* group A *Streptococcus,* and *Chlamydia* typically cause pneumonia in children from birth to age 3 months.
- *Streptococcus pneumoniae* and *Haemophilus influenzae* are typical causative agents in children ages 3 months to 5 years.
- RSV and other viruses are common causes of pneumonia in children ages 2 months to 5 years and causes pneumonia during the winter and spring.
- Parainfluenzae virus is a common cause in children ages 4 to 6 years and causes pneumonia during the fall.
- *Mycoplasma pneumoniae* affects children ages 5 to 12 and commonly causes pneumonia during the fall and winter.

Pathophysiology and classification
In all types of pneumonia, the lungs become inflamed and exudate accumulates within the alveoli.

Assessing and managing pneumonia

Pneumonia may be caused by such organisms as viruses, bacteria, mycoplasmas, rickettsiae, and fungi. This chart describes assessment findings and management of bacterial, viral, and mycoplasmal pneumonia.

TYPE	ASSESSMENT FINDINGS	MANAGEMENT
Viral pneumonia	• Insidious or sudden onset • Fever • Cough (may be productive or nonproductive) • Malaise	• Home management • Symptomatic measures, such as antipyretics, fluids, cool-mist vaporizer, and rest
Bacterial pneumonia	• Normally more severe than viral pneumonia • Sudden onset • Early signs: fever; headache; abdominal and chest pain; hacking, nonproductive cough; decreased breath sounds; and fine crackles • Late signs: productive cough, coarse crackles, and rhonchi • In severe cases: signs of respiratory distress, such as tachypnea, dyspnea, chest retractions, and hypoxia	• Home management: antipyretics, fluids, cool-mist vaporizer, rest, and oral antibiotics • Inpatient treatment (for children with respiratory distress or hypoxia): oral or rectal antipyretics, I.V. antibiotics, I.V. fluids, chest physiotherapy (to help break up consolidated exudate), oxygen (via nasal cannula or mist tent), and rest
Mycoplasmal pneumonia	• Insidious or sudden onset • Early signs: vague systemic signs and symptoms, such as fever, chills, headache, and malaise • Late signs: upper airway congestion, sore throat, nonproductive cough (which later becomes productive), and, possibly, fine crackles	• Home management • Antibiotics • Symptomatic measures: antipyretics, fluids, cool-mist vaporizer, and rest

Pneumonia may be classified by the portion of the lung affected:
• lobar pneumonia—consolidation of all or part of a lung lobe with exudate
• disseminated lobular pneumonia—patchy areas of infection involving both lungs, including the bronchi
• interstitial pneumonia—diffuse bronchiolitis and peribronchiolitis in both lungs, with inflammation of the alveolar walls.

Assessment and medical management

For clinical manifestations and treatment of viral, bacterial, and mycoplasmal pneumonia, see *Assessing and managing pneumonia.*

Nursing management

Nursing goals for the child with pneumonia include ensuring adequate hydration; promoting airway clearance and gas exchange; easing the work of breathing; and controlling fever.

To ensure adequate hydration, instruct parents to provide at least 8 to 10 glasses of clear fluids daily. If the child is hospitalized, encourage oral intake (if allowed) and maintain the I.V. fluid system.

To promote airway clearance and effective gas exchange, perform chest physiotherapy, as prescribed. Reposition the child at least every 2 hours to aid lung expansion and prevent stasis of pulmonary secretions. Administer supplemental oxygen, as prescribed. Give I.V. or oral fluids to help thin pulmonary secretions.

To ease the work of breathing, position the child comfortably for easy breathing (as described earlier in the section on "Bronchiolitis.") Provide frequent rest periods to help the child conserve energy for breathing.

To control fever, instruct the parents to administer acetaminophen if the child's temperature rises above 101.3° F (38.5° C).

Acute laryngotracheobronchitis

Acute LTB is an inflammation of the larynx, trachea, and bronchi. The most common cause of croup, acute LTB typically affects children under age 8 during the winter; it commonly is caused by a parainfluenzae virus.

Pathophysiology and assessment

Typically, acute LTB is preceded by an upper respiratory viral infection, which causes clear nasal discharge and nasal congestion. Symptoms progress slowly. The acute infection causes inflammation and subsequent narrowing of the larynx and trachea. With sufficient airway narrowing, the child has difficulty inspiring air. Inspiratory stridor, which sounds like high-pitched whistling, may result from partial obstruction of the trachea and larynx. The child also may have a barking cough or a hoarse cry. Other assessment findings include chest retractions, nasal flaring, tachypnea, and a low-grade fever.

Medical management

The child with minor signs and symptoms of acute LTB (such as periodic episodes of barking cough or stridor) may receive care at home. The physician may advise the parents to provide a cool-mist vaporizer and have the child inhale warm steam from a running shower to help ease respirations.

A child with continuous inspiratory stridor is hospitalized and uses a mist tent to help reduce airway inflammation and maintain a patent airway. Aerosolized racemic epinephrine (a bronchodilator) is prescribed if the child has significant airway obstruction. To support ventilation in a hypoxic child, oxygen is administered by nasal cannula or mist tent.

Because tachypnea increases fluid losses, the child with acute LTB has increased fluid requirements and typically receives I.V. fluids to maintain hydration. (Oral fluids are contraindicated because of the risk of aspiration.)

Nursing management

Ensuring a patent airway, easing the work of breathing, and maintaining hydration are the primary nursing goals for the child with acute LTB.

To ensure a patent airway, maintain the mist tent system. Keep the ice reservoir full to ensure high levels of cool humidity. Closely monitor the child's respiratory status. Immediately report signs of increased respiratory distress and impending total airway obstruction, such as rising heart and respiratory rates, worsening chest retractions, and increased restlessness or anxiety.

To help the child conserve energy to ease the work of breathing, alternate nursing care activities with frequent rest periods. Encourage parents to stay with the child to reduce anxiety.

To maintain adequate hydration, provide sufficient fluids and maintain the I.V. fluid system.

Acute epiglottitis

Acute epiglottitis is a potentially life-threatening inflammation of the epiglottis. Most common in children ages 3 to 8 during the winter, acute epiglottitis commonly results from *H. influenzae* infection.

Pathophysiology

The acute bacterial infection causes inflammation and potentially fatal obstruction of the epiglottis. With sufficient airway narrowing, the child has difficulty inspiring air.

Assessment

Acute epiglottitis has a sudden onset. Findings typically include inspiratory stridor, dysphagia (difficulty swallowing), drooling, high fever, tachycardia, tachypnea, and restlessness. Unlike acute LTB, acute epiglottitis does not cause coughing. The child typically assumes an upright position to aid breathing.

The diagnosis is confirmed by visual inspection of the child's throat, which appears red and inflamed, with a large, red, edematous epiglottis. However, because such inspection may cause complete airway obstruction, the throat is examined only if emergency equipment is available for intubation.

Medical management

Medical goals include maintaining a patent airway (through intubation, if necessary) and controlling the bacterial infection (for example, with I.V. antibiotic therapy).

Nursing management

To reduce airway inflammation, provide highly humidified air and administer I.V. medications, as prescribed. Continuously monitor the child for signs of increased respiratory distress.

Because acute epiglottitis can be fatal, be sure to provide support to the child and parents to ease anxiety and allay their fears.

Asthma

Also called reactive airway disease, asthma is a chronic disorder characterized by hypersensitivity of the trachea and bronchi. A leading cause of chronic illness in children, asthma typically first appears between ages 2 and 8.

Asthma affects more boys than girls. However, the severity of the disease is not related to sex.

Etiology

Both hereditary and allergic factors are suspected causes of asthma. The family or child may have a history of atopic disease, such as allergic rhinitis, eczema, or asthma.

Factors that may trigger an asthmatic episode include inhaled irritants (for example, smoke, fumes, or cold air), viral upper respiratory infections, and exercise.

Pathophysiology

During an acute asthmatic episode, the airways overrespond to stimuli (airway hypersensitivity). Associated pathophysiologic responses include mucosal edema, accumulation of thick bronchial secretions, and bronchial spasm. These events contribute to airway constriction (narrowing) and obstruction. Gas trapping occurs in areas obstructed by thick bronchial secretions.

Assessment

Clinical findings in the child with asthma occur in two stages—early and late. *Early* signs of asthma include:
- a hacking, nonproductive cough
- wheezing during expiration (The airways naturally shorten and contract during expiration; because they constrict more during an asthmatic episode, the child has most difficulty during the expiratory phase of respiration.)
- chest retractions (The child uses accessory muscles to exert greater force—in this case, during expiration.)
- dyspnea, which is most prominent during expiration
- a prolonged expiratory phase.
   Late signs of asthma include:
- audible wheezing during both inspiration and expiration
- coarse rhonchi and crackles
- ventilatory difficulty
- tachypnea
- decreased breath sounds
- hypoxia and hypercapnia
- anxiety and restlessness
- tachycardia
- difficulty speaking.

Diagnosis

The diagnosis of asthma rests on a family history of atopic disease, the child's physical findings, and characteristic abnormal pulmonary function test results. Asthmatic children have decreased peak expiratory flow rates even when otherwise free from respiratory difficulty.

Medical management

When asthma first manifests, the child is managed at home. To control acute bronchial spasm and edema, bronchodilators (via metered-dose inhaler) and nebulized or oral corticosteroids are prescribed. If symptoms persist, the child requires further medical attention. A child who fails to respond to conventional medical therapy for acute asthma develops status asthmaticus, which may lead to respiratory failure.

The goals of medical treatment during an asthmatic episode are to maintain airway patency, hydration, and ventilation. To maintain a patent airway, bronchodilators and corticosteroids may be administered.

To ensure hydration, the child receives I.V. fluids, which help thin bronchiolar secretions. The hypoxic child also receives oxygen to support ventilation.

Nursing management

Nursing goals include maintaining a patent airway, promoting gas exchange, and promoting easier breathing.

To maintain a patent airway, monitor the child's respiratory status and report signs of increased respiratory distress. Also monitor the effectiveness of drug therapy.

To promote gas exchange, monitor arterial oxygen saturation levels and administer supplemental oxygen (if prescribed). Ensure adequate hydration by providing fluids and maintaining the I.V. fluid system.

Hypoxia and difficulty breathing may make the child anxious and restless, further compromising the respiratory effort. To reduce anxiety and fear, provide a calm atmosphere. Explain all procedures to the child. Encourage parents to stay with the child. Before discharge, teach the child and parents asthma home-management skills. (See *Managing asthma at home: A teaching plan,* page 252.)

Cystic fibrosis

Cystic fibrosis is a hereditary disorder of the exocrine glands, causing those glands to produce abnormally thick mucus secretions. Transmitted by an autosomal recessive inheritance pattern, the disease shortens the life expectancy to a median of 27 years. Cystic fibrosis occurs predominantly in Caucasians and affects both sexes equally.

Pathophysiology and assessment

Abnormal amounts of thick mucus lead to problems in multiple body systems. Respiratory and gastrointestinal (GI) effects cause much of the morbidity associated with cystic fibrosis. (For GI, hematologic, reproductive, and integumentary effects, see *How cystic fibrosis affects other body systems,* page 253.)

In the respiratory system, mucus accumulates within the bronchioles, causing bronchial obstruction, ventilatory problems, and bacterial

Managing asthma at home: A teaching plan

A chronic disorder, asthma necessitates comprehensive teaching to help the child and family prevent and cope with acute asthmatic episodes. This chart lists teaching goals for the asthmatic child and family, along with corresponding content.

GOAL	TEACHING CONTENT
Prevent asthmatic episodes	• Avoid known allergens, especially smoke. • Monitor the child's pulmonary function at home. • Administer cromolyn sodium via metered-dose inhaler or nebulizer. (This drug interferes with the release of allergic mediators from bronchial mast cells, thereby preventing the secretion and release of histamine and reducing the stimulus for bronchospasm; however, it does not reverse bronchospasm once it begins.) • Ensure adequate hydration and administer inhaled bronchodilators when prodromal phase begins, before it progresses to an acute asthmatic episode. Prodromal symptoms include changes in peak flow values, nocturnal cough with no other symptoms of upper respiratory infection, irritability, and itching of the face, chest, and neck.
Teach the child over age 4 how to use a metered-dose inhaler (or other drug delivery device, such as Inspirese)	• Teach the child to shake the inhaler well before using. Then, have child exhale deeply, and activate medication during the next inhalation. Have child hold the breath for 5 to 10 seconds after activating, then exhale fully.
Improve the child's ventilatory effort	• Have the child perform breathing exercises—pursed-lip breathing and bubble blowing—to improve expiratory effort. • Also, have child engage in regular exercise (such as swimming or bicycle riding).

overgrowth. Signs of respiratory dysfunction include wheezing and a chronic, dry, nonproductive cough.

If bronchial obstruction leads to atelectasis, the patient exhibits decreased breath sounds, hypoxia, and hypercapnia. If bronchial infection arises, expect fever, productive cough, tachypnea, coarse rhonchi, and green or yellow sputum. Small pulmonary blebs may rupture spontaneously, causing pneumothorax. Rupture of small pulmonary capillaries leads to hemoptysis (blood-tinged sputum). Repeated pulmonary infections cause bronchial fibrosis. Increased pulmonary vascular resistance results in pulmonary hypertension and right-sided heart failure (cor pulmonale).

Cystic fibrosis also leads to obstructive emphysema accompanied by chronic hypoxia and hypercapnia. Long-term use of accessory muscles causes barrel chest. Chronic hypoxia results in finger clubbing.

Diagnosis

Genetic testing may identify asymptomatic carriers of cystic fibrosis. Prenatal diagnosis of cystic fibrosis also is possible through genetic testing of the parents and fetus.

Cystic fibrosis is assumed in any infant born with meconium ileus or in any child that exhibits failure to thrive and experiences repeated episodes of pneumonia. The sweat chloride test confirms the diagnosis

How cystic fibrosis affects other body systems

Besides causing serious respiratory effects, cystic fibrosis induces changes in other body systems.

Gastrointestinal system

Meconium ileus (mucus obstruction of the terminal ileus after birth) is the first obvious sign of cystic fibrosis in an infant. In an older child, thick mucus causes partial bowel obstruction, leading to nausea, colicky abdominal pain, and abdominal distention.

Mucus also obstructs the pancreatic ducts, thus preventing secretion of the digestive enzymes necessary for fat and protein digestion. Related signs include steatorrhea (greasy, bulky, foul-smelling stools caused by undigested fat in the stool), organic failure to thrive (caused by malabsorption of fats and proteins), and deficiency of the fat-soluble vitamins A, D, E, and K.

Hematologic system

Vitamin K deficiency may cause hypoprothrombinemia (deficiency of prothrombin, which is necessary for clotting). Therefore, a child with cystic fibrosis may bruise easily and have chronic mild anemia. Protein malabsorption and iron deficiency also contribute to anemia.

Reproductive system

Mucus obstructs the vas deferens in males and the cervix in females, causing fertility problems.

Integumentary system

The child's saliva and sweat contain abnormally large amounts of sodium and chloride, and the skin may taste salty. Excessive sweating (caused by hot weather, exercise, or fever) may lead to sodium depletion.

---

of cystic fibrosis. However, this test is done only in infants over age 6 months because younger infants do not produce enough sweat for the test to be valid.

Medical management

Medical goals for the child with cystic fibrosis are to promote airway clearance, control respiratory infections, and aid digestive function. Lung transplantation now is available for patients with advanced cystic fibrosis, thereby extending life expectancy and changing the goals for their social activities.

To promote airway clearance, the child receives adequate hydration to help thin bronchial secretions. Bronchodilators may be used to combat airway narrowing and help the child expel mucus. Breathing exercises and chest physiotherapy (at least four times daily) help to break up mucus obstructions and drain mucus from the bronchioles.

The child with an acute pulmonary infection receives I.V. and inhaled antibiotic therapy—typically, with third-generation synthetic penicillins or cephalosporins and aminoglycosides.

To promote digestive function, the child receives replacement pancreatic enzymes and vitamins and eats a low-fat, moderate-protein, high-carbohydrate diet. Total parenteral nutrition or nasogastric feedings may be given during sleeping hours to promote physical growth.

Nursing management

Nursing management of the child with cystic fibrosis includes promoting airway clearance, controlling pulmonary infection, ensuring adequate nutrition, and maximizing oxygenation.

To promote airway clearance, perform chest physiotherapy, as prescribed. The best time for chest physiotherapy is before meals. After chest physiotherapy is performed, encourage the child to breathe deeply and cough. To prevent stasis of pulmonary secretions, advise the child to change position at least every 2 hours.

To control pulmonary infection, administer I.V. medications, as prescribed. Because aminoglycosides may cause renal toxicity, collect urine samples and monitor laboratory studies of renal function, such as blood urea nitrogen and creatinine clearance values. Alert other health care personnel to draw peak and trough blood aminoglycoside levels, if the child is receiving this drug. A trough blood sample is drawn immediately before the dose is given; a peak sample, 30 to 60 minutes after the dose is given. Be sure to monitor peak and trough levels.

To promote adequate nutrition, administer pancreatic enzymes with every meal and snack. If the child has trouble swallowing the large capsules, sprinkle the capsule contents over a small portion of the child's food. Administer vitamins once daily. Help the child choose low-fat, high-carbohydrate foods, such as fruits, vegetables, pretzels, crackers, breads, cereals, and sherbet.

To maximize oxygenation, advise the child to perform activities as tolerated but to avoid exertion and fatigue, which increase oxygen demands. Be sure to provide emotional support to help the child and family cope with chronic illness.

STUDY ACTIVITIES

Short answer

1. How can oxygen be administered to a child with bronchiolitis?

_____

2. Differentiate the signs and symptoms of acute LTB from the signs and symptoms of acute epiglottitis.

_____

_____

_____

3. What are the three pathophysiologic responses associated with airway hypersensitivity in asthma?

_____

_____

4. How is cystic fibrosis diagnosed?

_____

_____

Matching related elements

Match the symptom on the left with its description on the right.

5. ___ Hemoptysis   **A.** Alveolar collapse

6. ___ Stridor   **B.** High-pitched whistling noise

7. ___ Dyspnea   **C.** Use of accessory breathing muscles

8. ___ Chest retractions   **D.** Labored breathing

9. ___ Atelectasis   **E.** Right-sided heart failure secondary to increased pulmonary vascular resistance

10. ___ Cor pulmonale   **F.** Blood-tinged sputum

Multiple choice

11. When assessing a child who has bronchiolitis, the nurse would expect which finding?
   A. Barking cough and stridor
   B. Finger clubbing
   C. Barrel chest
   D. Productive cough

12. Which information is most important for the nurse to include when formulating a teaching plan for a child with asthma?
   A. How to detect and treat symptoms early
   B. How to use Inspirex to expand lung volume
   C. How to perform chest physiotherapy
   D. How to ensure a high-carbohydrate diet

13. What is the main purpose of supplemental pancreatic enzymes for a child with cystic fibrosis?
   A. They promote adequate rest.
   B. They prevent intestinal mucus accumulation.
   C. They promote absorption of nutrients and fats.
   D. They prevent meconium ileus.

ANSWERS **Short answer**

   1. The child with bronchiolitis may receive oxygen by nasal cannula or mist tent.

2. Acute LTB has a slow onset and causes inspiratory stridor, a barking cough or hoarse cry, chest retractions, nasal flaring, tachypnea, and a low-grade fever. Epiglottis has a sudden onset and causes inspiratory stridor, dysphagia, drooling, high fever, tachycardia, tachypnea, and restlessness; cough is absent.

3. Pathophysiologic responses associated with airway hypersensitivity in asthma include mucosal edema, accumulation of thick bronchial secretions, and bronchial spasm.

4. Cystic fibrosis may be diagnosed prenatally through genetic testing of the parents and fetus. After birth, the sweat chloride test confirms the diagnosis.

Matching related elements

5. F

6. B

7. D

8. C

9. A

10. E

Multiple choice

11. D. Bronchiolitis causes a productive cough. A barking cough is more characteristic of acute LTB. Finger clubbing and barrel chest occur with chronic respiratory dysfunction, such as cystic fibrosis.

12. A. The nurse should teach the child and family how to recognize early signs of an impending asthmatic episode and how to manage the episode. Inspirex and chest physiotherapy are not used to manage asthma. The asthmatic child requires no dietary modifications, unless food allergies exist.

13. C. Pancreatic enzymes help the child digest fats and proteins. They have no effect on promoting rest or on preventing mucus accumulation or meconium ileus.

CHAPTER 19

Gastrointestinal disorders

OBJECTIVES After studying this chapter, the reader should be able to:

1. Describe the causes, pathophysiology, and clinical manifestations of dehydration in children.

2. Discuss medical and nursing management of the dehydrated child.

3. Identify the causes, pathophysiology, and clinical manifestations of vomiting, acute diarrhea, pyloric stenosis, Hirschsprung's disease, and inflammatory bowel disease.

4. Discuss medical and nursing management of children with these disorders.

OVERVIEW OF CONCEPTS The major function of the gastrointestinal (GI) system is to absorb, break down, and utilize nutrients for fuel and energy. In children, GI dysfunction occurs nearly as often as respiratory dysfunction.

Diarrhea and vomiting, two of the most common GI disorders, can cause major fluid and electrolyte losses, which may lead to serious fluid and electrolyte imbalances. To provide high-quality care for a child with these disorders, the nurse must be familiar with the principles of fluid and electrolyte balance as well as the pathophysiology of the specific imbalance. (For information on fluid and electrolyte balance, see Chapter 16, Management principles.)

This chapter delineates the pathophysiology, assessment, and management of dehydration, vomiting, and acute diarrhea. It explores two congenital disorders—pyloric stenosis and Hirschsprung's disease. Finally, the chapter investigates inflammatory bowel disease (IBD), a chronic disorder.

Dehydration In dehydration, excessive water is lost from body tissues. Also called fluid volume deficit, dehydration occurs secondary to several clinical disorders, including vomiting and diarrhea.

Pathophysiology and classification

Dehydration may be classified as isotonic, hypotonic, or hypertonic.

In *isotonic* dehydration, fluids and electrolytes are lost in equal proportions, but the patient maintains a normal serum sodium level (135 to 145 mEq/liter). Hypovolemic shock is a potential complication resulting from large fluid losses in isotonic dehydration.

In *hypotonic* dehydration, electrolytes are lost more rapidly than fluids, and the serum sodium level falls below 130 mEq/liter. Water then shifts into the intracellular spaces, further reducing extracellular fluid (ECF) volume. For this reason, hypotonic dehydration is more likely to cause hypovolemic shock than isotonic dehydration.

In *hypertonic* dehydration, fluid losses exceed electrolyte losses, and the serum sodium level is abnormally high (above 150 mEq/liter). Water shifts into the extracellular spaces, thereby increasing ECF volume. Therefore, hypertonic dehydration is less likely to cause hypovolemic shock than the other two forms of dehydration.

Assessment

Signs and symptoms of dehydration vary with the severity of the fluid loss. To estimate fluid loss, weigh the child daily, compare to baseline weight, and determine the percentage of weight lost. For example, the child with a 5% weight loss has 5% dehydration, which reflects mild dehydration. (For details on assessing the dehydrated child, see *Assessment findings in dehydration*.)

Medical management

The child with mild to moderate dehydration who is alert and able to ingest oral fluids receives an oral rehydration solution. Such a solution provides fluids and electrolytes (sodium, chloride, and potassium) in a balanced formula. Pedialyte and Lytren, for example, are available without a prescription at most drugstores and grocery stores.

For the child with isotonic or hypotonic dehydration, lost fluids are replaced over 24 hours (in addition to the child's usual fluid requirements). Half the amount of estimated fluids are replaced over the first 8 hours; the remaining half, over the next 16 hours. With hypertonic dehydration, lost fluids are replaced more slowly (over 48 hours) to avoid sudden decreases in the serum sodium level.

Children with severe or critical dehydration and those with moderate dehydration who cannot ingest fluids orally receive parenteral fluid therapy. Isotonic fluids, such as dextrose 5% in Ringer's lactated solution or dextrose 5% in 0.9% sodium chloride solution, are given according to the replacement principles described above. If necessary, potassium can be added to intravenous (I.V.) fluids once the child establishes sufficient urine output.

The physician may prescribe antiemetic agents (such as Compazine) if dehydration results from nausea and vomiting secondary to chemotherapy, administration of narcotic analgesia, or anesthesia.

Nursing management

Nursing goals for the dehydrated child include detecting changes in hydration, perfusion, and intravascular volume and providing replacement and maintenance fluids.

Assessment findings in dehydration

Signs and symptoms of dehydration vary according to the severity of the child's fluid volume deficit. To gauge the degree of dehydration, compare the child's weight to the baseline weight. For example, a child who loses 10% of baseline weight has 10%, or moderate, dehydration. This chart correlates assessment findings with the degree of dehydration.

ASSESSMENT FACTOR	MILD DEHYDRATION (5%)	MODERATE DEHYDRATION (10%)	SEVERE DEHYDRATION (15%)	CRITICAL DEHYDRATION (20%)
Heart rate	• Within normal limits	• Above normal	• Above normal	• Above normal
Blood pressure	• Within normal limits	• Within normal limits	• Low to normal	• Decreased, with low central venous pressure
Pulse	• Normal in quality	• Peripheral pulses 2+	• Peripheral pulses 1+	• Peripheral pulses 0
Capillary refill	• Less than 3 seconds	• More than 3 seconds	• More than 4 seconds	• More than 5 seconds
Skin	• Warm and pink	• Cool and pale	• Cool and mottled	• Cold and gray
Urine output	• Below 2 ml/kg/hour	• Below 1 ml/kg/hour	• Below 0.5 ml/kg/hour	• Absent (oliguria)
Mucous membranes	• Moist	• Dry; no tear formation	• Dry; no tear formation	• Parched; no tear formation
Neurologic findings	• Irritability	• Irritability	• Lethargy	• Decreased level of consciousness
Fontanels	• Flat	• Slightly depressed	• Sunken	• Sunken

To detect changes in the child's hydration status, monitor fluid intake and output carefully; check urine specific gravity; weigh the child daily; monitor skin turgor and moistness of mucous membranes; and check fontanels for bulging. Also, monitor crucial laboratory values— serum osmolarity, blood urea nitrogen (BUN), and serum sodium level. With dehydration, serum osmolarity increases and BUN level may rise. Depending on the form of dehydration, the child's serum sodium level may be normal, above normal, or below normal.

To monitor the child's perfusion status, check the heart rate, skin temperature and color, capillary refill time, and peripheral pulses. To monitor intravascular volume status, monitor the heart rate, blood pressure, and central venous pressure.

As prescribed, administer I.V. fluids. Calculate and replace ongoing fluid losses, as prescribed.

Vomiting Vomiting—the forcible expulsion of gastric contents —may be caused by an infection or other physiologic problems. Common causes of vomiting include gastroenteritis (inflammation of the stomach and intestines caused by bacterial or viral invasion or bacterial enterotoxins), appendicitis, intestinal obstruction, cancer chemotherapy, and emotional upset. Continued vomiting places the child at risk for dehydration, hyponatremia, hypokalemia, hypochloremia, and metabolic alkalosis.

Pathophysiology

The exact mechanism is unknown, but it appears to involve stimulation of the true vomiting center by the chemoreceptor trigger zone, cerebral cortex, hypothalamus, and midbrain via the sympathetic visceral, vagal visceral, and vestibulocerebellar afferent pathways.

Assessment

Vomiting typically is accompanied by nausea, tachycardia, sweating, and pallor. The content of the vomitus may have clinical significance. For example, fecal matter in the vomitus may indicate a lower bowel obstruction or peritonitis. Bright red blood or coffee-ground vomitus suggests GI bleeding; bile may indicate an obstruction.

Medical management

The physician determines and treats the underlying cause of vomiting. A viral or bacterial infection calls for fluid replacement therapy (as discussed in the section on "Dehydration" above) and, possibly, antibiotic therapy. If the child has severe vomiting, oral fluids are restricted to prevent further vomiting and I.V. fluids are administered. Vomiting caused by GI obstruction may necessitate surgery to correct the obstruction.

Nursing management

Assess the nature of the vomiting, including its onset, quality, and amount. Continuously monitor the child's fluid and electrolyte status.

Acute diarrhea

Acute diarrhea is an increase in the frequency of bowel movements. Stools are loose and may consist entirely of fluid. Acute diarrhea is most common in infants and young children.

Acute diarrhea in young children commonly is caused by a rotavirus. Other causes include toxins, IBD, parasites, and bacterial and other viral infections.

Pathophysiology

Frequent loose stools irritate the GI tract, causing inflammation and decreased nutrient absorption. Loss of fluids and bicarbonate in stools puts the child at risk for dehydration and metabolic acidosis.

Assessment

The child with acute diarrhea may have a fever, anorexia, irritability, and lethargy. The perianal area may become excoriated from contact with stool. With moderate to severe diarrhea, the child may become dehydrated.

Diagnosis rests on the child's signs and symptoms, a complete white blood cell (WBC) count, stool examination for occult blood, and stool culture. The stool also is inspected microscopically for fat, glucose, ova, parasites, and neutrophils.

Medical management

As indicated, the child with acute diarrhea is treated for dehydration. Some physicians prefer to restrict solid foods to allow the bowel to rest. To maintain fluid and electrolyte balance, the child receives an oral rehydration solution and other clear fluids. (Milk products are contraindicated during moderate or severe diarrhea.) With severe diarrhea, all oral fluids may be restricted and the child may receive fluids parenterally.

As diarrhea abates, the child takes clear fluids. Then, for the next few days, the BRATTY diet may be given. This diet consists of *B* for bananas, *R* for rice, *A* for applesauce, *T* for tea, *T* for toast, and *Y* for plain yogurt.

The child may resume the usual diet gradually if it is tolerated without a return of loose stools. Some infants cannot tolerate milk products after recovering from acute infectious diarrhea; they may receive soy-based products instead.

Nursing management

Nursing goals for the child with acute diarrhea include:
- providing fluids
- monitoring electrolyte balance
- preventing perineal irritation
- preventing the spread of infection
- conserving the child's energy and providing rest.

Provide fluids as described in the section on "Dehydration." Also monitor serum electrolyte values.

To prevent perineal irritation, thoroughly clean the child's perineum with mild soap and water after each bowel movement. Allow the area to air dry.

To prevent the spread of infection, place the hospitalized child on isolation precautions. If the child is at home, instruct the parents to isolate the child from friends and visitors.

To conserve the child's energy and provide rest, cluster nursing care activities and arrange for frequent rest periods and quiet time to reduce the child's metabolic demands.

Pyloric stenosis

Pyloric stenosis is an acute, congenital, obstructive disorder characterized by narrowing of the pyloric sphincter. This disorder is more common in males than females. Its precise cause has not been determined.

Pathophysiology

The pyloric sphincter at the outlet of the stomach becomes hypertrophic and narrows. The resulting obstruction prevents emptying of stomach contents into the small intestine.

Assessment

Signs of pyloric stenosis appear soon after birth. They include:
- vomiting shortly after a feeding, progressing to projectile vomiting; vomitus contains undigested formula or breast milk
- hunger behaviors, such as irritability and sucking vigorously on a pacifier or the fists
- weight loss
- visible peristaltic waves over the gastric area
- a palpable mass to the right of the umbilicus
- evidence of dehydration.

Laboratory findings typically include increased serum osmolarity; below normal serum sodium, chloride, and potassium levels; and arterial blood gas values indicating metabolic alkalosis.

Diagnosis rests on the infant's history and clinical findings. The pyloric muscle may be palpated as a small, olive-sized mass.

Medical management

Pyloric stenosis is corrected surgically to allow normal bowel function. Preoperatively, fluid and electrolyte balance are restored. The infant receives nothing by mouth (NPO); a nasogastric (NG) tube is inserted to provide gastric decompression.

Nursing management

Preoperative nursing goals including preventing further dehydration, restoring fluid balance, and preparing the child and parents for surgery.

To prevent further dehydration and restore fluid balance, see the section on "Dehydration" above. Also monitor the NG drainage system and note the amount and characteristics of drainage. Be sure to maintain patency of the NG tube. Prepare the child for surgery, as prescribed. (For information on preparing parents for a child's surgery, see Chapter 16, Management principles.)

After the child returns from surgery, provide care similar to that for any child who has undergone abdominal surgery (as discussed in Chapter 16, Management principles). Keep the infant on NPO status for 4 to 8 hours after the operation. As prescribed, initiate oral feedings, starting with clear fluids for the first 24 hours and advancing to full-strength formula. A child who can tolerate full, age-appropriate feedings is ready for discharge.

Hirschsprung's disease

Hirschsprung's disease is the congenital absence of autonomic parasympathetic ganglia in the smooth-muscle wall of the colon. The disorder is more common in males than females. Its exact cause is unknown.

Pathophysiology

Lack of ganglion cells prevents innervation to areas of the affected bowel, causing poor or absent peristalsis in the involved segment of the colon. Intestinal contents accumulate proximal to the affected bowel areas, thereby causing abdominal distention. The internal anal sphincter does not relax completely, causing incomplete evacuation of stool, liquids, and gas.

Assessment

Findings vary with the age at which the child's symptoms first appear. In a neonate, assessment may reveal failure to pass meconium, poor feeding, bile-stained vomitus, and abdominal distention. In an older infant, expect constipation; passage of ribbon-like, foul-smelling stool; abdominal distention; visible peristaltic waves; palpable fecal masses; anemia and hypoproteinemia secondary to malabsorption; and failure to thrive.

Diagnosis rests on clinical findings, including constipation. A barium enema reveals dilation of the proximal colon and narrowing of the distal colon. A rectal biopsy reveals lack of ganglia.

Medical management

The child with Hirschsprung's disease requires a temporary colostomy and resection of the affected bowel. Preoperative preparation includes a diet of clear fluids for 24 to 48 hours; bowel emptying with enemas or oral solutions; and reduction of the normal bowel flora with systemic antibiotics. Postoperative medical management resembles that for any child who has undergone abdominal surgery. The child is fitted with a colostomy appliance as soon as possible after surgery.

At approximately age 1, the child undergoes reanastomosis of the distal and proximal bowel.

Nursing management

After surgery, monitor the condition of the child's colostomy. Initially, the colostomy appears beefy-red, protruding, and edematous; a small amount of serous drainage is normal. A bluish colostomy indicates compromised blood supply to the exposed bowel loop; report this finding to the physician immediately. Over time, edema diminishes and the colostomy becomes pinkish-red.

Once bowel sounds return, provide a diet of clear fluids, then advance to a full diet, as appropriate for the child's age.

Prepare the parents for the appearance of the infant's colostomy. Reassure them that the stoma is not painful and will become less pronounced over time. Teach them how to perform colostomy care. Instruct them to change the colostomy appliance if it becomes loose or leaks. Advise them to clean the skin around the colostomy gently, using mild soap and water, and then apply a skin sealer and allow it to dry. Teach them to apply stoma paste around the base of the stoma, then gently press the appliance in place and secure it snugly.

Inflammatory bowel disease

IBD is a collective term for two chronic GI disorders—ulcerative colitis and Crohn's disease. These disorders share a similar etiology and cause similar signs and symptoms, although their pathophysiology and prognoses differ. The exact cause of IBD is unknown. Emotional stress seems to exacerbate signs and symptoms.

The incidence of IBD is higher among Caucasians, European and North American Jews, persons in higher socioeconomic groups, and those living in urban areas. Children with a positive family history also are at increased risk.

Typically, IBD has an onset during early adulthood. However, in approximately 15% of cases, onset occurs during childhood—typically, preadolescence.

Pathophysiology

In ulcerative colitis, inflammatory changes occur in the mucosal lining of the colon and rectum. The lining becomes ulcerated and cannot absorb nutrients, fluid, and electrolytes effectively.

Crohn's disease typically affects the terminal portions of the ileum. All layers of the intestinal mucosa become ulcerated. Unlike ulcerative colitis, in which the lesions are symmetric and continuous in the colon and rectum, the lesions characteristic of Crohn's disease are asymmetrical and patchy along the entire GI tract. Malabsorption is more common and more severe than in ulcerative colitis.

Both ulcerative colitis and Crohn's disease have been associated with an increased risk of bowel cancer.

Assessment

Signs and symptoms of ulcerative colitis and Crohn's disease differ somewhat.

Ulcerative colitis

Findings vary with the amount of bowel affected and whether the disease involves continuous colitis or a pattern of acute exacerbations and remissions. In a patient with continuous colitis, expect chronic diarrhea. In a patient who has acute exacerbations, expect severe, bloody diarrhea. Other assessment findings may include:
• rectal bleeding
• moderate weight loss during periods of diarrhea
• mild growth delays
• delayed sexual maturation.

Cramping, abdominal pain precedes diarrhea. The child may have 20 to 30 stools over a 24-hour period; diarrhea typically continues throughout the night. During acute exacerbations, the child is at risk for dehydration and metabolic acidosis. Malabsorption and GI bleeding may cause anemia.

Crohn's disease

This form of IBD causes mild to moderate diarrhea, intense and intermittent abdominal cramps aggravated by eating, anal or perineal fissures, anorexia, severe growth delays, and delayed sexual maturation. Acute dehydration and electrolyte disturbances are less common than in ulcerative colitis.

Diagnosis

IBD is diagnosed from the patient's history and clinical findings, radiography, endoscopy, and mucosal biopsy revealing an inflammatory response.

Medical management

Some children with IBD have a temporary colostomy to allow the bowel to rest. In ulcerative colitis, the entire area of the affected bowel may be resected and a permanent colostomy or ileostomy performed to halt the disease process and to prevent colon cancer.

In Crohn's disease, however, such surgery is avoided because removal of affected bowel areas may cause disease recurrence in other bowel regions. Also, surgery does not reduce the risk of colon cancer in patients with Crohn's disease.

Ulcerative colitis generally responds better than Crohn's disease to medical management. Drug therapy may include sulfasalazine to decrease exacerbations of the disease and corticosteroids to reduce the inflammatory response.

Dietary management is critical and aims to replace lost nutrients and correct nutritional deficits. Vitamin and mineral supplements are given. A severely malnourished child may need parenteral nutrition during acute exacerbations; a child with less severe signs and symptoms may receive enteral nutrition. During remission, the child eats a high-protein, high-calorie, low-fiber diet.

Nursing management

Nursing goals for the child with IBD include:
• preparing the child and family for surgery (as needed)
• decreasing diarrhea
• providing adequate nutrition
• ensuring sufficient rest
• teaching the child and parents about the disease and its management.
If surgery is scheduled, prepare the child and family for the surgical experience and for the colostomy or ileostomy.

During periods of severe diarrhea, the child is at risk for dehydration and metabolic acidosis. Give I.V. replacement fluids and electrolytes, as prescribed. To prevent severe dehydration and further mucosal damage, diarrhea must be alleviated. To rest the bowel, maintain the child's NPO status and administer corticosteroids, as prescribed.

During acute exacerbations, administer parenteral or enteral nutrition, as prescribed. Total parenteral nutrition (TPN) provides carbohydrates (in the form of concentrated, or hypertonic, glucose), protein, fat, and essential vitamins intravenously. Initially, the child may require insulin to help metabolize the concentrated glucose administered in TPN. Enteral nutrition delivers a high-protein, high-carbohydrate formula to the stomach via a nasogastric tube.

Before administering the enteral formula, make sure the tube is positioned properly in the stomach. Deliver the formula by slow drip, using an enteral feeding pump. Ensure a steady administration rate; a significant rate decrease or interruption in flow puts the child at risk for hypoglycemia.

Monitor the child's tolerance for the formula by observing for abdominal distention and checking the frequency and consistency of stools. To monitor the child's response to TPN, check temperature, weight, and urine glucose and serum electrolyte levels. Also, monitor the WBC count because TPN increases the risk of infection. Be sure to record fluid intake and output.

During remission, when the child can tolerate oral intake, provide a diet of high-protein, high-calorie foods, such as milk shakes, pudding, ice cream, and custards. Avoid giving raw fruits or vegetables and whole grain breads because the high fiber content may exacerbate IBD. Other poorly tolerated foods include nuts, popcorn, peas, beans, and highly seasoned or spicy foods.

If the child has a poor appetite, encourage the child to consume an adequate amount of food. Give small, frequent meals, which are tolerated better than three large meals a day. To reduce pain resulting from mouth ulcers (which are common in children with IBD), use topical anesthetics and provide bland foods.

During acute exacerbations, the child is physically exhausted because of water and nutrient depletion. Be sure to cluster nursing activities and provide a quiet, nonstimulating environment as well as frequent rest periods to promote rest.

Teach the child and parents about dietary management. Stress the importance of complying with drug and diet therapy, even during remissions. Provide emotional support to help the child adjust to the effects of chronic malnutrition—small stature, underweight, and delayed sexual development.

STUDY ACTIVITIES

Short answer

1. Compare and contrast isotonic dehydration, hypotonic dehydration, and hypertonic dehydration.

_____

_____

_____

2. Why is hypovolemic shock less likely to result from hypertonic dehydration than from isotonic or hypotonic dehydration?

_____

_____

_____

3. Describe the pathophysiology of Hirschsprung's disease.

_____

_____

_____

4. Compare and contrast the signs and symptoms of ulcerative colitis with those of Crohn's disease.

_____

_____

_____

Multiple choice

5. Which assessment finding most strongly suggests pyloric stenosis?
  A. Abdominal rigidity
  B. Substernal retractions
  C. Visible peristaltic waves
  D. Marked abdominal distention

6. Which assessment finding would the nurse expect in a child with 5% dehydration?
  A. Cool skin
  B. Increased perspiration
  C. Decreased urine output
  D. Increased heart rate

7. Which assessment finding is most common in children with ulcerative colitis?
  A. Profuse diarrhea
  B. Intense abdominal cramps
  C. Abdominal distention
  D. Anal fissures

8. What is the usual carbohydrate component of TPN?
  A. Hypertonic glucose solution
  B. Concentrated dextrose solution
  C. High-calorie formula
  D. Low-fiber foods

ANSWERS   **Short answer**

1. In isotonic dehydration, fluids and electrolytes are lost in equal proportions but the patient maintains a normal serum sodium level (135 to 145 mEq/liter). In hypotonic dehydration, electrolytes are lost more rapidly than fluids, and the serum sodium level falls below 130 mEq/liter. In hypertonic dehydration, fluid losses exceed sodium losses, and the serum sodium level is abnormally high (above 150 mEq/liter).

2. Hypovolemic shock is less likely to result from hypertonic dehydration because water shifts into the extracellular spaces, thereby increasing ECF volume.

3. In Hirschsprung's disease, lack of ganglion cells prevents innervation to areas of the affected bowel, causing poor or absent peristalsis in the involved segment of the colon. Intestinal contents accumulate proximal to the affected bowel areas, thereby causing abdominal distention. The internal anal sphincter does not relax completely and causes incomplete evacuation of stool, liquids, and gas.

4. In ulcerative colitis, the patient typically has rectal bleeding; cramping abdominal pain preceding diarrhea; severe, bloody diarrhea during acute exacerbations; chronic diarrhea with continuous colitis; moderate weight loss during periods of diarrhea; mild growth delays; and delayed sexual maturation.

In Crohn's disease, the patient has mild to moderate diarrhea, intense and intermittent abdominal cramps aggravated by eating, anal or perineal fissures, anorexia, severe growth delays, and delayed sexual maturation.

Multiple choice

5. C. Visible peristaltic waves are the most characteristic sign of pyloric stenosis.

6. C. The child with 5% dehydration has a decreased urine output (below 2 ml/kg/hour). Cool skin and an increased heart rate are associated with more severe dehydration. The dehydrated child does not perspire.

7. A. Ulcerative colitis causes profuse diarrhea. The other choices are seen more commonly in Crohn's disease.

8. A. A hypertonic (concentrated) glucose solution provides the carbohydrates in TPN.

CHAPTER 20

Cardiovascular disorders

OBJECTIVES   After studying this chapter, the reader should be able to:

  1. Discuss the causes, pathophysiology, and clinical manifestations of congestive heart failure.

  2. Describe medical and nursing management of the child with congestive heart failure.

  3. Discuss the causes, pathophysiology, and clinical manifestations of congenital heart disease.

  4. Describe medical and nursing management of the child with congenital heart disease.

OVERVIEW OF CONCEPTS   Caring for a child with a cardiovascular disorder requires a sound knowledge of hemodynamic principles and cardiovascular pathophysiology. This chapter explores two types of cardiovascular disorders—congestive heart failure (CHF) and congenital heart disease—and focuses on the nursing management of children with these conditions.

Congestive heart failure   CHF is an abnormal condition characterized by the heart's inability to pump adequate blood to the systemic circulation in order to meet the body's metabolic needs. CHF arises secondary to other diseases.

Etiology

The causes of CHF are varied. However, four general etiologic conditions been identified—volume overload, pressure overload, decreased contractility, and high cardiac output demand.

  Volume overload results from:

• increases in circulating systemic volume (preload), such as from accidental fluid overload, overhydration, and renal failure

• increases in right atrial or ventricular volume, such as from congenital heart disease with left-to-right shunting (as in ventricular or atrial septal defect) and regurgitant valvular heart disease.

  Pressure overload is caused by increased systemic or pulmonary vascular resistance (afterload), such as from coarctation of the aorta, cystic fibrosis (which causes pulmonary hypertension), and systemic hypertension.

Decreased contractility occurs when the heart cannot pump effectively, such as in cardiomyopathy (in which cardiac muscle is weakened), severe anemia (which causes myocardial ischemia), acidemia, and electrolyte disturbances (such as hypokalemia, hypoglycemia, hypocalcemia, and hypomagnesemia).

High cardiac output demand occurs when the body's need for oxygenated blood exceeds the heart's output even though blood volume may be normal. Causes include sepsis, severe anemia, and hyperthyroidism.

Pathophysiology

When the body's demand for an increased blood volume occurs, the heart initially attempts to supply the increased demand through these compensatory mechanisms:

- The sympathetic nervous system (SNS) stimulates sympathetic fibers, thereby causing an increase in the heart rate and force of myocardial contraction to boost cardiac output. Tachycardia and cardiomegaly (enlargement of the heart muscle) result.
- The SNS also stimulates cholinergic fibers, resulting in sweating and peripheral vasoconstriction. Peripheral vasoconstriction causes venous return to increase.
- In response to the initial decreased cardiac output and the subsequent drop in renal blood flow, aldosterone and antidiuretic hormone (ADH) are released, causing sodium and water retention. This, in turn, boosts blood volume, venous return, and cardiac output.

Unless the underlying condition is corrected, however, these compensatory mechanisms eventually fail—and CHF occurs.

Classifications

Theoretically, CHF falls into two classifications: right-sided CHF and left-sided CHF. Clinically, however, these disease forms rarely can be separated because each side of the heart affects the other; when one side fails, the other side functions poorly.

Right-sided CHF occurs when the right ventricle cannot pump blood into the pulmonary artery and then to the lungs. Blood accumulates in the right ventricle, eventually causing blood to pool in the venous circulation. This, in turn, induces systemic venous hypertension and congestion.

Left-sided CHF occurs when the left ventricle cannot pump blood into the aorta and then to the rest of the body. Blood accumulates in the left ventricle, eventually causing blood to pool in the left atrium and the pulmonary vein; this causes pulmonary hypertension and congestion.

Assessment

General signs and symptoms of CHF, which reflect impaired myocardial function, include:

- tachycardia

- sweating
- fatigue
- restlessness
- anorexia
- galloping rhythm (resulting from ventricular dilatation)
- cardiomegaly.

In right-sided CHF, also expect:

- hepatomegaly (liver enlargement)
- ascites (fluid accumulation in the peritoneal space)
- edema (fluid accumulation in the soft tissues)
- weight gain (secondary to edema)
- pleural effusion (fluid accumulation the pleural spaces)
- distended neck and peripheral veins (in children over age 2).

With left-sided CHF, the patient also may exhibit:

- dyspnea
- cough
- tachypnea
- chest retractions
- orthopnea (difficulty breathing while lying down)
- cyanosis
- wheezing
- crackles
- rhonchi.

Because left-sided CHF decreases the cardiac output, also expect decreased blood pressure, weak peripheral pulses, cool and pale extremities, and oliguria (decreased urine output).

CHF may impair a child's nutritional status, thereby altering physical growth. As the metabolic demands of the failing heart increase, calories and energy are diverted to the heart in an attempt to maintain its function. Thus, these calories are unavailable for general growth. With chronic CHF, the child may have organic failure to thrive. (For information on assessing failure to thrive, see Chapter 14, Child abuse and maltreatment.)

Diagnosis

CHF commonly can be diagnosed from clinical findings. Chest X-rays show an enlarged heart, echocardiography reveals impaired myocardial function, and electrocardiography detects changes indicating ventricular hypertrophy.

Medical management

Specific therapy depends on the child's clinical problems.

Pulmonary congestion. A child with pulmonary edema, concurrent respiratory infections, or pulmonary hypertension typically receives supplemental oxygen. By increasing the amount of oxygen available during inspiration, oxygen administration may improve tissue oxygenation.

Venous congestion. A child with venous congestion may receive diuretics (such as furosemide, spironolactone, or chlorothiazide) to remove accumulated fluid and sodium, as well as an angiotensin-converting enzyme (ACE) inhibitor (such as captopril or enalapril) to block the effects of aldosterone and thus prevent sodium and water reabsorption. To treat acute CHF, the physician may restrict fluids.

Impaired cardiac function. The child receives digoxin to reduce the heart rate and increase the strength of myocardial contraction. To induce vasodilation and decrease afterload, an ACE inhibitor may be prescribed to block the effects of renin and angiotensin.

Nursing management

Nursing goals for the child with CHF include improving tissue oxygenation, easing respiratory distress, promoting fluid loss, enhancing cardiac output, reducing cardiac demands, and promoting physical growth.

To improve tissue oxygenation and ease respiratory distress, elevate the head of the bed, or place an infant in an infant seat. Administer humidified oxygen, as prescribed. Encourage turning, coughing, and deep breathing in an older child. Monitor the child's skin color, respiratory rate, breath sounds, quality and quantity of respiratory secretions, and blood oxygen saturation or arterial blood gas values.

To promote fluid loss, administer diuretics and ACE inhibitors, as prescribed, and maintain fluid restrictions. Monitor for therapeutic and adverse effects of diuretics. (See *Drugs used to treat congestive heart failure.*) Also monitor the child's weight; inappropriate weight gain suggests fluid retention.

To reduce cardiac demands, cluster nursing care to allow frequent rest periods and encourage the child to engage in quiet activities. Try to avert prolonged crying spells and prolonged feeding sessions.

To promote physical growth, provide sufficient calories to meet the child's metabolic needs. As prescribed, provide high-calorie, low-sodium supplements. Feed by gavage or gastrostomy, if necessary, because these methods require less energy than prolonged bottle-feeding.

Congenital heart disease

Congenital heart disease refers to a structural or functional abnormality or defect of the heart or the great vessels that exists from birth. The condition, which may take various forms, may manifest at birth or may not be apparent until later.

Etiology

Specific causes of congenital heart disease have not been identified. However, its incidence is greater in infants with Down syndrome and Turner's syndrome as well as in those born to women over age 40, insulin-dependent diabetic mothers, and women who used alcohol or drugs during pregnancy.

Drugs used to treat congestive heart failure

A child with congestive heart failure may receive any of the drugs described below.

DRUG	USE	NURSING CONSIDERATIONS
digoxin (Lanoxin)	A cardiac glycoside used to increase cardiac output; it increases the force of myocardial contraction, decreases heart rate, and increases renal perfusion (indirectly improving urine output).	• Count patient's apical pulse for 1 full minute before administering. Withhold medication if apical pulse is below 100 beats/minute in infants up to age 3 months, below 80 beats/minute in infants ages 3 months to 2 years, below 70 beats/minute children ages 2 to 12 years, and below 60 beats/minute in children over age 12. • When giving digitalizing doses, place child on cardiac monitor to observe for desired effects, such as prolonged PR interval and decreased apical pulse. • Monitor serum potassium level. Hypokalemia increases the risk of digitalis toxicity. • Monitor for signs and symptoms of drug toxicity: nausea, vomiting, anorexia, bradycardia, and arrhythmias.
captopril (Capoten), enalapril (Vasotec)	An angiotensin-converting enzyme (ACE) inhibitor used to increase cardiac output and promote diuresis. It blocks the action of angiotensin I and angiotensin II, causing vasodilation; pulmonary and systemic vasodilation enhances pulmonary blood flow and cardiac output. This drug also enhances renal perfusion (thus improving urine output) and blocks action of aldosterone (thereby decreasing fluid retention by the kidneys).	• Monitor for adverse effects: hypotension with captopril or enalapril; allergic reactions and fever with captopril. • Do not administer concomitantly with potassium supplements; ACE inhibitors do not promote renal excretion of potassium.
furosemide (Lasix)	This loop diuretic is used to promote diuresis; it blocks renal reabsorption of sodium and water and causes chloride and potassium excretion.	• Record patient's fluid intake and output. • Monitor for dehydration; furosemide is a potent diuretic. • Monitor serum potassium, chloride, and bicarbonate values. • Monitor for adverse effects: nausea, diarrhea, ototoxicity, hypokalemia, and postural hypotension. • Encourage patient to consume foods rich in potassium (such as bananas, orange juice, and green leafy vegetables). If necessary, give potassium supplements.
chlorothiazide (Diuril)	A thiazide diuretic, this drug promotes diuresis by decreasing renal reabsorption of sodium, potassium, chloride, bicarbonate, and water.	• Monitor for adverse effects: nausea, weakness, muscle cramps, hypokalemia, and acidosis. • Monitor serum potassium and bicarbonate levels. • Encourage patient to consume foods rich in potassium. If necessary, give potassium supplements.
spironolactone (Aldactone)	This potassium-sparing diuretic promotes diuresis by blocking the action of aldosterone, thereby decreasing sodium and water reabsorption by the kidneys.	• Monitor for adverse effects: ataxia, hyperkalemia, and drowsiness. • Do not administer potassium supplements; spironolactone does not promote renal excretion of potassium.

Pathophysiology, classification, and assessment

Congenital heart disease may be classified according to the altered hemodynamics caused by the particular anomaly. Clinical manifestations vary with the hemodynamic consequences.

Congenital heart disease also may be classified as acyanotic or cyanotic. In acyanotic defects, unoxygenated blood from the right side of the heart and oxygenated blood from the left side do not mix. In cyanotic defects, unoxygenated and oxygenated blood do mix.

Acyanotic anomalies that cause increased pulmonary blood flow

These anomalies—atrial septal defect, ventricular septal defect, patent ductus arteriosus (PDA), and endocardial cushion defect—are characterized by a defect in the septal wall or an abnormal connection between the pulmonary artery and the aorta. The defect or abnormal connection allows blood to flow from the left side of the heart, where pressure is higher, to the right side, where pressure is lower. Increased blood volume on the right side boosts pulmonary blood volume but reduces cardiac output.

These anomalies cause increased pulmonary blood volume, which may lead to pulmonary congestion. Signs and symptoms of pulmonary congestion include dyspnea, cough, tachypnea, chest retractions, orthopnea, wheezing, crackles, and rhonchi.

Atrial septal defect. An opening in the atrial septal wall causes blood to flow from the left atrium through the opening into the right atrium. Increased right atrial volume is ejected into the right ventricle and pulmonary artery.

A small atrial septal defect generally is well tolerated. Auscultation reveals a crescendo-decrescendo systolic ejection murmur and wide, fixed splitting of the second heart sound (S_2). CHF and pulmonary congestion are rare.

Ventricular septal defect. An opening in the ventricular wall causes blood to flow from the left ventricle into the right ventricle. Increased right ventricular volume is ejected into the pulmonary artery. This is the most common acyanotic heart defect; a high percentage of these cases resolve on their own.

A large ventricular septal defect typically causes early signs of pulmonary congestion (discussed above). Auscultation may reveal a loud, harsh, pansystolic murmur. Respiratory infections are common. The heart's increased metabolic demands may lead to failure to thrive.

PDA. In this defect, the ductus arteriosus—a fetal structure connecting the aorta and pulmonary artery—fails to close after birth. This causes blood to flow from the aorta, where pressure is higher, through the ductus to the pulmonary artery, where pressure is lower.

Clinical findings include failure to thrive and signs of pulmonary congestion and infection. In some children, however, the only sign is a pansystolic, machinery-like murmur.

Endocardial cushion defect. Defective endocardial cushion development causes openings in the lower atrial septal wall and upper ventricular septal wall as well as atrioventricular valve defects. Blood flows from the left atrium and ventricle through the openings into the right atrium and ventricle, increasing pulmonary blood volume.

Also called atrioventricular canal defect, endocardial cushion defect is the most common cardiac anomaly in infants with Down syndrome. Pulmonary congestion is the classic sign. Auscultation reveals a systolic murmur.

Acyanotic anomalies that cause obstruction of systemic blood flow

In these anomalies, obstruction of the systemic blood flow increases pressure in the left ventricle and aorta proximal to the obstruction site. Aortic pressure decreases, causing a drop in cardiac output distal to the obstruction site. Clinical manifestations vary with the specific anomaly.

Coarctation of the aorta. In this anomaly, aortic narrowing reduces cardiac output. The narrowing may be located proximal (preductal), distal (postductal), or at the level (juxtaductal) of the ductus arteriosus. If the narrowing occurs proximal to the ductus, systemic circulation to the lower half of the body comes from the right ventricle, through the patent ductus to the aorta. If the narrowing occurs distal to the ductus, collateral circulation develops during fetal life to supply systemic circulation to the lower half of the body.

Severe aortic coarctation manifests at infancy, causing evidence of CHF and severe systemic hypoperfusion, such as weak peripheral pulses, decreased urine output, and cool and pale extremities. With less severe coarctation, signs may not arise until later, and may include hypertension of the upper extremities, bounding radial and brachial pulses, weak femoral pulses, and a heart murmur. Hypertension may cause headache and epistaxis (nosebleed). The lower extremities may be cooler than the upper extremities.

Aortic stenosis. In this anomaly, progressive aortic stenosis, or narrowing, leads to diminished cardiac output and left ventricular and atrial hypertension. Pulmonary congestion may follow.

Clinical findings, such as signs of systemic hypoperfusion and CHF, may be severe at birth. Less severe aortic stenosis may not manifest until later, when the child exhibits exercise intolerance secondary to decreased cardiac output.

Pulmonic stenosis. Narrowing of the pulmonic valve reduces blood flow to the lungs. With severe narrowing, pulmonary blood flow is sustained by aortic blood flowing through the PDA to the pulmonary artery. Right ventricular hypertension may lead to CHF and systemic venous congestion. Reduced pulmonary blood flow may cause systemic hypoxia and cyanosis.

Clinical findings in a child with pulmonic stenosis may include dyspnea and fatigue (resulting from decreased pulmonary blood flow), as well as signs of systemic venous congestion.

Cyanotic anomalies that cause decreased pulmonary blood flow

In these anomalies, obstruction of pulmonary blood flow causes increased pressures on the right side of the heart. An associated atrial or ventricular septal defect allows blood to flow from the right side, where pressure is higher from the obstructed pulmonary flow, to the left side, where pressure is lower. Consequently, unoxygenated blood flows from the right side to the left side of the heart.

Because unoxygenated blood flows directly to the left side and is ejected into the systemic circulation, signs of systemic hypoxia arise. Cyanosis—especially upon exertion—is the most common sign of mild hypoxia. Severe hypoxia produces fatigue upon mild exertion (including during feeding), tachypnea, dyspnea, and failure to thrive. Signs of chronic hypoxia include finger and toe clubbing as well as polycythemia (a compensatory increase in the number of red blood cells that aims to improve tissue oxygenation). Polycythemia increases the risk of thrombus formation.

Tetralogy of Fallot. This anomaly consists of four separate defects: ventricular septal defect, pulmonic stenosis, an overriding aorta or dextroposition of the aorta, and right ventricular hypertrophy.

Signs of tetralogy of Fallot range from mild cyanosis with mild pulmonary artery obstruction to severe cyanosis with severe pulmonary artery obstruction and significant shunting of blood from the right ventricle via the ventricular septal defect to the left ventricle.

Tricuspid atresia. In this anomaly, the tricuspid valve fails to develop, causing obstruction of blood flow from the right atrium to the right ventricle. Thus, unoxygenated blood flows from the right atrium through the foramen ovale (an opening in the septum between the right and left atria in the fetal heart) to the left atrium. A PDA permits pulmonary blood flow. A small ventricular septal defect also may be present, allowing left ventricular blood to enter the right ventricle for ejection into the pulmonary artery. Decreased pulmonary blood flow is the usual consequence.

Tricuspid atresia typically causes cyanosis at birth. Depending on the size of the ductus arteriosus, cyanosis may be mild to severe. Tachypnea and dyspnea also occur.

Cyanotic anomalies that cause increased pulmonary blood flow

In these anomalies, mixing of unoxygenated blood from the right side of the heart with oxygenated blood from the left side causes systemic hypoxia. Pulmonary blood flow increases, and pulmonary congestion and systemic hypoxia occur.

Total anomalous pulmonary venous return. In this defect, pulmonary veins return oxygenated blood to the right atrium (rather than the left atrium), where it mixes with deoxygenated blood. Some of this blood flows through an associated atrial septal defect to the left atrium, where it is ejected to the left ventricle and aorta. The remaining venous return is ejected into the right ventricle and pulmonary artery, increasing the pulmonary blood flow. With sufficient pulmonary flow and return, minimal desaturation of systemic blood occurs.

However, if pulmonary venous return is obstructed, oxygenated pulmonary venous return cannot enter the right atrium. This diminishes shunting of blood across the atrial septal defect, leading to decreased cardiac output and systemic hypoxia. The child has CHF, severe cyanosis, and respiratory distress.

With unobstructed pulmonary venous return, the child typically has signs of pulmonary congestion and respiratory infection. Mild cyanosis also may occur.

Truncus arteriosus. In this defect, the child has one rather than two great vessels; the single vessel serves both the pulmonary and systemic circulations. Most children also have a ventricular septal defect.

Because systemic resistance exceeds pulmonary vascular resistance, increased amounts of blood flow to the pulmonary vasculature, thereby causing pulmonary congestion and decreased aortic output. A large ventricular septal defect allows pressures to equalize between the ventricles, resulting in mixing of oxygenated and deoxygenated blood.

Truncus arteriosus causes signs and symptoms of pulmonary congestion. Cyanosis may not appear because of the excessive pulmonary blood flow.

Transposition of the great arteries. In this anomaly, the pulmonary artery arises from the left ventricle and the aorta arises from the right ventricle, creating two separate circulatory systems. For the child to survive, the left and right sides of the heart must communicate, such as through an atrial or ventricular septal defect or a PDA. An atrial septal defect or PDA allows oxygenated blood to flow from the left to the right side of the heart, for ejection into the systemic circulation. A ventricular septal defect permits unoxygenated blood from the right ventricle to flow to the left ventricle, causing increased blood volume in the left ventricle and pulmonary artery.

With a small atrial septal defect or PDA, little oxygenated blood can enter the right side of the heart and systemic circulation; consequently, the child has severe cyanosis and CHF. With a large ventricular septal defect, signs of pulmonary congestion occur.

Hypoplastic left heart syndrome. In this defect, the left ventricle is underdeveloped, causing inefficient left ventricular emptying and decreased cardiac output. Blood flow from the pulmonary artery through the PDA to the aorta sustains the systemic circulation.

Clinical findings include cyanosis (as desaturated blood from the pulmonary artery enters the aorta), tachypnea, CHF, and systemic hypoperfusion.

Diagnosis

Congenital heart disease may be suspected in any infant born with a heart murmur or with cyanosis that persists despite supplemental oxygen administration. Echocardiography may reveal a structural heart defect. The child undergoes cardiac catheterization for definitive identification of the specific anomaly. (See *Cardiac catheterization in children*.)

Medical management

Medical goals for the child with congenital heart disease include:
• controlling CHF and improving cardiac function (as described in the section on "Congestive heart failure")
• maintaining a PDA in a child depending on this structure for systemic or pulmonary blood flow; typically, this is accomplished by administering prostaglandin E to the pulmonary artery via a catheter
• correcting the defect surgically. Surgical procedures vary with the specific anomaly. For example, a simple atrial or ventricular septal defect may be repaired surgically by closing the septal opening with a natural or synthetic patch. Other defects call for different procedures. (For more information, consult a standard pediatric textbook.)

Nursing management

Nursing goals for the child with uncorrected congenital heart disease vary with the specific anomaly. For all such children, the nurse should promote physical growth and development. Additional goals for several common defects are outlined below.
• For the child with atrial or ventricular septal defect, PDA, coarctation of the aorta, or aortic stenosis: Promote cardiac output.
• For the child with ventricular septal defect, endocardial cushion defect, PDA, total anomalous pulmonary venous return, or truncus arteriosus: Reduce respiratory distress and signs of pulmonary congestion.
• For the child with pulmonary stenosis or another anomaly causing right-sided heart failure: Promote fluid loss.
For nursing measures specific to each goal, see the section on "Congestive heart failure."

Children with cyanotic anomalies experience fatigue and exercise intolerance because of insufficient oxygen to meet metabolic demands. These children generally can monitor their own activity level and will rest when needed.

For the infant, who may become exhausted from feeding, limit feeding sessions to 20 minutes. If needed, schedule more frequent feedings to provide sufficient calories for growth. For the bottle-fed infant, use a soft nipple to decrease the energy required to suck.

Cardiac catheterization in children

In an infant or a child with congenital heart disease, the physician may perform cardiac catheterization to obtain information about structural heart defects, blood flow and pressures within the systemic and pulmonary circulations, and oxygen content in the various heart chambers and vessels.

Procedure

After administering local anesthesia to numb the insertion site, the physician threads the catheter through the infant's right or left femoral artery or vein into the heart chambers. (The antecubital fossa may be used in an older child.) Injecting dye into the catheter permits visualization of heart vessels and chambers. Heparin may be given to reduce the risk of thrombus (clot) formation. After obtaining all the required information, the physician removes the catheter.

Preprocedural nursing care

As prescribed, withhold fluids and solid foods for 4 hours before cardiac catheterization. Prepare the parents and child for the procedure. For the child, use developmentally appropriate materials and strategies (as discussed in Chapters 15, Illness Concepts, and Chapter 16, Management principles). Explain the purpose of the procedure to the parents. Discuss the information to be obtained from this test and describe the technique, possible adverse outcomes, and the care the child will receive before and after the procedure. Immediately before the procedure, insert an I.V. line, as prescribed.

Postprocedural nursing care

After cardiac catheterization, monitor the child's vital signs every 15 minutes for the first hour, then every hour until discharge. Do not take blood pressure on the affected extremity.

Observe the pressure dressing at the catheter insertion site for swelling, bleeding, and drainage. If bleeding occurs, apply firm pressure. A sandbag should be placed over the dressing for 12 hours; 24 hours after the procedure, the pressure dressing may be removed and replaced with a dry 2″ × 2″ gauze pad, which is taped in place.

Suspect diminished venous return if the affected extremity is bluish and warm and has good pulses. To increase venous return, raise the extremity. As prescribed, offer fluids and monitor the child's urine output.

Also, watch for signs of such complications as thrombophlebitis, pulmonary embolism, bradycardia, bleeding, reaction to the dye (indicated by flushing, arrhythmias, headache, restlessness, nausea, laryngeal edema, and decreased renal perfusion), infection, arterial spasms, arrhythmias, cerebrovascular accident, cardiac perforation, and hypoxemia.

Palpate the child's pulses in the affected extremity. Diminished pulses distal to the catheter site, a cool and pale extremity, and prolonged capillary refill may signal arterial obstruction; report any of these findings to the physician.

The child is discharged after recovering fully from the procedure—typically, 24 hours after catheterization. (An inpatient is returned to the floor 1 to 2 hours after the procedure.) When preparing for discharge, teach the parents that the child can resume regular activity. Advise them to report a fever over 101.3° F (38.5° C), as well as redness, swelling, or drainage at the catheter insertion site. Instruct them to change the groin dressing if it becomes soiled.

STUDY ACTIVITIES

Short answer

1. Explain why the child with CHF may have altered physical growth.

_____

_____

_____

2. What are the four structural abnormalities associated with tetralogy of Fallot?

_____

_____

3. What is the purpose of performing cardiac catheterization in a child with congenital heart disease?

_____

_____

Matching related elements

Match the term on the left with its definition on the right.

4. ___ Ascites   **A.** Difficulty breathing while lying down

5. ___ Pleural effusion   **B.** Enlargement of the liver

6. ___ Cardiomegaly   **C.** Fluid accumulation in the peritoneal space

7. ___ Hepatomegaly   **D.** Enlargement of the heart

8. ___ Edema   **E.** Fluid accumulation in the pleural space

9. ___ Orthopnea   **F.** Decreased urine output

10. ___ Oliguria   **G.** Fluid accumulation in the soft tissues

Multiple choice

11. Melinda, age 4 months, is admitted for evaluation of suspected congenital heart disease. Upon assessment, the nurse detects a strong, bounding radial pulse coupled with a weak femoral pulse. Which congenital anomaly would the nurse suspect?

    A. PDA
    B. Coarctation of the aorta
    C. Ventricular septal defect
    D. Truncus arteriosus

12. Cardiac catheterization is most likely to cause which of the following problems?

A. Arrhythmias

B. Rapidly rising blood pressure

C. Hypostatic pneumonia

D. CHF

13. Robert, age 2 months, is admitted with CHF. During assessment, the nurse would expect to find:

A. Widened pulse pressure

B. Bounding peripheral pulses

C. A gallop heart rhythm

D. Bradycardia

ANSWERS

Short answer

1. As the metabolic demands of the failing heart increase, calories and energy are diverted to the heart in an attempt to maintain its function. Thus, these calories are unavailable for general growth. With chronic CHF, the child may have failure to thrive.

2. Tetralogy of Fallot is characterized by a ventricular septal defect, pulmonic stenosis, an overriding aorta or dextroposition of the aorta ventricular septal defect, and right ventricular hypertrophy.

3. Cardiac catheterization is performed to obtain information about structural heart defects, blood flow and pressures within the systemic and pulmonary circulations, and oxygen content in the various heart chambers and vessels.

Matching related elements

4. C

5. E

6. D

7. B

8. G

9. A

10. F

Multiple choice

11. B. Coarctation of the aorta causes signs of peripheral hypoperfusion (such as a weak femoral pulse) and a bounding radial pulse. These signs are uncommon in the other choices.

12. A. Arrhythmias may follow cardiac catheterization. The other responses are not typical complications of this procedure.

13. C. CHF may cause a gallop rhythm in children. The other responses are not associated with CHF.

CHAPTER 21

Hematologic disorders

OBJECTIVES
After studying this chapter, the reader should be able to:
1. Discuss the causes, pathophysiology, and clinical manifestations of anemia, sickle cell disease, and hemophilia.
2. Identify laboratory tests used to diagnose hematologic dysfunction.
3. Describe medical and nursing management of children with anemia, sickle cell disease, and hemophilia.

OVERVIEW OF CONCEPTS
Hematologic dysfunction in children usually results from deficiencies of the formed elements of the blood—red blood cells (RBCs), white blood cells, and platelets—or deficiencies of the coagulation factors. This chapter explores the most common hematologic disorders in children—anemia, sickle cell disease, and hemophilia.

Anemia
A symptom rather than a disease, anemia is characterized by an abnormally low hemoglobin level in the RBCs. It is the most common hematologic problem in children.

Pathophysiology
Anemia may reflect any one (or more) of three basic processes:
• decreased hemoglobin or RBC production
• increased RBC destruction (hemolysis)
• blood loss.
Hemoglobin within the RBCs carries oxygen. Therefore, if the RBC volume or hemoglobin level decreases, less oxygen is available to body tissues. Ultimately, tissue hypoxia occurs.

Classification
Anemia may be classified according to RBC size or the hemoglobin content of RBCs. The mean corpuscular volume (MCV) laboratory test can determine RBC size.
RBC size. Anemia may be categorized as normocytic, microcytic, or macrocytic, according to the size of the RBCs.
   In normocytic anemia, RBCs are normal in size, with a MCV of 75 to 95 million/μm^3. Causes of normocytic anemia include condi-

tions characterized by abnormal bone marrow function (such as leukemia), acute blood loss, or hemolysis (such as sickle cell disease).

In microcytic anemia, RBCs are smaller than normal and MCV measures less than 75 million/μm^3. Microcytic anemia reflects impaired hemoglobin production, as in iron deficiency and poisoning. (For information on iron-deficiency anemia and lead poisoning, see Chapter 7, The toddler and family.)

In macrocytic anemia, RBCs are larger than normal, and MCV exceeds 95 million/μm^3. This form of anemia results from a deficiency of vitamin B_{12} or folate.

Hemoglobin content. Based on hemoglobin content, anemia may be normochromic or hypochromic. In normochromic anemia, RBCs have a normal hemoglobin content, resulting in a normal RBC color. In microchromic anemia, RBCs have a decreased hemoglobin content, causing them to appear pale. The mean corpuscular hemoglobin (MCH) and the mean corpuscular hemoglobin concentration (MCHC) test evaluate the the quantity of hemoglobin in RBCs.

Assessment

When anemia develops suddenly (as with acute hemorrhage), acute cardiovascular signs, such as tachycardia and heart murmurs, arise. Congestive heart failure (CHF) may follow.

Anemia is better tolerated when it develops slowly because the body is better able to adapt. With gradual onset, signs and symptoms (which reflect tissue hypoxia) include muscle weakness; fatigue; exercise intolerance; and paleness of the skin, mucous membranes, and conjunctivae. Central nervous system (CNS) changes associated with anemia include headache, dizziness, irritability, slowed thought processes, and decreased attention span.

Chronic anemia may occur secondary to certain disorders, such as sickle cell anemia. A child with chronic anemia has growth retardation and delayed sexual maturation, which results from chronic tissue and cellular hypoxia. Anemia may be suspected during an assessment or based on clinical findings; laboratory values can confirm a diagnosis of anemia.

Medical management

Medical therapy aims to correct the underlying cause of anemia. For example, the child who has suffered an acute blood loss receives blood transfusions. The child with an iron deficiency receives iron supplements and nutritional counseling.

Nursing management

The primary nursing goal for the child with anemia is to reduce tissue oxygen requirements. Because physical exertion increases these requirements, have the child avoid strenuous activity and rest when fatigued. For the child with severe anemia, enforce bed rest, as prescribed, and assist with activities of daily living as needed. To promote rest, suggest or provide diversional activities, such as television viewing and reading.

Emotional stress also increases tissue oxygen demands. Therefore, try to prevent prolonged crying spells. For an infant, provide a pacifier and hold and rock the child. Encourage the parents to stay with the child during hospitalization.

Sickle cell disease

Sickle cell disease refers to a group of autosomal recessive genetic disorders called hemoglobinopathies. These disorders are caused by substitution of valine for glutamine within the deoxyribonucleic acid (DNA) molecule.

Sickle cell trait and sickle cell disease are the most common hemoglobinopathies in North America. They occur primarily in African Americans.

Pathophysiology and assessment

Normal adult hemoglobin (Hgb A) is replaced completely or partially by a different type of hemoglobin—Hgb S, fetal hemoglobin (Hgb F), or Hgb C. This causes RBCs to become fragile and distorted. In sickle cell trait and sickle cell anemia, Hgb S replaces Hgb A.

Sickle cell trait occurs when a child inherits one gene for Hgb S and one gene for Hgb A. Approximately 55% of the child's RBCs contain Hgb A. Because of the high percentage of normal hemoglobin in their RBCs, children with sickle cell trait normally are asymptomatic. However, under conditions of extreme deoxygenation, they may suffer acute, episodic conditions called sickle cell crises.

Sickle cell anemia occurs when a child inherits two Hgb S genes. The disorder is transmitted by an autosomal recessive inheritance pattern (discussed in Chapter 2, Pediatric nursing concepts). A chronic disorder, sickle cell anemia is characterized by moderate anemia. RBCs containing Hgb S have a shortened life span. The child's RBC count decreases because the bone marrow cannot produce sufficient RBCs to meet the body's needs. Chronic normocytic, normochromic anemia then develops, with the hemoglobin level typically ranging from 7 to 9 g/dl. Under normal conditions, the child can compensate for the moderate anemia, and symptoms may be limited to growth retardation and fatigue upon physical exertion. The child also is susceptible to infection.

However, acute symptoms develop during exacerbations or crises, when RBCs containing Hgb S become sickle-shaped. Conditions that may cause sickling include acidosis, dehydration, and decreased arterial oxygen tension (such as from physiologic stress caused by infection, surgery, anesthesia, strenuous and prolonged physical exertion, high altitudes, or emotional stress). Sickle-shaped RBCs become tangled within the vascular system. Blood viscosity increases, and smaller capillaries become clogged.

In young infants with sickle cell anemia, RBCs contain 60% to 80% Hgb F. Because Hgb F does not sickle, sickle cell anemia is not apparent until Hgb S becomes present in sufficient quantities—typically, by age 6 months.

Sickle cell crisis

Many children with sickle cell disease suffer periodic sickling episodes called sickle cell crises. Such crises can take several forms—vaso-occlusive crisis, splenic sequestration crisis, or aplastic crisis.

Vaso-occlusive crisis occurs when sickle-shaped RBCs clump within vessels, causing acute tissue ischemia (hypoxia) in multiple organs. Signs of acute tissue ischemia appear mainly in the bones, joints, and abdomen, causing severe pain. Joints may become swollen and the abdomen may become distended. A child under age 2 may have hand-foot syndrome—pain and swelling over the soft tissues of the hands and feet. The child is predisposed to osteomyelitis (bone infection).

RBC clumping during vaso-occlusive crisis affects these organs:

- *Liver and spleen.* Congested with sickle-shaped cells, the liver and spleen become enlarged (hepatosplenomegaly) and tender. With repeated infarcts (acute arterial blockages), liver and spleen cells are destroyed and replaced by fibrotic tissue. The liver becomes cirrhotic and may fail. The spleen cannot filter bacteria from the blood, thereby leaving the child vulnerable to infection.
- *Kidneys.* Repeated infarcts of the glomerular capillaries lead to hematuria (blood in the urine), poor urine concentrating ability, and enuresis (urine incontinence, especially at night).
- *CNS.* Chronic anemia may lead to irritability, slowed thought processes, and a decreased attention span. Acute ischemia may cause cerebrovascular accident (stroke).
- *Skin.* Thrombosis and decreased peripheral circulation may lead to chronic leg ulcers.

Splenic sequestration crisis occurs when large amounts of blood pool within the spleen. This causes hypovolemia (a drop in circulating blood volume) and profound anemia. Hypovolemic shock may follow.

Aplastic crisis develops when the bone marrow cannot produce enough RBCs to provide tissues with adequate oxygen. An infection typically triggers increased RBC hemolysis, and the bone marrow eventually fails to produce sufficient RBCs. Profound anemia develops.

Diagnosis

Several laboratory tests may be used to diagnose sickle cell anemia. Hemoglobin electrophoresis, which separates and measures the various forms of hemoglobin, provides definitive diagnosis of sickle cell anemia because it "fingerprints" the protein by the pattern formed on the paper.

The sickle cell test—also known as the hemoglobin S test, the HGB,S test, or the Sickledex screening test—reveals whether RBCs contain Hgb S. A positive result indicates sickle cell trait or sickle cell disease. However, test results may not be reliable in a child with a hemoglobin level below 10 g/dl or in infants under age 6 months, who have insufficient Hgb S levels.

A peripheral blood smear may reveal sickled RBCs. However, during periods of normal oxygenation, the RBCs of children with sickle cell anemia are normal in shape, causing misleading test results.

Medical management

Medical goals include preventing sickling episodes, treating sickle cell crises, and guarding against infection.

To prevent sickling, the child must maintain adequate oxygenation and hydration. (For details, see "Nursing management" below.) A child who has recurring splenic sequestration crises may undergo a splenectomy.

During sickle cell crisis, the goal of therapy is to prevent further sickling, such as by minimizing oxygen demands and promoting hemodilution. The child is placed on bed rest to preserve energy and decrease oxygen demands. The physician orders oral and intravenous (I.V.) fluids at 50% above normal maintenance requirements, as well as I.V. pain medications. Other measures may include bicarbonate administration to treat acidosis, blood transfusions to treat profound anemia, and supplemental oxygen to treat CHF.

To prevent infection, pneumococcal, *Haemophilus influenzae* Type B, and meningococcal vaccines are given. The child also may receive prophylactic oral penicillin.

Nursing management

Nursing goals for the child with sickle cell anemia include:
- preventing sickling episodes
- increasing tissue perfusion and oxygenation during sickle cell crisis
- relieving pain during sickle cell crisis
- helping the child and family adjust to the effects of a chronic disease.
  (For a discussion of chronic illness in children, see Chapter 15, Illness Concepts.)

To prevent sickling episodes, provide comprehensive teaching to the parents and child. (For details, see *Teaching the family how to prevent sickling episodes.*)

To increase tissue perfusion and oxygenation during a sickle cell crisis, use measures to prevent further sickling and decrease the child's oxygen demands. For example, administer I.V. fluids as prescribed, encourage oral fluid intake, maintain bed rest, provide diversional activities, administer antibiotics (if prescribed for infection), and encourage the parents to stay with the child to reduce emotional stress.

To relieve pain during a sickle cell crisis, administer pain medications, as prescribed, and evaluate the child's response. Use non-pharmacologic pain relief methods as appropriate for the child's age. Apply heat to painful joints.

Teaching the family how to prevent sickling episodes

Comprehensive instruction by the nurse can help prevent sickling episodes in a child with sickle cell anemia. Although the teaching points below are geared to the parents, the nurse may direct teaching to the child as well, depending on the child's age. Be sure to cover these points:

- Make sure the child receives sufficient fluids.
- Stay alert for signs and symptoms of dehydration. Do not use urine output to monitor the child's hydration status, because a child with sickle cell anemia cannot conserve water. Instead, observe for dry skin or dry mucous membranes.
- Protect the child from known sources of infection.
- Call the physician at the first sign of illness, such as elevated temperature, vomiting, or diarrhea.
- Have the child avoid strenuous physical activity.
- Minimize emotional stress, including prolonged crying episodes.
- Have the child avoid high altitudes.

Hemophilia

Hemophilia refers to a group of disorders characterized by excessive bleeding. These disorders are transmitted by an X-linked recessive inheritance pattern that causes deficiency of one of the coagulation factors. The most common types of hemophilia are hemophilia A (Factor VIII deficiency, or classic hemophilia) and hemophilia B (Factor IX deficiency, or Christmas disease). Most hemophiliacs have the severe form of hemophilia A.

Pathophysiology

In hemophilia A, Factor VIII is present but defective. In hemophilia B, Factor IX may be present but is defective or deficient. In both disorders, the dysfunctional clotting factors prevent normal coagulation and cause inappropriate and prolonged bleeding.

Assessment

A child with the severe form of hemophilia A has spontaneous bleeding even in the absence of trauma. Bleeding follows minor falls and scrapes, vigorous toothbrushing, and needle sticks. A child with the moderate form of hemophilia A experiences prolonged bleeding only after significant injury, such as deep lacerations. With the minor form, the child typically is asymptomatic, except after severe trauma or surgery.

Bleeding may occur in any area of the body, and bruising is common. Hemarthrosis—bleeding into joints—can lead to crippling joint deformities. Most commonly, it affects the ankle, knee, and elbow joints. Early signs of hemarthrosis are minor joint pain and stiffness in the affected joint. Later signs include moderate to severe pain; warmth, redness, and swelling of the affected joint; and loss of the usual range of motion (ROM). Epistaxis (nosebleed), hematuria (blood in the urine), and life-threatening intracranial hemorrhages also may occur.

Diagnosis

Diagnosis may rest on the child's history of bleeding episodes. Laboratory tests used to diagnose hemophilia include:
- partial thromboplastin time (PTT), which measures abnormalities of clotting Factors I, II, V, VIII, IX, X, and XII
- thromboplastin generation test, which differentiates among deficiencies of the various clotting factors.

Medical management

Medical therapy aims to prevent spontaneous bleeding. The physician prescribes I.V. administration of the deficient clotting factor. Parents (and children over age 8) are taught to administer the clotting factor at home. Today, blood products are unlikely to transmit human immunodeficiency virus (HIV) and other diseases because of improved blood screening and decontamination procedures. However, more than 70% of hemophiliac children who received blood products before 1989 acquired HIV from these products.

Supportive medical therapy depends on the child's symptoms. For hemarthrosis, ice packs are applied and affected joints are immobilized during active bleeding. Once active bleeding stops, ROM exercises to the affected joint help maintain normal joint function. A regular exercise program can strengthen muscles surrounding the joints, thus limiting hemarthrosis.

Corticosteroids are given to reduce inflammation. For severe joint pain, the physician may prescribe acetaminophen (with or without codeine) or meperidine (for short-term use only). Aspirin and other nonsteroidal anti-inflammatory drugs are avoided because of their adverse effects on platelet function. Ibuprofen, however, has proven to be safe and effective for pain management.

The physician may prescribe antifibrinolytic agents, such as aminocaproic acid, to treat mouth or tongue lacerations and before tooth extractions. The child with hematuria needs an increased fluid intake.

Nursing management

Nursing goals for the hemophiliac child include preventing bleeding episodes, minimizing active bleeding, preventing joint deformities, and helping the child and family adjust to the effects of a chronic disease (as described in Chapter 15, Illness concepts.)

To prevent bleeding episodes, teach the parents and child how to administer the prescribed clotting factor at home. Also teach them how to prevent injury. Urge the parents to safeguard the house, such as by removing sharp objects and keeping chairs away from counters to prevent the child from climbing and falling. Advise parents to supervise the child during outside play to reduce the risks associated with falls.

With an older child, emphasize that contact sports are prohibited. Encourage safe alternatives, such as bicycle riding (with a helmet) and swimming.

To minimize the risk of hemorrhage, teach the child to use a soft-bristled toothbrush and a water irrigation device, set on low, to clean the teeth. Teach an adolescent to use an electric shaver rather than a razor blade for shaving. Inform the parents that the child must avoid intramuscular injections and venipunctures and should not take aspirin and guaifenesin (contained in many over-the-counter cough remedies).

During periods of active bleeding, administer replacement clotting factors, as prescribed. Apply firm pressure to the injury site for 10 to 15 minutes. Elevate the injury site above heart level and immobilize the joint. Apply cold to the injury site for the first 24 hours. Once active bleeding stops, administer passive ROM exercises. Encourage the child to engage in a medically prescribed exercise program.

Teach the child and family measures to minimize active bleeding, such as ice and direct pressure. Also teach them how to recognize occult (hidden) bleeding, such as bleeding into joints. Early signs of bleeding into joints include mild pain and stiffness. Also teach them to look for hematuria; black stools (which indicate slow gastrointestinal bleeding); hematemesis (bloody or dark brown emesis, which signals gastric bleeding); and severe headache, slurred speech, and lethargy, which may signal intracranial hemorrhage.

To prevent joint deformities, teach the parents and child how to recognize early signs of bleeding into joints.

STUDY ACTIVITIES

Short answer

1. Differentiate among microcytic, macrocytic, and normocytic anemia.

_____

_____

_____

2. Why does sickle cell anemia lead to chronic anemia?

_____

_____

_____

Matching related elements
Match the term on the left with its definition on the right.

3. ___ Osteomyelitis		**A.** RBC destruction
4. ___ Hemolysis		**B.** Nosebleed
5. ___ Infarct		**C.** Acute arterial blockage
6. ___ Hemarthrosis		**D.** Bone infection
7. ___ Epistaxis		**E.** Bleeding into a joint

Multiple choice
8. What is a major nursing goal for the child with hemophilia?
   A. Increasing tissue perfusion
   B. Preventing bleeding episodes
   C. Promoting tissue oxygenation
   D. Controlling pain

9. To detect hemarthrosis promptly in a child with hemophilia, the nurse should observe for which early sign?
   A. Decreased peripheral pulses
   B. Active bleeding
   C. Joint stiffness
   D. Hematuria

ANSWERS

Short answer
1. In microcytic anemia, RBCs are smaller than normal and MCV is below 75 million/μm^3. In macrocytic anemia, RBCs are larger than normal and MCV exceeds 95 million/μm^3. In normocytic anemia, RBCs are normal in size and MCV ranges from 75 to 95 million/μm^3.

2. In sickle cell anemia, RBCs containing Hgb S have a shortened life span. The child's RBC count decreases because the bone marrow cannot produce sufficient RBCs to meet the body's needs. A chronic normocytic, normochromic anemia then develops.

Matching related elements
   3. D
   4. A
   5. C
   6. E
   7. B

Multiple choice
8. B. A child with hemophilia is prone to bleeding episodes. Therefore, a primary nursing goal is to prevent bleeding episodes.

9. C. Joint stiffness is an early sign of hemarthrosis. Bleeding into joints cannot be observed directly. Pulses are not affected in hemarthrosis. Hematuria might indicate urinary bleeding.

CHAPTER 22

Immunologic disorders

OBJECTIVES

After studying this chapter, the reader should be able to:

1. Describe the causes, pathophysiology, and clinical manifestations of systemic lupus erythematosus, juvenile rheumatoid arthritis, rheumatic fever, and Kawasaki disease.

2. Discuss medical and nursing management of patients with the above disorders.

3. Describe the cause, transmission modes, pathophysiology, and clinical manifestations of human immunodeficiency virus (HIV) infection.

4. Describe medical and nursing management for patients with HIV infection.

OVERVIEW OF CONCEPTS

When the complex processes of the immune system malfunction, a person's immune response may become exaggerated, misdirected, or depressed. Immunologic disorders fall into three general categories—hypersensitivity disorders, characterized by an exaggerated or inappropriate immune response; autoimmunity disorders, characterized by a misdirected immune response; and immunodeficiency disorders, characterized by a depressed immune response.

Immunologic dysfunction may affect a child in various ways. Minor disorders, such as allergic rhinitis, cause discomfort but are managed easily. Some serious disorders, such as systemic lupus erythematosus (SLE) and HIV infection, are debilitating and incurable.

This chapter focuses on management of children with immunologic disorders. It presents general information on autoimmunity and immunodeficiency. Then it discusses selected immune-related disorders—SLE, juvenile rheumatoid arthritis (JRA), rheumatic fever, Kawasaki disease, and HIV infection.

Autoimmunity and immunodeficiency

In autoimmune disorders, the body makes antibodies against its own healthy, normal cells, thereby leading to tissue damage and multisystemic dysfunction. Although the precise cause of the misdirected immune response is unknown, experts have linked certain autoimmune disorders with genetic factors, bacteria, viruses, and drugs. Autoimmune disorders in children include SLE, JRA, insulin-dependent diabetes mellitus (which is discussed in Chapter 23, Endocrine disorders), and acute poststreptococcal glomerulonephritis (which is discussed in Chapter 24, Renal disorders).

In immunodeficiency disorders, the depressed or absent immune response makes the patient highly susceptible to infection. An immunodeficiency disorder may be primary, involving a defect in an immune system component, or secondary, resulting from an underlying disease or other factor that impairs the immune response.

Systemic lupus erythematosus

SLE is a chronic, incurable, and potentially fatal inflammatory disease of the connective tissues. Its cause is unknown. SLE is more common in females and blacks. In children, the disease is more likely to occur during early adolescence.

The prognosis for long-term survival has improved. Today, most children with SLE live more than 5 years after diagnosis. Earlier and more aggressive treatment has diminished the incidence of life-threatening renal disease—the most common cause of death in children with SLE.

Pathophysiology and clinical manifestations

In SLE, widespread inflammation occurs and typically involves multiple body systems. Initially, most children have arthritis-like symptoms and complain of moderate to severe joint pain. Small joints are affected more commonly than large joints. A butterfly-shaped rash may appear over the cheeks and the bridge of the nose.

Systemic manifestations of SLE include fever, malaise, fatigue, nausea, diarrhea, weight loss, photosensitivity, and oral and nasopharyngeal ulcers. (For details on the systemic effects of SLE, see *How SLE affects body systems.*)

Diagnosis

SLE is diagnosed from clinical and laboratory findings. A definitive diagnosis requires at least four of the following findings:
- butterfly-shaped rash
- discoid rash
- photosensitivity
- oral or nasopharyngeal ulcers
- arthritis in more than two joints
- pleuritis or pericarditis
- seizures or psychosis
- renal disease (as indicated by proteinuria or cellular casts)
- hematologic disease (hemolytic anemia, leukopenia, lymphopenia, or thrombocytopenia)
- immunologic dysfunction (as indicated by positive anti-double-stranded DNA, positive anti-Smith antibodies, or false-positive VDRL for more than 6 months)

How SLE affects body systems

Systemic lupus erythematosus (SLE) may cause clinical manifestations in multiple body systems.

Cardiopulmonary system
- Endocarditis (inflammation of the inner lining of the heart)
- Myocarditis (inflammation of the heart muscle)
- Pericarditis (inflammation of the pericardium)
- Pleuritis (inflammation of the pleural lining)

Central nervous system
- Behavioral changes
- Headache
- Psychosis
- Seizures

Hematologic system
- Hemolytic anemia

- Leukopenia (below normal white blood cell count)
- Thrombocytopenia (below normal platelet count)

Integumentary system
- Alopecia (hair loss)
- Scaly rash
- Urticaria (hives)

Renal system
- Hemolytic uremia
- Nephritis
- Renal failure

- presence of antinuclear antibodies (ANAs).

Medical management

Treatment of SLE is supportive and varies with the degree of systemic involvement. The physician typically prescribes a corticosteroid and tapers the drug to the lowest effective dose that suppresses symptoms. In most children, corticosteroid therapy induces remission of acute symptoms. Antimalarial drug therapy, such as hydroxychloroquine sulfate (Plaquenil), may be used to relieve SLE-induced arthritis.

To manage arthritic symptoms, the physician prescribes aspirin or ibuprofen. A child with hypertension, which may arise secondary to renal disease or corticosteroid therapy, also receives antihypertensive drugs.

Because sunlight seems to aggravate SLE, the child must stay out of direct sunlight and use sunscreen when outside. To minimize fatigue, which can exacerbate SLE, the physician may recommend one or two daytime rest periods in addition to least 8 hours of sleep at night.

Nursing management

Nursing goals include helping the child and family adapt to the effects of a chronic disease (as discussed in Chapter 15, Illness concepts) and preventing exacerbations and complications of the disease.

Instruct the child to avoid direct sunlight and to wear a broad-rimmed hat or a baseball cap to protect the face from sunlight. Teach the child to apply sunscreen to all areas that will be exposed to direct sunlight.

For the adolescent, SLE may present additional problems. Skin rashes and adverse corticosteroid effects, such as weight gain, fluid retention, and "moon face," may cause body-image disturbances—which are particularly disturbing during adolescence. The need for adequate rest may interfere with the adolescent's school, work, and recreational activities.

To minimize these problems, advise the adolescent to monitor activities to learn how much and which activities seem to trigger exacerbations of the disease. To help the adolescent maintain remission and prevent acute exacerbations, stress the importance of complying with drug therapy. Be aware that the unpleasant adverse effects of corticosteroids may decrease compliance.

Because emotional stress may exacerbate SLE, teach the adolescent how to recognize escalating stress levels as well as techniques for managing stress. Encourage the child to express feelings about the disease. If appropriate, recommend a support group for teenagers with SLE or chronic diseases.

Juvenile rheumatoid arthritis

JRA is an autoimmune disease affecting the connective tissue in joints. The exact trigger of the autoimmune response is unknown.

Disease onset peaks between ages 1 and 3 and again between ages 8 and 11. JRA is more common in females than males; however, the systemic form of JRA affects males and females equally.

Classification

JRA may be systemic, pauciarticular, or polyarticular. Systemic JRA, the rarest type, affects any joints. In systemic JRA, initial symptoms may occur in other body systems; only 20% of children have joint pain at time of diagnosis. Symptoms may include fever, malaise, rash, pleuritis, pericarditis, splenomegaly, and hepatomegaly. In pauciarticular JRA, the most common type, arthritis affects less than five joints, typically the lower extremities; in polyarticular JRA, it affects more than five joints, simultaneously and generally on both sides of the body.

Few children with pauciarticular JRA test seropositive for rheumatoid factor; most are positive for ANAs.

Polyarticular JRA may be subdivided according to whether the patient tests seronegative or seropositive for rheumatoid factor. Seronegative children suffer less disability, respond better to treatment, and have a better prognosis.

Pathophysiology and clinical manifestations

Inflammation starts in the synovial membrane of the joint, causing pain, functional loss, and deformity. All children with JRA experience joint stiffness in the morning and after inactive periods as well as mild to moderate intermittent pain and swelling over affected joints. Some children have localized overgrowth in affected joints, causing discrepancies in limb length. Some are short in stature.

With systemic JRA, the child initially has a high, spiking fever which may last several weeks or more, along with intermittent joint pain and swelling. An erythematous macular rash ("rheumatoid rash") typically appears on the trunk. A severe normocytic, normochromic anemia commonly develops, and some children may develop pleuritis, pericarditis, or myocarditis. Laboratory findings show absence of rheumatoid factor and ANAs. Later, symptoms of chronic polyarticular arthritis may develop.

Pauciarticular JRA causes swelling of one or more large joints (most commonly the knee, rarely the hip), joint stiffness, and unilateral growth discrepancies (particularly in children ages 1 to 2). Pain and fever are absent. The older child with pauciarticular JRA has asymptomatic, large-joint involvement in the lower extremities (most commonly the knee, sometimes the hip), a progressive decline in joint and motor function, decreased exercise capacity, and malaise. Some children have systemic manifestations, such as weight loss, fever, anorexia, and eye inflammation (uveitis).

Polyarticular JRA typically affects the small joints of the hands and feet, although large joints also may be involved. Some children have mild fever and mild anemia; all children have some degree of disability resulting from joint dysfunction. Disability may range from minimal (the child can perform all activities of daily living without assistance) to severe (the child is wheelchair-bound).

Medical management

Because JRA cannot be cured, treatment is supportive. To reduce inflammation and pain, the physician prescribes high doses of aspirin (80 to 100 mg/kg/day) or another nonsteroidal anti-inflammatory drug (NSAID). Systemic signs, such as fever and anorexia, typically respond to aspirin. If NSAIDs are ineffective, the physician may prescribe gold salts or other antirheumatic drugs. Corticosteroids are indicated for a child with severe complications, such as pericarditis. Corticosteroid eye drops are used to treat uveitis.

Dry or moist heat, such as from a warm bath or shower, reduces morning joint stiffness. Physical therapy and regular exercise promote mobility and reduce deformity.

Nursing management

Nursing goals for the child with JRA include promoting physical mobility, relieving pain, and helping the child and family adapt to living with a chronic disease.

To promote physical mobility, urge the parents and child to comply with drug therapy. Instruct parents to apply heat to stiff joints. Encourage the child to engage in a physical therapy program as well as regular physical and recreational activities—especially swimming. Advise parents to encourage the child to perform as many self-care activities as possible.

To help relieve the child's pain, stress the importance of compliance with drug therapy. Instruct parents to apply heat to joints before the child exercises to reduce exercise-related discomfort and to have the child take short rest breaks to reduce discomfort from sore joints.

The child with JRA may be at risk for body image disturbances related to noticeably swollen joints and limited physical mobility. Such disturbances may prevent the child from engaging in recreational activities with peers. To help the child cope with this problem, suggest physical activities, such as swimming or biking, that the child can participate in comfortably. Encourage the child to express feelings about the disease. Recommend a support group to help the child deal with the stress of living with a chronic, disabling disease.

Rheumatic fever

Rheumatic fever is an inflammatory disease that may follow an untreated Group A beta-hemolytic streptococcal infection— typically, streptococcal pharyngitis. Rheumatic fever is thought to be the most common cause of acquired heart disease in children. The most serious manifestation of rheumatic fever is carditis. Children who do not experience carditis at the onset of the disease generally recover completely.

Rheumatic fever typically affects children ages 6 to 16, with peak incidence occurring in ages 8 to 10. Like streptococcal pharyngitis, rheumatic fever commonly occurs during the late winter and early spring.

Rheumatic fever was common in the United States until the early 1970s, when its incidence declined sharply. However, recent data show a rising incidence.

Pathophysiology and clinical manifestations

Immune system hyperactivity to streptococcal antigens seems to play a key role in rheumatic fever. In untreated streptococcal pharyngitis, streptococcal bacteria release large amounts of toxins, which spread throughout the body. The resulting inflammatory process affects the heart, joints, skin, and central nervous system.

Signs and symptoms of rheumatic fever appear 2 to 6 weeks after untreated streptococcal pharyngitis. The initial acute disease phase lasts approximately 2 to 3 weeks. The acute phase is followed by a proliferative phase which may involve the heart. (For signs and symptoms, see *Assessment findings in rheumatic fever.*) Cellular aggregates, called Aschoff bodies, localize in the mitral valve area causing fibrosis and scarring which may lead to permanent cardiac damage.

Recurrent episodes of acute rheumatic fever may cause rheumatic heart disease, in which an autoimmune reaction in heart tissue damages heart muscle and valves. The patient may develop such disorders as mitral or aortic regurgitation or stenosis. Whether chronic rheumatic heart disease develops depends on the degree of initial carditis and the number of recurrences of acute rheumatic fever.

Assessment findings in rheumatic fever

Assessment findings vary and depend on the site of involvement, severity of the attack, and stage at which child is first seen. The findings typically involve the heart, joints, skin, and central nervous system. Polyarthritis (tender, painful joint swelling and stiffness) and carditis (inflammation of the heart muscle) are the most common manifestations. Polyarthritis may be migratory (moving from joint to joint), typically lasts approximately 3 weeks, and leaves no permanent disability.

Carditis, which commonly involves the heart valves, may lead to heart failure. Suggestive findings include a heart murmur and an increased heart rate. Mild carditis resolves within 2 weeks; severe carditis may persist for up to 6 months.

Other assessment findings in children with rheumatic fever may include:

- a low-grade fever (101° to 102° F [38.3° to 38.8° C])
- malaise
- fatigue
- weight loss

- arthralgia (joint pain without swelling or stiffness)
- subcutaneous nodules (firm, nontender, moveable masses palpable over the extensor surfaces of the elbows, knees, knuckles, ankles, scalp, or spine) which typically appear several weeks after onset onset of rheumatic fever and are closely associated with carditis.

Erythema marginatum, another common finding, is a slightly red, raised, nonpruritic macular rash on the trunk and inner aspects of the extremities. The rash shows central clearing and may extend outward to form rings. It may come and go, and is most noticeable after skin exposure to warmth or moist heat.

Some children also have chorea (St. Vitus' dance), characterized by involuntary, purposeless movements of facial and arm muscles and possibly accompanied by moods swings and personality changes. Most common in prepubertal girls, chorea may arise long after the initial infection. It lasts from a few weeks to few months.

Diagnosis

Diagnosis of rheumatic fever rests on the following criteria:

- the presence of two major signs of the disease (polyarthritis, carditis, subcutaneous nodules, erythema marginatum, or chorea) *or*
- the presence of one major sign plus two minor clinical or laboratory findings (arthralgia, fever, leukocytosis, elevated erythrocyte sedimentation rate [ESR], C-reaction protein test, or a prolonged PR interval on electrocardiogram [ECG]) *plus*
- evidence of a recent group A streptococcal disease (scarlet fever, a positive throat culture, or elevated antistreptolysin-O antibodies).

Medical management

Treatment of rheumatic fever is supportive and includes bed rest (when carditis is present), penicillin to treat the infection, and aspirin to relieve joint pain. Physical activity is limited until the child's heart rate returns to the baseline value. To prevent recurrences of acute rheumatic fever, the physician typically prescribes monthly intramuscular penicillin injections or twice-daily doses of oral penicillin. Prophylactic treatment continues for at least 5 years.

Nursing management

Nursing goals include providing symptomatic relief and preventing disease recurrences. Implement prescribed medical treatments. As prescribed, use aspirin and heat to relieve stiff, aching joints. Counsel the child and family about the importance of complying with aspirin and penicillin therapy as well as the need to maintain bed rest (if necessary). To limit the child's physical activity, provide diversional activities.

Once the acute phase is over, stress the need to comply with prophylactic drug therapy to prevent recurrences and the risk of permanent heart disease. Additional prophylactic antibodies are given prior to dental, upper respiratory, or urologic procedures.

Kawasaki disease

Kawasaki disease is an acute inflammatory disorder characterized by multisystemic vasculitis (inflammation of the vascular system). Presumably, it results from immunologic hypersensitivity to an unidentified virus.

Kawasaki disease was first recognized in children of Japanese origin and is most common in children of Japanese and Korean ancestry. However, the disorder occurs worldwide, usually striking before age 2. Most children recover fully. However, chronic cardiac disease may develop in patients with initial cardiac complications.

Pathophysiology and clinical manifestations

The hyperimmune response leads to extensive inflammation within the vascular system. This disease has three main phases—acute, subacute, and convalescent—and each phase has its own set of clinical manifestations.

Acute phase

During this phase, which starts abruptly and lasts about 7 to 10 days, the child is extremely irritable. Kawasaki disease is diagnosed in any child with at least five of the following signs:
• fever lasting at least 5 days; the temperature may reach up to 104° F (40° C).
• changes in extremities, such as purplish discoloration of the palms and soles and edema of the hands and feet
• erythematous rash
• cervical lymphadenopathy
• bilateral conjunctival inflammation
• oral mucosal changes—reddened, dry, cracking lips; "strawberry" tongue; or oropharyngeal erythema.
Vasculitis within the gastrointestinal system causes anorexia, abdominal pain, diarrhea, and nausea. Most children have tachycardia, and some have a gallop rhythm. Aseptic meningitis, hepatic dysfunction, pericarditis, and myocarditis also may occur. Laboratory findings include an elevated white blood cell (WBC) count and an above normal ESR.

Subacute phase

During this phase, which begins about 7 to 10 days after first symptoms appear, fever abates, and arthralgia and polyarthritis may occur. Desquamation (peeling of the uppermost skin layer) occurs over the palms, soles, and fingertips. Although it may look bad, desquamation is painless.

Irritability and anorexia persist during this phase. The child may develop arrhythmias or signs of congestive heart failure (CHF). Laboratory findings include an elevated ESR an elevated platelet count (thrombocytosis).

Convalescent phase

During this phase, which begins when symptoms have ended, echocardiography may reveal coronary aneurysm (which may rupture). Myocardial infarction also may occur. (In some patients, these problems occur during the subacute phase.) Within 6 to 8 weeks, the ESR returns to normal and the convalescent phase is over.

Medical management

Treatment is supportive. Medical goals include treating signs and symptoms and detecting systemic complications, such as carditis and coronary aneurysm. Typically, the physician prescribes aspirin in doses up to 100 mg/kg/day to reduce inflammation and inhibit platelet formation, then lowers the dosage to 10 mg/kg/day once fever subsides. Aspirin therapy continues throughout the convalescent phase and may extend for up to 1 year after diagnosis to prohibit platelet aggregation and subsequent coronary thrombosis.

To help prevent coronary artery abnormalities, the child receives gamma globulin. Corticosteroids are avoided because they seem to promote aneurysm development. The child with CHF receives digoxin and diuretics.

Typically, the child is hospitalized during the acute phase of Kawasaki disease to allow close monitoring for cardiac or hepatic dysfunction. The child with no cardiac abnormalities may be discharged at the end of this phase, but requires close outpatient monitoring to detect cardiac dysfunction, which sometimes does not arise until the subacute or convalescent phase.

Nursing management

Nursing goals include monitoring the child for complications, providing comfort measures, ensuring sufficient fluid intake, and teaching parents about home management.

Carefully monitor the child for signs of cardiac complications, such as CHF, arrhythmias, and pericarditis. Maintain continuous ECG monitoring, and periodically check ECG tracings for arrhythmias. Observe for signs of CHF, such as gallop rhythm, worsening tachypnea, an increased respiratory rate, crackles, edema, and decreased urine output. Carefully record the patient's fluid intake and output.

To relieve discomfort from rash and edema, apply cool, moist cloths to the appropriate areas. Provide passive range-of-motion exercises if arthritis develops; this may be easiest to do during the child's bath. To reduce irritability during the acute phase, maintain a quiet environment. Reassure the parents that irritability results from the disease and not from the child's personality.

Anorexia, cracked lips, and mouth sores may make the child extremely reluctant to eat or drink. Providing mouth care and lip balm may bring temporary relief, thereby allowing the child to drink. Lubricate the child's lips to ease dryness and cracking. To ensure adequate fluid intake, provide such foods as ice pops, ice chips, and gelatin. Encourage the child to consume enough fluids to meet baseline requirements. However, because of the risk of CHF, be sure to prevent overhydration.

Before discharge, advise parents that the child needs close outpatient monitoring. Inform them that irritability is likely to persist for 2 to 3 weeks (possibly up to 8 weeks) after discharge. Tell them to expect peeling of the child's soles and palms, which generally occurs during the second and third weeks, and reassure them that it is painless. Inform parents that the child must not receive live vaccines until 3 months after gamma globulin administration.

HIV infection

HIV infection commonly leads to acquired immunodeficiency syndrome (AIDS). HIV is transmitted via blood and blood products, body secretions (semen and breast milk), organs, and maternal-fetal blood transfer (a pregnant woman to her fetus). A fetus with an HIV-infected mother has a 25% to 30% chance of acquiring HIV.

Although maternal-fetal transmission accounts for most pediatric AIDS cases, children also may acquire AIDS from infected blood products or donor organs. However, improved blood screening methods have significantly reduced HIV transmission by these modes. Adolescents may acquire AIDS through unprotected sex or intravenous (I.V.) drug use.

Pathophysiology and clinical manifestations

HIV infects human CD4 (T4 helper/inducer) lymphocytes. The virus may not be evident for years—up to 2 years with neonatally acquired disease and up to 7 years in children infected through other means. However, early infections do occur. During the asymptomatic period, the child is considered HIV-positive.

Once the virus becomes active, it destroys helper T cells. HIV infection also destroys or renders ineffective other components of the immune system. Eventually, severe immunodeficiency develops, leaving the child vulnerable to frequent and unusual infections and malignancies.

Clinical manifestations of AIDS in children are not identical to those occurring in adults; they also vary with the child's age. (For a comparison of signs and symptoms in neonates and older children, see *Clinical indicators of HIV infection.*)

Clinical indicators of HIV infection

Assessment findings in children with HIV infection may vary with the child's age. In a neonate, expect any of the following:
- lymphadenopathy
- persistent diarrhea
- failure to thrive
- persistent or recurrent candidiasis (oral thrush)
- chronic otitis media
- lymphoid interstitial pneumonia
- thrombocytopenia
- recurrent bacterial sepsis
- hepatosplenomegaly
- encephalopathy
- loss of developmental milestones.

Older children and adolescents with AIDS may have:
- fever
- lymphadenopathy
- encephalopathy
- weight loss
- opportunistic infections, such as *Pneumocystis carinii* pneumonia
- thrombocytopenia
- nephrotic syndrome.

An adolescent also may have a prodromal period before developing AIDS. This prodromal period is characterized by weight loss, fever, malaise, lymphadenopathy, and diarrhea. Kaposi's sarcoma, common in adults with AIDS, is rare in children.

Diagnosis

Two tests may be used to determine if a child is HIV-positive—the enzyme-linked immunosorbent assay (ELISA), which determines antibody response to the HIV virus, and the Western blot test, which detects antibodies to the virus. However, other criteria must be met to establish the diagnosis of AIDS.

Diagnosing HIV infection in an infant is difficult because transfer of maternal antibodies causes a positive ELISA or Western blot test in all infants born to HIV-infected women. However, not all of these children actually are infected with the virus. In uninfected infants, antibodies passively acquired from the mother decrease and are undetectable by age 15 months. In contrast, HIV-infected infants show a persistent or rising HIV antibody level. (For details on diagnosis, see *Diagnosing AIDS in children*, page 302.)

Medical management

AIDS is incurable and ultimately fatal. Treatment may include zidovudine (AZT) and didanosine; these drugs inhibit replication of HIV within cells and seems to slow progression of the disease.

Preventing infection is critical in managing HIV infection. The physician typically prescribes prophylactic antibiotics, such as co-trimoxazole (Bactrim or Septra) and pentamidine, to help prevent *Pneumocystis carinii* pneumonia, an opportunistic infection. Monthly gamma globulin administration may decrease the overall incidence of bacterial infection. HIV-positive children who acquire chicken pox receive acyclovir.

Nutritional supplements also are prescribed. A severely undernourished child may require nasogastric feedings or total parenteral nutrition.

Diagnosing AIDS in children

The Centers for Disease Control and Prevention (CDC) has issued guidelines for diagnosing pediatric acquired immunodeficiency syndrome (AIDS). In children under age 15 months, the diagnosis of AIDS is based on the confirmed presence of human immunodeficiency virus (HIV) in blood or tissues, or the presence of HIV antibody, or evidence of immunodeficiency and AIDS indicator diseases. In children over age 15 months, the diagnosis of AIDS is based on the confirmed presence of HIV in blood or tissues, or the presence of HIV antibody, or AIDS indicator diseases. Indicator diseases include the following:

- *Pneumocystis carinii* pneumonia
- multiple severe bacterial infections
- lymphoid interstitial pneumonia
- Kaposi's sarcoma
- oral candidiasis
- extrapulmonary cryptococcosis
- diarrhea lasting more than 1 month
- cytomegalovirus (CMV) infection (CMV retinitis, colitis, or pneumonia)
- herpes simplex pneumonitis, esophagitis, or cutaneous ulcer
- lymphoma
- toxoplasmosis
- multifocal leukoencephalopathy
- nonpulmonary *Mycobacterium avium-intracellulare* infection
- *Mycobacterium tuberculosis* infection
- *Strongyloides* superinfection
- syphilis that does not respond to therapy
- recurrent pneumococcal or *Salmonella* bacteremia
- atypical lymphoma
- decreased levels of CD4 cells.

CDC. "Classification System for Human Immunodeficiency Virus (HIV) Infection in Children Under 13 Years of Age." In *Morbidity and Mortality Weekly Report,* 1(15): April 24, 1987.

Children with HIV should receive the usual childhood vaccinations. However, they should receive inactivated polio virus instead of oral polio virus and should receive pneumonia vaccines at age 2 and influenza vaccinations at age 6 months and then yearly.

Nursing management
Nursing goals for the child with HIV infection or AIDS include:
- prevent secondary infection
- promote typical childhood development
- provide sufficient calories for growth
- help the child and family adapt to the effects of a chronic, incurable disease. (For details, see Chapter 15, Illness concepts.)

Infections pose a life-threatening risk. Counsel the parents about the need to comply with prophylactic drug therapy. Teach them how to recognize early signs of opportunistic infection, such as fever and malaise, and to notify the physician immediately if they occur. Teach the child and parents basic measures to prevent infection, such as good personal hygiene, careful hand washing, proper food preparation, and avoidance of persons with known infections.

Like all children, the child with HIV infection or AIDS should participate in age-appropriate activities. Encourage the child to engage in social groups and noncontact sports. If necessary, act as an advocate to help the child gain entry into social or sport groups. Advise parents that the child should attend school, but should stay home during measles and chicken pox outbreaks.

The child with AIDS may need up to twice the normal caloric requirements for his or her age. Advise parents to provide small, frequent, high-calorie meals and snacks. To increase the child's caloric intake, suggest milk shakes, pudding made with whole milk, and egg custard.

STUDY ACTIVITIES

Short answer

1. Summarize the pathophysiology of autoimmune disorders.

_____

_____

2. Describe the rash that typically appears in children with SLE.

_____

3. What causes the hypertension associated with SLE?

_____

4. Identify at least two factors that exacerbate SLE.

_____

5. Risa, age 10, has JRA. To improve her physical mobility, the nurse formulates the following nursing diagnosis: _Impaired physical mobility related to arthritis._ The expected outcomes are that Risa participates in activities of daily living and engages in physical exercise (as tolerated). Identify four nursing interventions that would help achieve these outcomes.

_____

_____

_____

Matching related elements
Match the finding on the left with its definition on the right.

6. ___ Alopecia   **A.** Below normal platelet count

7. ___ Thrombocytopenia   **B.** Hives

8. ___ Urticaria   **C.** Hair loss

9. ___ Leukopenia   **D.** Below normal WBC count

Multiple choice

10. What is the primary purpose of administering corticosteroids to a child with SLE?
- **A.** To combat inflammation
- **B.** To prevent infection
- **C.** To prevent platelet aggregation
- **D.** To promote diuresis

11. When obtaining the history of a child with suspected rheumatic fever, which information would the nurse consider most important?
- **A.** A 3-day history of fever
- **B.** Disinterest in food
- **C.** A recent history of pharyngitis
- **D.** A 2-day history of vomiting

12. Gil, age 5, is about to be discharged after treatment for acute rheumatic fever. Which statement by his parents would indicate that the nurse's discharge teaching has been effective?
- **A.** "We will keep Gil in bed for at least 7 days."
- **B.** "We will give Gil penicillin twice a day."
- **C.** "We will measure Gil's blood pressure every day."
- **D.** "We will keep Gil on corticosteroid therapy."

13. To detect potential complications of Kawasaki disease, the nurse should:
- **A.** Auscultate the child's breath sounds
- **B.** Place the child on a cardiac monitor
- **C.** Monitor the child's blood pressure
- **D.** Assess the child's skin daily

14. Ms. Saggert, who is HIV-positive, recently delivered a daughter. She asks if her newborn has AIDS. Which response would be most appropriate?
- **A.** "Don't worry about that now. It's too soon to tell."
- **B.** "Chances are she'll be OK because you don't have AIDS."
- **C.** "She may have acquired HIV during the pregnancy. We won't know for sure until she is older."
- **D.** "All infants of HIV-positive mothers are infected with HIV. However, symptoms usually don't appear for years."

ANSWERS   **Short answer**

1. In autoimmune disorders, the body makes antibodies against its own normal, healthy cells, leading to tissue damage and multisystemic dysfunction.

2. In children with SLE, a butterfly-shaped rash develops over the cheeks and the bridge of the nose.

3. Hypertension associated with SLE arises secondary to renal disease or corticosteroid therapy.

4. Factors that exacerbate SLE include fatigue, emotional stress, and sunlight.

5. Stress the importance of complying with drug therapy. Instruct Risa's parents to apply heat to stiff joints. Encourage Risa to engage in a physical therapy program as well as regular physical and recreational activities. Advise Risa's parents to encourage her to perform as many self-care activities as possible.

Matching related elements

6. C

7. A

8. B

9. D

Multiple choice

10. A. Corticosteroids are used to combat inflammation. Antibiotics prevent infection and aspirin helps prevent platelet aggregation. Diuresis is not associated with SLE.

11. C. A recent history of pharyngitis is the most important factor in establishing the diagnosis of rheumatic fever. Although a child with rheumatic fever may have a history of fever or vomiting or may seem disinterested in food, these assessment findings are not specific to this disease.

12. B. A child recovering from acute rheumatic fever must receive prophylactic penicillin for at least 5 years. Bed rest is not indicated once the acute phase ends. Monitoring blood pressure and administering corticosteroids are not appropriate in this situation.

13. B. Kawasaki disease sometimes causes cardiac complications, including arrhythmias. Although the other options are important, placing the child on a cardiac monitor is crucial in detecting such complications.

14. C. Diagnosing AIDS in newborns is difficult because all newborns of HIV-positive mothers initially test positive for HIV antibodies (from transfer of maternal antibodies). However, not all actually are infected with HIV. The infant of an HIV-positive woman has a 25% to 30% chance of developing HIV.

CHAPTER 23

Endocrine disorders

OBJECTIVES   After studying this chapter, the reader should be able to:

   1. Describe the function of the thyroid, adrenal, and pituitary glands and the islets of Langerhans in the pancreas.

   2. Describe the causes, pathophysiology, clinical manifestations, and management of congenital and juvenile hypothyroidism, Graves' disease, Addison's disease, Cushing's syndrome, diabetes insipidus, and syndrome of inappropriate antidiuretic hormone.

   3. Describe the causes, pathophysiology, and clinical manifestations of insulin-dependent diabetes mellitus.

   4. Discuss medical and nursing management of the child with newly diagnosed insulin-dependent diabetes mellitus.

   5. Describe the causes, clinical manifestations, and management of hypoglycemia, hyperglycemia, and diabetic ketoacidosis in children with insulin-dependent diabetes mellitus.

OVERVIEW OF CONCEPTS   The endocrine system is a network of ductless glands and other structures that secrete hormones into the bloodstream, thereby influencing the function of specific target organs. In conjunction with the nervous system, the endocrine system controls and integrates the body's metabolic activities. Endocrine glands include the thyroid gland, adrenal glands, pituitary gland, parathyroid glands, pancreas, and gonads (ovaries and testes).

   Endocrine dysfunctions generally are classified as hypofunction, hyperfunction, inflammation, and tumor. Because endocrine dysfunction does not always cause obvious physical signs, children with endocrine disorders may not appear ill. However, most childhood endocrine disorders are chronic, and the child and family must learn to adapt to living with a chronic disorder.

   This chapter reviews the functions of selected endocrine glands. Then, it explores selected endocrine disorders that occur in children—hypothyroidism, Graves' disease, Addison's disease, Cushing's syndrome, diabetes insipidus, syndrome of inappropriate antidiuretic hormone (SIADH), and insulin-dependent diabetes mellitus (IDDM). The chapter also highlights management of IDDM.

Thyroid dysfunction Like other endocrine glands, the thyroid gland is under the influence of the hypothalamus and pituitary gland. The hypothalamus produces thyrotropin-releasing hormone (TRH), which stimulates the production of thyroid-stimulating hormone (TSH) from the pituitary gland. TSH, in turn, triggers release of thyroid hormone from the thyroid gland. Thyroid hormones, which include triiodothyronine (T_3) and thyroxine (T_4), regulate the rate of metabolism for all body systems and are necessary for brain, bone, and tooth growth. They also promote mobilization of fats and gluconeogenesis (formation of carbohydrates from noncarbohydrate molecules).

Primary thyroid dysfunction results from dysfunction within the gland itself; secondary thyroid dysfunction results from dysfunction of the hypothalamus or pituitary gland.

Congenital hypothyroidism

This disorder results from a deficiency of thyroid hormone secretion during fetal development or early infancy. Congenital hypothyroidism is the most common primary thyroid disease in children.

Possible causes of congenital hypothyroidism include genetic factors, maternal treatment of thyroid disease, and defective thyroid hormone synthesis. Sometimes, the cause remains unknown.

Pathophysiology

Embryonic development of the thyroid gland appears to be defective in children with congenital hypothyroidism. Some children are born with no thyroid gland (thyroid aplasia); others, with only a partial gland. The latter initially may have sufficient thyroid hormone.

Insufficient circulating thyroid hormone severely limits the child's physical growth and intellectual development. The disorder affects all cellular functions and slows most physiologic functions.

Assessment

When signs are present at birth, they typically include a large posterior fontanel; an umbilical hernia; persistent physiologic jaundice; poor feeding; lethargy; minimal crying; extended sleeping; below-normal to low-normal temperature and heart rate; and cool and mottled extremities. However, these signs are subtle and may be missed.

By age 6 months, the infant develops classic signs of hypothyroidism: slowed physical growth, a large and protruding tongue, coarse facial features, poor feeding, constipation, hypotonia, and a hoarse cry. Infants treated by age 3 months may have normal intellectual development (a mean IQ of 90). Those who are not treated by age 6 months have severe, irreversible mental retardation. Older children exhibit mental deficiency, stunted growth, and bone and muscle dystrophy.

Diagnosis. All neonates delivered in American hospitals undergo mandatory screening for metabolic disorders, including congenital hypothyroidism. Those with low serum T_4 concentrations, undergo additional laboratory studies. The diagnosis of congenital hypothyroidism rests on a below-normal serum T4 level with a high serum TSH level.

Medical management

The medical goal is to help the child maintain an adequate level of circulating thyroid hormone. This is accomplished through daily thyroid hormone replacement in the form of levothyroxine sodium. To prevent further delays in cognitive development, the child begins full-dose therapy immediately.

Nursing management

Teach the parents appropriate home-management skills. Inform them that the child needs lifelong thyroid hormone replacement therapy. Caution them that the infant may show behavioral changes once this therapy begins, including an increased activity level, increased crying, and decreased sleeping. Advise parents that the child will require periodic medical evaluation. Teach them how to recognize the signs of thyroid hormone deficiency (fatigue, sleepiness, constipation, anorexia, and weight gain) and thyroid hormone excess (increased heart rate, restlessness, insomnia, diarrhea, and weight loss).

Juvenile hypothyroidism

Juvenile (acquired) hypothyroidism is hypothyroidism that occurs after age 2. Causes of the disorder include radiation therapy, iodine deficiency, and autoimmune responses.

Pathophysiology

Because thyroid hormones are responsible for normal metabolic function of all body systems, juvenile hypothyroidism impairs the child's physical growth. However, unlike congenital hypothyroidism, juvenile hypothyroidism does not impair intellectual processes.

Assessment

Signs and symptoms of juvenile hypothyroidism vary with the child's age at onset of the disease. Slowing of growth is the primary sign. The earlier the onset, the more severely the disorder affects physical growth. In a younger child, expect initial slowing of growth, progressing to failure to grow in stature. The child shows an abnormal weight gain pattern, moving from a lower percentile for weight and age to a higher percentile. Obesity sometimes is the first sign of hypothyroidism in a child.

Other signs and symptoms of juvenile hypothyroidism include a slow pulse; coarse, dry skin; constipation; fatigue; increased sleep requirements; a "puffy" appearance; and inactivity.

Diagnosis. Thyroid function tests reveal whether hypothyroidism is primary or secondary. Bone scans may determine how long the thyroid gland has been dysfunctional and help identify growth delays.

Medical management

The physician prescribes thyroid hormone replacement therapy. Because the child has adjusted to low levels of circulating thyroid hormone, immediate full-dose therapy would cause toxic effects—increased heart rate, insomnia, restlessness, irritability, and diarrhea. Therefore, therapy starts with low doses and gradually progresses to full doses.

After treatment begins, most children show accelerated growth. However, many children remain somewhat small in stature.

Nursing management

Provide appropriate teaching to the child and parents, as described earlier in the section on "Congenital hypothyroidism."

Graves' disease

The most common form of hyperthyroidism, Graves' disease is a metabolic imbalance that results from thyroid gland hyperfunction. The disorder typically strikes adolescents, and affects more girls than boys. Causes of Graves' disease include genetic and immunologic factors.

Pathophysiology

Thyroid hyperfunction causes oversecretion of thyroid hormone, leading to increased metabolic function of all body systems.

Assessment

Graves' disease has a gradual onset. Signs and symptoms include voracious appetite, weight loss, insomnia, restlessness, hyperactivity, irritability, tachycardia, hypertension, excessive sweating, tremors, and brisk reflexes. Hyperactivity and restlessness may impair the child's academic performance.

Palpation may reveal an enlarged thyroid gland (goiter). Exophthalmos (bulging eyes)—common in adults with Graves' disease—is relatively rare in children.

Diagnosis. Laboratory studies reveal normal TSH and elevated T_4 levels. To determine thyroid size, the patient may undergo ultrasonography, a nuclear scan, or both.

Medical management

Treatment aims to reduce thyroid activity. The physician prescribes oral propylthiouracil or methimazole—thyroid hormone antagonists that suppress excess thyroid hormone production. This therapy continues for 1 to 2 years. Normal metabolic function returns within 6 weeks after therapy begins. If excess thyroid function persists, another 2-year course of therapy may be prescribed. The child also may receive propranolol to control tachycardia.

If drug therapy proves ineffective, partial thyroid removal may be an option. However, the physician and family must consider the risks of surgery and of inadequate thyroid removal (which causes continued hyperthyroidism) or excessive thyroid removal (which results in hypothyroidism).

If drug therapy proves ineffective and surgery is not an option, the physician may prescribe radioactive iodine therapy. Radioactive iodine settles in the thyroid gland and destroys thyroid tissue, thus reducing thyroid hormone secretion. The child may need repeated doses to obtain desired effects. In some children, radioactive iodine therapy causes hypothyroidism.

Nursing management

The nursing goal is to help manage symptoms of Graves' disease. To help the child cope with the heightened energy demands caused by accelerated metabolism, recommend that the child take several rest periods during the day. Instruct parents to maintain a quiet, nonstimulating environment during rest periods. Advise them to restrict the child's physical energy demands and discourage active play.

Because hyperthyroidism causes heat intolerance, instruct the child to wear cool, loose clothing and avoid warm or humid environments.

Adrenal dysfunction

The adrenal gland has two main sections—the cortex and the medulla. The adrenal cortex secretes three types of hormones: mineralocorticoids, androgens, and glucocorticoids.

Mineralocorticoids, including aldosterone, are controlled by the renin-angiotensin system. Renin, an enzyme, is secreted into the blood by the kidneys in response to decreased arterial pressure or blood volume. Renin converts angiotensinogen to angiotensin I, then angiotensin II. Increased angiotensin levels stimulate the adrenal cortex to secrete aldosterone, which triggers sodium and water reabsorption by the kidneys. As sodium is reabsorbed, potassium is excreted.

Androgens play a role in the development of secondary sex characteristics, reproductive organs, and bones. Glucocorticoids (cortisol and corticosterone) are controlled by corticotropin, which is produced by the anterior pituitary gland. Besides playing a part in fat, protein, and carbohydrate metabolism, glucocorticoids stimulate gluconeogenesis (leading to hyperglycemia); suppress inflammatory, allergic, and immune responses; promote sodium and water retention; and aid the body's response to stress.

The adrenal medulla produces epinephrine and norepinephrine, catecholamines that cause vasoconstriction. Epinephrine also triggers the fight-or-flight response.

Hypoactivity of the adrenal cortex causes Addison's disease; hyperactivity of the adrenal cortex leads to Cushing's syndrome.

Addison's disease

A primary hypofunction of the adrenal gland, Addison's disease is characterized by decreased mineralocorticoid, glucocorticoid, and androgen secretion. It typically results from an adrenal tumor or autoimmune destruction of the adrenal gland. Addison's disease is relatively rare in children.

Pathophysiology and clinical manifestations

Addison's disease has a slow onset. Decreased levels of circulating adrenocortical hormones cause hyperpigmentation, salt craving (caused by excess sodium loss), and fasting hypoglycemia (caused by diminished gluconeogenesis). During times of increased emotional or physical stress, acute adrenal insufficiency may cause such symptoms as muscle weakness, weight loss, and hypotension (caused by water loss) as well as irritability and hypoglycemia.

Diagnosis. A diagnosis of Addison's disease is confirmed by a below normal plasma cortisol level.

Medical management

The physician prescribes replacement corticosteroids, including a glucocorticoid, such as hydrocortisone, and a mineralocorticoid, such as fludrocortisone acetate (Florinef). The patient must take these drugs daily, with additional glucocorticoid doses during periods of increased stress.

Nursing management

Inform the parents that the child needs lifelong daily corticosteroid therapy, with supplemental glucocorticoids during times of increased stress. Teach them how to recognize adverse effects of glucocorticoids, such as gastric irritation, insomnia, and weight gain. Advise parents to minimize stress at home.

Cushing's syndrome

Cushing's syndrome refers to a group of clinical abnormalities caused by excessive levels of adrenocortical hormones or related corticosteroids and, to a lesser extent, androgens and aldosterone.

Etiology

Cushing's syndrome typically results from excess corticotropin production and subsequent hyperplasia of the adrenal cortex. Causes of corticotropin overproduction include pituitary hypersecretion, a corticotropin-producing tumor in another organ, and administration of synthetic glucocorticoids or corticotropin. Cushing's syndrome also may result from a cortisol-secreting adrenal tumor (which commonly is benign). In infants, adrenal carcinoma is the typical cause of the disorder.

Assessment

Signs and symptoms of Cushing's syndrome reflect excessive amounts of circulating cortisol. Typically, fat collects in the patient's face ("moon face"), neck, and trunk. (For other specific assessment findings, see *Signs and symptoms of Cushing's syndrome,* page 312.)

Diagnosis. Clinical findings may suggest Cushing's syndrome. Laboratory tests typically reveal an excessive plasma cortisol level, fasting hyperglycemia, hypokalemia, alkalosis, and excessive 24-hour urine levels of 17-hydroxycorticosteroids and 17-ketosteroids.

Signs and symptoms of Cushing's syndrome

Expect the following clinical manifestations in a child with Cushing's syndrome:
- Abnormal fat distribution in the face ("moon face"), neck, upper back, and trunk
- Purple striae on skin
- Muscle wasting (thin extremities and weakness) caused by increased protein catabolism
- Poor wound healing caused by increased protein catabolism
- Increased susceptibility to infection caused by immunosuppression
- Masculinization in a female (hirsutism, acne, deepening of the voice, and amenorrhea) caused by excessive androgen production
- Hypertension caused by salt and water retention
- Osteoporosis caused by increased renal calcium excretion
- Peptic ulcer caused by increased gastric acid production
- Mental or emotional disturbances, such as psychosis, irritability, insomnia, depression, and euphoria
- Weight gain caused by water retention.

The dexamethasone suppression test confirms the diagnosis. In children with Cushing's syndrome, dexamethasone fails to suppress plasma cortisol levels.

Medical management

Treatment depends on the underlying cause of Cushing's syndrome. A child with an adrenal tumor undergoes bilateral adrenalectomy, followed by lifelong glucocorticoid and mineralocorticoid replacement therapy. A child with a pituitary tumor has surgery or radiation therapy, followed by replacement of growth hormone as well as hormones secreted by endocrine glands under the control of the pituitary gland (the thyroid and adrenal glands). To minimize adverse effects, the physician may prescribe daily morning doses of cortisone.

Nursing management

Nursing measures depend on the cause of the disorder and the treatment plan. A child with Cushing's syndrome that is caused by cortisone therapy may have an altered body image (from abnormal fat distribution and weight gain). Encourage this child to discuss concerns and feelings about weight gain. Advise the child to wear loose clothing to disguise fat around the waist and upper back. If Cushing's syndrome is caused by a tumor, surgical removal and replacement therapy are necessary. The child and parents will need instructions about hormonal replacement therapy.

Posterior pituitary dysfunction

The posterior pituitary gland secretes antidiuretic hormone (ADH) and oxytocin in response to the hypothalamus. ADH stimulates the kidneys to conserve water; oxytocin stimulates uterine contractions and plays a role in lactation.

ADH deficiency causes diabetes insipidus, a condition characterized by high urine output. Excessive ADH release causes SIADH.

Diabetes insipidus

Characterized by extreme polyuria (frequent urination) and polydipsia (excess thirst), diabetes insipidus results from deficient ADH secretion or production (may be caused by a pituitary tumor) or from inability of the renal tubules to respond to ADH.

Diabetes insipidus most commonly follows neurologic injury or surgery. Sometimes it is genetic, having been transmitted by an autosomal recessive inheritance pattern.

Pathophysiology

Without sufficient ADH secretion, filtered water is excreted in the urine instead of being reabsorbed. This leads to diuresis.

Assessment

Diabetes insipidus has a sudden onset. The child is extremely thirsty, consumes large amounts of water, and urinates frequently. Nocturia (nighttime urine production) and nocturnal enuresis (nighttime loss of bladder control) are common. The child may have signs of mild dehydration, such as 5% weight loss, dry mucous membranes, elevated serum osmolarity, and a slightly elevated serum sodium level.

Diagnosis. Initially, urine and serum tests are performed, including electrolytes, blood urea nitrogen, creatinine, sodium, and osmolarity.

The water deprivation test confirms diabetes insipidus. Because this test poses risks, the child is hospitalized and responses are monitored carefully. In this test, the child is deprived of fluids, and hourly measurements record urine output, body weight, urine osmolality or specific gravity, and plasma osmolality. Fluid deprivation continues until the child loses 3% of body weight or has severe postural hypotension. Hourly measurements of urine volume and specific gravity continue after administration of aqueous vasopressin; patients with diabetes insipidus respond to exogenous vasopressin as evidenced by decreased urine output and increased urine specific gravity.

Medical management

The physician attempts to correct the underlying cause of diabetes insipidus. Treatment typically involves daily ADH replacement therapy, which continues until the disorder disappears. Desmopressin acetate (DDAVP) typically is administered by nasal spray.

Nursing management

Teach the child and parents about DDAVP therapy. Instruct them to check for signs of a therapeutic response—stable weight, normal urine output, and normal thirst patterns. Advise parents to give the child free access to fluids.

Syndrome of inappropriate antidiuretic hormone

A form of posterior pituitary hyperfunction, SIADH is characterized by excessive ADH release, which upsets the body's fluid and electrolyte balances. Causes of SIADH include neurologic injury, brain tumors, and certain drugs.

SIADH is a transient disorder. In most children, pituitary gland function returns to normal within a few days. However, because complications of SIADH can be fatal, prompt recognition and treatment are mandatory.

Pathophysiology and clinical manifestations

Excessive ADH production causes water reabsorption by the kidneys, leading to mild to moderate fluid volume excess (hypervolemia).

Clinical and laboratory evidence of SIADH includes decreased urine output, weight gain, increased urine specific gravity, decreased serum osmolarity, and decreased serum sodium level. Fluid and electrolyte disturbances may lead to anorexia and neurologic changes, including lethargy, confusion, and seizures. SIADH is diagnosed from clinical findings.

Medical management

The medical goal is to reduce hypervolemia and restore a normal serum sodium level. Fluids are restricted to two-thirds of the maintenance requirement. Such restriction decreases intravascular volume and raises the serum sodium level by decreasing water volume (relative to sodium level).

Nursing management

Closely monitor the patient's fluid intake and output and urine specific gravity for changes. Also, assess the patient's heart rate, blood pressure, and neurologic status for signs of fluid overload.

Pancreatic dysfunction

The pancreas contains endocrine tissue called the islets of Langerhans, which contain beta cells. These cells secrete insulin, a hormone crucial to the transport of glucose, fat, and protein into muscle and fat cells. Insulin also prevents fat mobilization from fat cells and promotes storage of glucose as glycogen in the liver and muscles. Insulin deficiency or absence causes diabetes mellitus.

Alpha cells of the islets of Langerhans secrete glucagon, which counters the action of insulin. Glucagon stimulates gluconeogenesis, causing the serum glucose level to rise. Delta cells of the islets produce somatostatin, which presumably regulates insulin and glucagon release.

Diabetes mellitus

Diabetes mellitus is a disorder of absolute or relative insulin deficiency or resistance. The most common endocrine disorder in children, diabetes mellitus is characterized by disturbances in carbohydrate, protein, and fat metabolism.

Although three major forms of diabetes mellitus are recognized, the following discussion is limited to insulin-dependent diabetes mellitus (IDDM), also known as Type I diabetes mellitus, which arises during childhood.

Etiology
Multiple factors, including genetic, autoimmune, and environmental factors, are thought to cause destruction of beta cells, resulting in insulin deficiency.

Pathophysiology and clinical manifestations
In IDDM, lack of insulin causes glucose to remain in the bloodstream, leading to an increased serum glucose level (hyperglycemia). The high glucose concentration increases serum osmolarity. In an attempt to dilute the hyperosmotic serum, extravascular fluid shifts to the vascular spaces.

When the glucose concentration exceeds 180 mg/dl, the kidneys excrete the excess glucose along with large volumes of water (osmotic diuresis). Thus, polyuria and polydipsia are significant, early signs of IDDM. Mild indications of dehydration typically follow these two signs.

Because glucose is unavailable, the body breaks down fat reserves for energy use. The liver converts fat to glucose through gluconeogenesis—a process that further increases the serum glucose level. The liver converts free fatty acids (FFAs), by-products of fat breakdown, to ketone bodies (acids). Excessive ketone bodies cause acidosis and may lead to ketoacidosis. Ketonuria (presence of urine ketones) reflects use of FFAs for energy. If metabolic acidosis occurs, Kussmaul's respirations (characterized by increased respiratory rate and depth) occur, reflecting the body's attempt to compensate by eliminating carbon dioxide. Metabolic acidosis may lead to nausea, vomiting, and abdominal pain.

Protein also is broken down for energy. The liver converts protein to glucose, further increasing the serum glucose level. As protein stores become depleted, the child's appetite increases (polyphagia) in an attempt to restore protein. However, increased carbohydrate intake exacerbates hyperglycemia. Muscle wasting and weight loss occur. (For a summary of signs and symptoms of IDDM, see *Assessment findings in IDDM,* page 316.)

Diagnosis. IDDM may be suspected from the child's history and clinical findings. The physician diagnoses IDDM if the child has a fasting blood glucose level above 120 mg/dl or a random blood glucose level above 200 mg/dl in conjunction with typical signs and symptoms.

Medical management
Treatment of IDDM requires a multidisciplinary approach, with the dietitian and diabetes nurse educator playing important roles. Typically, the child requires insulin therapy, dietary modifications, and an exercise program.

Assessment findings in IDDM

In the child with insulin-dependent diabetes mellitus (IDDM), clinical and laboratory results may reveal:
- polyuria caused by osmotic diuresis
- glucosuria caused by increased glucose load
- polydipsia caused by osmotic diuresis and dehydration
- nocturnal enuresis caused by osmotic diuresis
- polyphagia caused by decreased carbohydrate, fat, and protein metabolism
- weight loss caused by osmotic diuresis and muscle wasting
- fatigue and malaise caused by dehydration
- nausea, vomiting, and abdominal pain caused by acidosis when diabetic ketoacidosis (DKA) is present
- fruity breath odor caused by acetone in the breath when DKA is present.

Insulin therapy. Insulin therapy, the primary treatment, aims to maintain a normal or near-normal blood glucose level and prevent episodes of hypoglycemia and hyperglycemia. The child's insulin requirement is determined by blood glucose monitoring. However, insulin needs are affected by individual patient factors; for example, illness, inactivity, emotional stress, and puberty increase insulin needs; physical exercise decreases insulin needs.

Insulin may be given in two or more daily injections or by continuous subcutaneous infusion. Most children require a combination of short-acting (regular) insulin and intermediate-acting (NPH or lente) insulin, which is given before breakfast and before dinner. Others fare better with one daily dose of long-acting (ultralente) insulin, accompanied by injections of short-acting insulin before each meal. (For details on the various types of insulin, see *Types of insulin.*)

The child's blood and urine glucose levels must be monitored to evaluate the effectiveness of insulin therapy. Because the diabetes nurse educator normally teaches the child and family how to monitor these levels, the appropriate techniques are discussed in the section on "Nursing management" below.

To evaluate long-term diabetes control, glycosylated hemoglobin levels may be measured—especially in children with hard-to-control IDDM. These levels reflect the child's average blood glucose level during the previous 2 to 3 months.

Dietary modifications. Nutritional needs of the child with IDDM resemble those of any child. The diet must provide sufficient calories to allow for energy expenditure and physical growth.

However, the child with IDDM must avoid concentrated sugar to prevent hyperglycemia. Fat intake must be restricted to 30% of total daily calories. Carbohydrates should account for 55% to 60% of total daily calories; proteins, 15% to 20%.

Types of insulin

The patient with insulin-dependent diabetes mellitus requires exogenous insulin to compensate for insufficient or absent production of endogenous insulin. Insulin is available in various forms, which differ mainly in onset, peak, and duration of action.

TYPE OF INSULIN	ONSET	PEAK	DURATION
Short-acting (regular)	30 minutes to 2 hours	3 to 4 hours	4 to 6 hours
Intermediate-acting	4 to 6 hours	8 to 14 hours	20 to 24 hours
Long-acting	4 to 8 hours	10 to 30 hours	24 to 36 hours

Unlike children with normal insulin secretion, the child with IDDM does not secrete sufficient insulin in response to dietary intake. Therefore, meals, snacks, and insulin administration must be planned carefully, with food intake coordinated with insulin administration to allow optimal timing and effect of insulin doses. The child must eat meals at set times, and must eat between-meal snacks to prevent hypoglycemia.

The dietitian helps the child and family plan for the child's nutritional needs, designing a program of meals and snacks that provides a balanced diet and includes foods from all the food groups. To make sure the child consumes roughly the same number of calories each day and derives similar calories and nutrients from meals and snacks, the dietitian and patient may use exchange lists, which consist of foods with similar carbohydrate, protein, and fat content. The patient can substitute one food for any other food in the same list without altering nutrient intake.

Exercise. Because exercise lowers the blood glucose level, all children with IDDM should exercise regularly. However, intense physical activity, such as prolonged periods of running, swimming, or other sport, may reduce blood glucose to a dangerous level. To maintain an adequate blood glucose level, the child must modify food intake during prolonged exercise, such as by eating additional snacks.

Before exercising, the child checks the blood glucose level. If it is below 100 mg/dl, the child consumes a pre-exercise snack; a level between 100 and 250 mg/dl does not warrant additional food intake. If the blood glucose level exceeds 250 mg/dl, the child must check for urine ketones (typically using the urine dipstick method). If ketones are absent, the child may perform the planned exercise without additional food intake. If ketones are present, the child must administer insulin and abstain from exercise until ketones disappear.

Sick-day guidelines. During illness, stress hormones (epinephrine and corticosteroids) stimulate gluconeogenesis, thereby causing the blood glucose level to rise and increasing the child's insulin requirements. For this reason, blood glucose must be monitored more frequently during illness. Depending on the result, the insulin dosage may need to be adjusted.

Hypoglycemia management. An abnormally low blood glucose level lower than 60 mg/dl, hypoglycemia may result from such factors as delayed, skipped, or inadequate meals or an increase in physical activity without additional food intake. Hypoglycemic episodes are common even in children with well-controlled diabetes.

Hypoglycemia has a sudden onset. Signs and symptoms include nervousness, irritability, difficulty concentrating, headache, dizziness, hunger, pallor, diaphoresis, tachycardia, and tremors. The blood glucose level typically falls below 60 mg/dl. (Other laboratory values are within normal limits.) If left untreated, hypoglycemia may lead to seizures and coma.

To reduce the frequency and minimize the effects of hypoglycemic episodes, the child and parents must learn to recognize symptoms of hypoglycemia. If possible, they should measure the child's blood glucose level to confirm hypoglycemia.

Treatment of hypoglycemia consists of prompt ingestion of 10 to 15 g of a simple carbohydrate, such as milk (8 oz), fruit juice (4 oz), soda (6 oz), or Insta-Glucose (available commercially). (Although candy also raises the blood glucose level rapidly, it should be used only as a last resort because some children may fake a hypoglycemic episode to receive candy.) After ingesting a simple carbohydrate, the patient ingests a complex carbohydrate (such as bread or cereal) to maintain the blood glucose level.

Symptoms should start to subside within 5 minutes of carbohydrate ingestion. If they persist, the child should consume another carbohydrate in 10 to 15 minutes.

Hyperglycemia management. Characterized by a blood glucose level above 250 mg/dl, hyperglycemia is common in children with IDDM. Hyperglycemic episodes may result from ingestion of concentrated carbohydrates, overeating, or illness. Persistent hyperglycemia reflects poor diabetes control, as from puberty-related hormonal changes or insufficient insulin administration.

Hyperglycemia has a gradual onset. Signs and symptoms include lethargy, confusion, weakness, thirst, flushed skin, polyuria, polydipsia, and diminished reflexes. Initially, laboratory values may be normal (except blood glucose). If left untreated, hyperglycemia may progress to diabetic ketoacidosis (DKA). See *How to manage hyperglycemia* for information on hyperglycemia management.

DKA management. An acute, life-threatening complication of uncontrolled IDDM, DKA accounts for most IDDM-related hospital admis-

How to manage hyperglycemia

To help prevent diabetic ketoacidosis and other complications of diabetes mellitus, make sure the child and parents know how to detect hyperglycemia and know what to do if it occurs. Review the following guidelines:

- If the child's blood glucose level measures above 140 mg/dl but below 250 mg/dl and urine is negative for ketones, monitor blood glucose and urine ketones every 4 hours. Notify the physician if hyperglycemia persists.
- If the child's blood glucose level is above 250 mg/dl but below 400 mg/dl and urine is negative for ketones, monitor blood glucose and urine ketones every 4 hours and increase the child's water intake. Notify the physician if hyperglycemia persists.
- If the child's blood glucose level exceeds 400 mg dl and urine is negative for ketones, give the child short-acting insulin, increase the child's water intake, and monitor blood glucose and urine ketones every 4 hours. Notify the physician if hyperglycemia persists.
- If the child's blood glucose level exceeds 200 mg/dl and urine is positive for ketones, administer short-acting insulin, monitor blood glucose and urine ketones every 2 hours, increase the child's water intake, and notify the physician.

sions. This disorder is characterized by hypovolemia, electrolyte imbalance, extreme hyperglycemia, and breakdown of FFAs, which causes acidosis. If left untreated, DKA may lead to coma.

The child with DKA may have 10% (moderate) dehydration, severe metabolic acidosis, hyponatremia, and hypokalemia. The blood glucose level exceeds 250 mg/dl and sometimes rises as high as 800 mg/dl. (For details on DKA and its management, see *Assessing and managing DKA*, page 320.)

Nursing management

Nursing goals for the child with IDDM differ according to whether DKA is present.

Management of IDDM (without DKA). Nursing goals for the child with newly diagnosed IDDM include:

- restoring a normal blood glucose level (80 to 140 mg/dl)
- teaching the child and parents about diabetes management
- helping the child and parents adjust to living with a chronic disease. (For more information on caring for the child with a chronic disease, see Chapter 15, Illness concepts.)

The immediate goal is to restore the blood glucose level to normal. Measure the child's blood glucose level; based on the value, administer insulin as prescribed. To evaluate the effectiveness of insulin therapy, closely monitor and document blood glucose and urine ketone levels. Also implement the prescribed dietary management plan. Carefully monitor the child's dietary intake, and make sure the child consumes meals and snacks at the prescribed times. Assess for signs and symptoms of hypoglycemia and hyperglycemia.

Assessing and managing DKA

Most common in patients with undiagnosed insulin-dependent diabetes mellitus, diabetic ketoacidosis (DKA) results from uncontrolled hyperglycemia. It is characterized by osmotic diuresis, which leads to dehydration and hypovolemia. Inadequate renal perfusion causes renal dysfunction, retention of hydrogen ions, and metabolic acidosis.

Assessment
Initially, the child exhibits signs of hyperglycemia, followed by evidence of increasing dehydration and hypovolemia (dry mucous membranes, tachycardia, and weak peripheral pulses) and acidosis (abdominal pain, nausea and vomiting, fruity breath odor, and deep, rapid respirations). Laboratory tests reveal a blood glucose level above 250 mg/dl; significant levels of urine and blood ketone bodies; a low bicarbonate level; arterial pH below 7.30; and elevated serum sodium, hematocrit, and hemoglobin values (resulting from hemoconcentration secondary to hypovolemia).

Management
As prescribed, administer insulin intravenously to decrease the blood glucose level, and provide fluid and electrolyte therapy to correct dehydration, hypovolemia, electrolyte disturbances, and acidosis. Monitor blood glucose and urine ketones hourly. Once metabolic acidosis resolves and peristalsis returns, provide oral intake and administer subcutaneous insulin, as prescribed.

To meet the family's extensive teaching needs, provide information about the pathophysiology of IDDM and the role of insulin in disease management. Encourage the child and parents to ask questions. Provide answers and clarify any misconceptions.

Describe the various insulin preparations. Based on the child's management plan, explain the action, peak effects, and duration of each type of insulin prescribed. Demonstrate procedures for mixing, drawing up, and administering insulin. Describe appropriate injection sites (lateral surface of the upper arms, anterior and lateral surfaces of the thighs, lateral aspects of the abdomen, and upper outer quadrant of the buttocks). Have the child choose two or three injection sites. Emphasize that the child should rotate these sites to prevent hypertrophy which may result from overuse of a single site.

Teach the parents insulin injection techniques, and ask them to demonstrate these techniques. If appropriate, teach the child how to self-administer insulin. The age at which a child can learn self-administration techniques varies. Some children as young as age 8 can learn these techniques; by age 12, most children can self-administer insulin. Instruct the parents or child to inject insulin 30 to 60 minutes before meals, at approximately the same time each day.

To help evaluate the effectiveness of insulin therapy, teach the parents and child (if appropriate) how to monitor blood and urine glucose levels. (Most children ages 8 and over can learn how to monitor blood glucose.) Initially, instruct them to measure the child's blood glucose level at least four times a day—before each meal and snack. Explain home monitoring systems. Demonstrate blood sampling techniques and procedures for obtaining accurate results, and have the parents or child provide a return demonstration.

Also teach the parents and child how to monitor for urine ketones. Instruct them to check urine for ketones whenever the child's blood glucose level exceeds 250 mg/dl as well as during periods of illness or vomiting (a sign of ketoacidosis).

In conjunction with the dietitian, explain the principles of dietary management. Describe each food group, and list specific foods in each group. Emphasize that the child must not eat concentrated carbohydrates. Suggest such alternatives as sugar-free drinks, juices, and jelly. Review the prescribed meal plans. Explain how to use exchange lists for meal planning. Stress that the child must eat meals and snacks at consistent times each day.

Teach the child and parents about the importance of exercise. Explain that regular exercise aids the day-to-day management of IDDM by lowering the blood glucose level. Instruct parents to measure and record the child's blood glucose level before and after exercise when the child begins an exercise program (such as swimming, running, or other organized sport). Based on blood glucose levels, the physician may recommend supplemental food intake before or during exercise. Caution the child and parents to avoid injecting insulin into a recently exercised body part (such as an arm or leg) because increased blood flow to muscles during exercise enhances insulin absorption and may lead to hypoglycemia.

Explain sick-day guidelines to the child and parents. Instruct parents to monitor the child's blood glucose level every 4 to 6 hours during illness because hyperglycemia is more likely occur. Tell parents to administer the usual insulin doses even if the child has a poor appetite.

Review the signs and symptoms of hypoglycemia with the child and parents. Make sure the parents know what to do if hyperglycemia occurs. Advise them to obtain a blood glucose level at the first indication of hypoglycemia, and to give the child 10 to 15 g of a concentrated carbohydrate if the blood glucose level is below 60 mg/dl. Because the hypoglycemic child may be unable to follow instructions or obtain food unassisted, emphasize that another person should be responsible for giving the carbohydrate to the child. Instruct parents to check the child's blood glucose level 15 minutes after carbohydrate ingestion. If it is still less than 60 mg/dl, the child should ingest another 10 to 15 g of carbohydrate. If the blood glucose level exceeds 60 mg/dl, parents should give the child a complex carbohydrate.

Explain how diet, exercise, insulin, and hypoglycemia are interrelated. Teach the parents how to modify the child's diet or exercise program in response to changes in blood glucose levels. Suggest that the parents or child carry a concentrated simple carbohydrate (such as hard candy) at all times in case hypoglycemia occurs.

Also, review the signs and symptoms of hyperglycemia with the child and parents. Instruct them to obtain a blood glucose level at the first indication of hyperglycemia; explain that a value above 250 mg/dl indicates severe hyperglycemia. Review hyperglycemia treatment guidelines with the family. (See *How to manage hyperglycemia*, page 320.)

Explain how diet, illness, puberty, insulin, and hyperglycemia are interrelated. Stress the importance of eliminating concentrated carbohydrates from the child's diet. Review the principles of illness management. Explain that puberty may increase insulin requirements.

Also review the signs and symptoms of DKA. Instruct the parents to bring the child to the emergency room if they suspect DKA.

Management of IDDM and DKA. For the child admitted to the hospital with DKA, nursing goals include:
• restoring a normal blood glucose level (80 to 140 mg/dl)
• restoring fluid and electrolyte balance
• preventing recurrences of DKA.

Administer insulin by continuous infusion, as prescribed. To evaluate insulin effectiveness, monitor the child's blood glucose level every hour. As prescribed, administer intravenous (I.V.) fluids to maintain fluid balance and renal function. Once kidney function has been restored, add potassium to the I.V. solution, as prescribed.

Acidosis resolves gradually as the blood glucose level falls and the kidneys excrete ketone bodies. Once the blood glucose level returns to normal and the child no longer is acidotic, administer insulin subcutaneously and have the child resume oral intake, as prescribed.

Monitor fluid intake and output hourly. Evaluate the child's fluid status carefully by checking vital signs every 2 hours, inspecting mucous membranes and skin turgor every 4 hours, and weighing the child daily. Review the child's laboratory values (pH, bicarbonate, serum sodium, and serum potassium levels) daily.

Once the child's condition stabilizes, try to determine what caused DKA. Ask the child and parents about such possible triggers as recent illness or missed insulin doses. If illness precipitated DKA, review sick-day guidelines with the family. If insulin doses were skipped deliberately, explore the reason for this. Reinforce the importance of complying with insulin therapy and the dietary management plan. If necessary, ask a family member to assume responsibility for monitoring the child's blood glucose levels and administering insulin.

STUDY ACTIVITIES

Short answer

1. What is the primary sign of juvenile hypothyroidism?

_____

2. List at least five clinical manifestations of Graves' disease.

_____

_____

3. What are three adverse effects of corticosteroid therapy?

_____

4. Explain why illness may lead to hyperglycemia in the child with IDDM.

_____

_____

5. Bobby, age 7, has DKA. To help restore his fluid and electrolyte balance, the nurse formulates the following nursing diagnosis: *High risk for fluid volume deficit related to osmotic diuresis.* The expected outcomes are that Bobby maintain a urine output of 2 ml/kg/hour and a urine specific gravity of 1.006 to 1.020; exhibit moist mucous membranes and normal skin turgor; maintain vital signs and laboratory values within normal limits; and resume his preadmission weight. Identify three nursing interventions that would help achieve these outcomes.

_____

Matching related elements

Match the hormone on the left with its function on the right.

6. ___ Thyroid hormone   **A.** Promotes glucose transport into cells

7. ___ Mineralocorticoid   **B.** Promotes normal fat, protein, and glucose metabolism

8. ___ Corticosteroid   **C.** Stimulates the renal reabsorption of sodium

9. ___ Insulin   **D.** Regulates the metabolic rate

Multiple choice

10. In a child with juvenile hypothyroidism, which assessment finding would the nurse expect?

    A. Recent weight loss

    B. Goiter

    C. Tachycardia

    D. Insomnia

11. The nurse administers DDAVP to a child with diabetes insipidus. Which assessment finding indicates a positive response to this therapy?
  A. Decreased urine output
  B. Increased blood glucose level
  C. Decreased blood pressure
  D. Reduction of nausea

12. The nurse prepares to give short-acting insulin to a diabetic child with hyperglycemia. To evaluate the effectiveness of insulin therapy, when should the nurse measure the child's blood glucose level?
  A. Immediately before administering insulin
  B. 15 minutes after administering insulin
  C. 1 hour after administering insulin
  D. 4 hours after administering insulin

ANSWERS **Short answer**

  1. The primary sign of juvenile hypothyroidism is slowing of growth.
  2. Clinical manifestations of Graves' disease include voracious appetite, weight loss, insomnia, restlessness, hyperactivity, irritability, tachycardia, hypertension, excessive sweating, tremors, and brisk reflexes.
  3. Adverse effects of corticosteroid therapy include gastric irritation, weight gain, and insomnia.
  4. During illness, stress hormones are released. These hormones stimulate gluconeogenesis, thereby causing hyperglycemia.
  5. Administer I.V. fluids, as prescribed. Record Bobby's fluid intake and output hourly. Monitor the moistness of mucous membranes, skin turgor, and vital signs. Evaluate Bobby's weight and laboratory values daily.

Matching related elements

  6. D
  7. C
  8. B
  9. A

Multiple choice

10. B. Juvenile hypothyroidism also results in weight gain and a slow heart rate, not weight loss and a fast heart rate (tachycardia). Sleepiness rather than insomnia would be present.
11. A. The primary action of DDAVP is to stimulate water reabsorption by the kidneys. Therefore, decreased urine output signals a positive response to DDAVP therapy. DDAVP has no effect on blood pressure, glucose levels, or nausea.
12. C. The action of short-acting insulin peaks 30 minutes to 2 hours after administration. The nurse should check the child's blood glucose level during this period, such as 1 hour after insulin administration.

CHAPTER 24

Renal disorders

OBJECTIVES   After studying this chapter, the reader should be able to:

1. Describe the causes, pathophysiology, and clinical manifestations of glomerulonephritis and nephrotic syndrome.

2. Discuss medical and nursing management of children with glomerulonephritis and nephrotic syndrome.

3. Identify the causes, pathophysiology, and clinical manifestations of acute renal failure and chronic renal failure.

4. Discuss medical and nursing management of children with renal failure.

OVERVIEW OF   The kidneys are crucial in maintaining the body's fluid and electrolyte
CONCEPTS   balances. Renal dysfunction may upset these balances and result in serious consequences in other body systems. For this reason, the nurse who cares for children with renal disorders must understand renal pathophysiology and its systemic effects.

This chapter explores selected renal disorders in children—glomerulonephritis, nephrotic syndrome, acute renal failure (ARF), and chronic renal failure (CRF). For each disorder, it discusses the causes and underlying pathophysiology, identifies assessment findings, and delineates medical and nursing management.

Glomerulonephritis   Glomerulonephritis is a noninfectious inflammation of the glomerulus of the kidney. The disorder may be primary or may arise secondary to a systemic disease, such as systemic lupus erythematosus (SLE) or sickle cell disease.

Classification

Several forms of glomerulonephritis have been identified. Acute glomerulonephritis sometimes results from systemic disease. However, it typically occurs as acute poststreptococcal glomerulonephritis (APSGN), an autoimmune disorder arising after a bout with untreated streptococcal pharyngitis. APSGN is the most common form of glomerulonephritis in children. Generally, acute glomerulonephritis is self-limiting and resolves spontaneously within a few weeks.

Anticipating complications of APSGN

The predominant form of glomerulonephritis in children, acute poststreptococcal glomerulo-nephritis (APSGN) may lead to the following complications:

- hypertensive encephalopathy, as manifested by headache, dizziness, nausea and vomiting, vision disturbances, and seizures
- acute cardiac decompensation and heart failure, indicated by tachycardia, tachypnea, crackles, and dyspnea
- acute renal failure, which causes such early signs as severe oliguria or anuria, elevated blood urea nitrogen level, and hyperkalemia.

Rapidly progressive glomerulonephritis may occur secondary to drug toxicity or to acute glomerulonephritis (rare). Sometimes, the cause is unknown. This form of glomerulonephritis leads to CRF within months.

Chronic glomerulonephritis results from autoimmune mechanisms. It may follow a series of acute exacerbations of preexisting renal disease; some patients, however, have no history of renal disease. The disorder develops fairly slowly, and symptoms may appear only after loss of considerable renal function. It progresses to CRF and eventually to end-stage renal disease (ESRD).

Pathophysiology

In APSGN, antibodies develop in response to streptococcal infection and attack glomerular cells, causing kidney enlargement and edema. As glomerular inflammation and obstruction impair glomerular filtration, water and electrolytes accumulate within the vascular system. Hypervolemia and edema follow. (For complications of APSGN, see *Anticipating complications of APSGN*.)

Assessment

Signs and symptoms of APSGN arise suddenly—1 to 2 weeks after streptococcal infection. They include:

- general malaise
- anorexia
- fatigue
- weight gain
- hypertension
- headache
- periorbital and peripheral edema
- urinary changes, such as moderate proteinuria, moderate hematuria, dark urine, and oliguria (decreased urine output)
- increased urine specific gravity.

The acute phase of APSGN typically lasts 4 to 10 days but may persist for up to 3 weeks. During this phase, the child is lethargic. Weight and blood pressure may fluctuate and blood pressure may become danger-ously high.

Increased urine output is the first sign that the child's condition is improving. As urine output increases, weight starts to drop. Within a few days, massive diuresis occurs. Blood pressure returns to normal as excess water is excreted.

Diagnosis

A diagnosis of APSGN is made based on evidence of recent streptococcal infection, a positive throat culture, or a positive antistreptolysin titer as well as glomerular disease confirmed by hematuria, proteinuria, and red blood cell (RBC) casts.

Medical management

APSGN warrants supportive treatment. A child with adequate urine output, minimal edema, and normal or mildly elevated blood pressure may receive care at home. A child with moderate to severe hypertension, oliguria, and moderate to severe edema is admitted to the hospital for observation.

The medical goal is to detect and treat complications. Fluid balance is monitored closely. The physician typically prescribes furosemide (Lasix) if the child has significant fluid overload, as indicated by severe edema, severe hypertension, tachycardia, crackles, and tachypnea. However, furosemide has limited value in treating uncomplicated acute glomerulonephritis because decreased glomerular filtration prevents most sodium from reaching the distal tubules.

Depending on the child's condition, other measures may include:
- digoxin therapy to treat acute cardiac decompensation
- antihypertensive therapy to treat persistent moderate to severe hypertension
- dietary sodium and potassium restrictions to relieve significant edema and oliguria
- protein restriction to correct elevated blood urea nitrogen (BUN) level
- fluid restriction to treat pronounced oliguria
- antibiotic therapy to treat active streptococcal infection. (However, antibiotic therapy does not alter the course of glomerulonephritis.)

Nursing management

Nursing goals for the child with APSGN include:
- detecting changes in fluid balance
- preventing further fluid retention
- preventing injury caused by complications of hypervolemia.

To detect changes in fluid balance, weigh the child daily, measure fluid intake and output, record urine specific gravity, and stay alert for changes in edema.

To prevent further fluid retention, restrict dietary sodium, administer furosemide, and maintain fluid restrictions, as prescribed.

To prevent injury caused by complications of hypervolemia, administer antihypertensives, as prescribed, and record the patient's blood pressure every 4 hours. Monitor the patient's cardiovascular and pulmonary status, including heart rate, peripheral pulses, respiratory rate, and lung sounds, every 4 hours. Administer digoxin, as prescribed. Also evaluate the patient's neurologic status, observing for headache and lethargy.

Nephrotic syndrome

The most common glomerular disorder in children, nephrotic syndrome is characterized by marked proteinuria, hypoproteinemia (as evidenced by low serum albumin level), hyperlipidemia, and edema. Nephrotic syndrome may occur in patients with glomerular disorders or renal vein thrombosis. Sometimes it arises as a complication of a systemic disease, such as amyloidosis, diabetes mellitus, SLE, or multiple myeloma. Although the exact cause of nephrotic syndrome is unknown, immunologic responses have been implicated.

Classification

Nephrotic syndrome is classified as primary when localized to the glomerulus and secondary when resulting from the destructive glomerular effects of other disorders.

Minimal-change nephrotic syndrome (MCNS), the most common form of primary nephrotic syndrome, accounts for about 85% of nephrotic syndrome cases. MCNS affects males more than females. Typically, it follows a pattern of acute exacerbations alternating with periods of remission. Approximately 75% of children achieve final remission by adolescence. The other forms of nephrotic syndrome carry a less favorable prognosis. Other forms of primary nephrotic syndrome include congenital nephrotic syndrome (an inherited type) and chronic glomerulonephritis (various types of glomerulonephropathy). Secondary nephrotic syndrome refers to renal involvement that results from other disease or such causes as bacterial or viral infections, neoplasms, multisystemic disorders (SLE or diabetes mellitus), heredity (sickle cell anemia), toxins, or drugs.

Pathophysiology

The pathophysiology of MCNS is not well understood. For some reason, glomerular capillaries become permeable to protein. Large amounts of protein are excreted in the urine, leading to hypoproteinemia (a decrease in plasma proteins). Hypoproteinemia, in turn, causes the plasma oncotic pressure to fall, allowing intravascular fluid to shift to the extravascular (interstitial) spaces. Consequently, blood volume decreases, profound edema occurs, and the patient gains weight.

The decrease in blood volume triggers release of antidiuretic hormone (ADH), which in turn causes water reabsorption by the kidneys. This contributes further to edema. Decreased blood volume also activates the renin-angiotensin system, stimulating aldosterone release. Aldosterone causes renal water and sodium reabsorption, which further worsens edema.

Assessment

All forms of nephrotic syndrome cause similar signs and symptoms. However, the clinical course, response to treatment, and prognosis differ. The discussion below applies to MCNS, the most common form.

In most children, a viral infection, such as an upper respiratory infection, precedes MCNS symptoms. However, researchers do not believe such infections actually cause nephrotic syndrome.

Clinical manifestations of nephrotic syndrome, including edema, arise rather slowly. Commonly, periorbital and facial edema are apparent in the morning and subside during the day. Abdominal distention and peripheral edema may occur later in the day. Labial and scrotal edema also are common. As the syndrome progresses, generalized profound edema (anasarca) may develop.

The patient has pallor, fatigue, and a slow but steady weight gain (resulting from fluid retention and edema). Intestinal edema causes anorexia and diarrhea. Urine volume decreases, and urine becomes frothy and dark amber in color. Urine specific gravity rises, and massive proteinuria occurs. Blood pressure remains normal or drops slightly, resulting from decreased circulating blood volume. The patient is predisposed to infections—probably resulting from corticosteroid therapy and poor nutritional status.

Laboratory findings include hypercholesterolemia (caused by increased hepatic synthesis of lipids), hypoalbuminemia, and elevated hematocrit and hemoglobin values (caused by hemoconcentration).

Diagnosis

Nephrotic syndrome is diagnosed from clinical manifestations and from hypercholesterolemia, hypoalbuminemia, and proteinuria in the absence of hematuria and hypertension. A renal biopsy determines the form of nephrotic syndrome.

Medical management

Treatment aims to reduce urinary protein excretion, relieve edema, and prevent relapse. Corticosteroid therapy typically decreases urinary protein excretion. For full resolution of proteinuria, the child may need to continue corticosteroid therapy for up to 1 month; the dosage is tapered once proteinuria and edema disappear.

To reduce severe edema, the physician prescribes furosemide; metolazone may be used in combination with furosemide. Albumin is used for those patients with persistent edema, vascular insufficiency, or oliguria or anuria that lasts several days. A plasma protein, albumin causes interstitial fluid to shift into the vascular spaces. Administering furosemide concomitantly with albumin promotes diuresis. However, this therapy has little effect on stopping the renal excretion of protein.

During the acute phase, the physician commonly prescribes a low-sodium diet to limit edema and also may restrict water intake.

To minimize acute exacerbations in a child predisposed to frequent relapses, the physician may prescribe long-term, low-dose corticosteroid therapy. Every-other-day administration minimizes the effects of prolonged corticosteroid therapy, such as obesity, delayed growth, hypertension, increased risk of infection, and gastrointestinal (GI) irritation. Cyclophosphamide (Cytoxan), an immunosuppressant drug, also has proven effective in reducing the relapse rate.

Nursing management
During the acute phase of nephrotic syndrome, nursing goals include:
• detecting changes in the patient's fluid status
• preventing fluid retention
• preventing infection
• preventing skin breakdown
• improving the patient's nutritional status
• promoting adequate rest
• promoting a positive self-concept.

To detect changes in fluid status and prevent fluid retention, document the child's fluid intake and output, urine specific gravity, and urine protein levels. Weigh the child and measure abdominal girth daily; an increase in either indicates fluid retention. Monitor the child's heart rate, pulse quality, and blood pressure every 4 hours. Increased heart rate, reduced pulse quality, and decreased blood pressure may indicate intravascular fluid volume deficit (hypovolemia). As prescribed, administer corticosteroids. Give albumin and diuretics, as prescribed, and maintain fluid and salt restrictions.

During albumin therapy, the child is at risk for hypervolemia resulting from sudden fluid shifts into the intravascular spaces. To detect hypervolemia, monitor vital signs hourly and auscultate the lungs for crackles, which indicate pulmonary edema. Weigh the child before and after therapy; expect weight to drop. To promote urine output, administer diuretics, as prescribed. Carefully document urine output; expect diuresis.

To prevent infection, protect the child from known sources of infection. Monitor the white blood cell count, and take the child's temperature every 8 hours.

To prevent skin breakdown, monitor the skin for redness and breakdown. Place sheepskin or a low-air-loss mattress under the child. Change the child's position every 2 hours. Keep the skin dry, especially at the skin folds. Apply powder to reduce friction on the skin, and avoid using tape on the skin. Provide loose clothing. Use saline wipes to clean edematous eyelids. Provide support for an edematous scrotum.

To improve the child's nutritional status, let the child select foods, within dietary constraints. Be aware that the child in remission can eat a full regular diet. To provide age-appropriate and favorite foods, obtain help from the dietary department or the parents. Provide foods in an attractive setting. Sit with the child during meals, or encourage the parents to do so.

To promote adequate rest, maintain bed rest during periods of severe edema. Provide quiet activities and a quiet, nonstimulating environment. Provide access to diversional activities, such as a television or radio.

Body changes stemming from edema and corticosteroid therapy put the child at risk for a disturbed body image. To promote a positive self-concept, encourage the patient to discuss feelings about appearance. Stress the positive aspects of the child's appearance. Discuss clothing options to camouflage weight gain. Provide positive feedback for the child's grooming efforts. Encourage the child to participate in peer-related activities.

Acute renal failure

ARF occurs when the kidneys suddenly lose their ability to regulate excretory function. Although relatively uncommon in children, ARF can be fatal.

ARF can be reversible or irreversible. Reversible ARF begins with a low-output phase marked by oliguria, which lasts from a few days in infants and younger children to a few weeks in older children. Next, a period of diuresis, called the high-output phase, occurs; it begins suddenly and lasts up to a week. The child recovers fully within 6 months of diagnosis.

With irreversible ARF, the child develops CRF and requires lifelong support (as discussed in the section on "Chronic renal failure" below).

Etiology

Various clinical conditions may lead to ARF. These conditions may be prerenal, intrarenal, or postrenal. Prerenal causes are most common in children and are characterized by decreased renal perfusion; such conditions include hypovolemia, hypotension, hypoxia, and renal vascular obstruction.

Intrarenal causes include renal diseases (such as acute glomerulonephritis, nephrotic syndrome, and hemolytic uremia syndrome) and exposure to renal toxins (such as certain antineoplastic and anti-inflammatory agents, certain anesthetics and heavy metals, and dyes used in radiographic studies).

Postrenal causes of ARF include such obstructive conditions as renal calculi, tumors, and congenital structural anomalies.

Pathophysiology

In ARF, a severe drop in the glomerular filtration rate impedes urine production and electrolyte excretion. (For details on the pathophysiology, see *Understanding the pathophysiologic effects of ARF,* page 332.)

Understanding the pathophysiologic effects of ARF

In the child with acute renal failure (ARF), a decreased glomerular filtration rate leads to the following changes:
- reduced urine output, fluid retention, and increased intravascular fluid volume (hypervolemia). These changes, in turn, cause generalized edema and hypertension. The child also is at risk for pulmonary and cerebral edema and congestive heart failure.
- inappropriate secretion of antidiuretic hormone, which exacerbates fluid retention
- decreased excretion of electrolytes and body wastes, causing the blood urea nitrogen and serum creatinine levels to rise. Inadequate excretion of excess hydrogen ions leads to metabolic acidosis; inadequate excretion of excess potassium ions causes hyperkalemia, setting the stage for cardiac arrhythmias. Failure to excrete excess phosphorus leads to hyperphosphatemia and hypocalcemia, putting the child at risk for neuromuscular irritability and decreased clotting time.

Potential complications of ARF include hyperkalemia and its consequences, acute cardiac decompensation, and cerebral encephalopathy.

Assessment

Clinical manifestations of ARF appear suddenly and include:
- oliguria (urine output below 50 ml/24 hours)
- lethargy (caused by electrolyte disturbances)
- nausea and vomiting (caused by electrolyte disturbances)
- edema (caused by fluid retention)
- hypertension (caused by increased intravascular volume).

Laboratory findings include an elevated BUN, increased plasma creatinine level, metabolic acidosis, hyponatremia, hyperkalemia, and hypocalcemia.

Diagnosis

ARF is diagnosed from clinical and laboratory findings described above.

Medical management

The physician reviews the patient's history to determine the underlying cause of ARF. Besides measures to correct the underlying cause, treatment includes supportive therapy and measures to prevent or manage complications. In some cases, ARF resolves once the underlying cause is treated. For example, fluid volume replacement rapidly improves kidney function in ARF caused by severe hypovolemia.

Supportive therapy

Supportive therapy may involve multiple measures.

Urine output monitoring. An indwelling (Foley) catheter may be inserted to measure hourly urine output. Some patients require an external collection device to prevent urinary tract infection.

Fluid therapy. The patient with prerenal ARF receives fluid replacement therapy, which generally restores urine output within 2 hours. A child who does not produce urine but is adequately hydrated (as reflected by clinical and laboratory findings) may receive a diuretic to induce urine production. Continued failure to produce sufficient urine (more than 1 ml/kg/hour) requires fluid restriction.

Fluids also are restricted in children with intrarenal or postrenal ARF. These children receive only enough fluids to replace sensible and insensible losses. A central venous line may be inserted to monitor intravascular fluid volume status.

Once the high-output phase of ARF begins, the physician orders fluids and electrolytes to prevent dehydration and electrolyte depletion.

Electrolyte management. The physician restricts the child's oral and intravenous (I.V.) intake of sodium, chloride, and potassium to prevent further electrolyte excesses.

Nutritional support. The child with ARF needs adequate nutrition to reduce the effects of tissue catabolism and to repair the kidneys. The physician prescribes a diet high in carbohydrate and low in protein, sodium, and potassium. If persistent nausea and anorexia limit the child's caloric consumption, parenteral nutrition may be necessary.

Hypertension management. To lower the child's blood pressure, the physician restricts fluids (to reduce the fluid load) and prescribes antihypertensive drugs.

Preventing and managing complications

Complications of ARF may be life-threatening and must be detected and treated promptly.

Hyperkalemia. Hyperkalemia may cause cardiac arrhythmias and cardiac arrest. Frequent electrocardiograms (ECGs) and serum potassium monitoring can detect these problems early. To prevent hyperkalemia, the physician eliminates potassium from I.V. fluids and oral intake and corrects metabolic acidosis.

The child with a serum potassium level approaching 7 mg/dl or with suggestive ECG changes requires prompt corrective measures, such as administration of calcium gluconate, sodium bicarbonate, or 50% glucose with insulin. However, these therapies bring only transient improvement. Longer-acting therapies, such as sodium polystyrene sulfonate (Kayexalate) therapy or dialysis, must be instituted. Given orally or rectally, Kayexalate binds with potassium, promoting its removal from the body. Dialysis removes excessive electrolytes and water from the body (it is discussed later in the section "Chronic renal failure").

Hypertensive encephalopathy. The child with encephalopathy is extremely irritable, complains of headache, and may experience seizures. The physician prescribes I.V. antihypertensives to lower the blood pressure quickly.

Anemia. This condition may arise secondary to the shortened RBC life span associated with uremia and decreased RBC production (which results from decreased erythropoietin production). The child with a hemoglobin value below 6 mg/dl may receive blood transfusions. However, transfusions increase the risk of volume overload.

Cardiac failure and pulmonary edema. To treat these complications which result from hypervolemia, the physician restricts fluid and sodium intake to decrease fluid volume. Digoxin, normally excreted by the kidneys, is contraindicated because the child with ARF is at increased risk for digitalis toxicity.

Nursing management

Nursing goals for the child with ARF include:
- detecting changes in fluid status
- preventing further fluid retention
- implementing measures to remove excess fluid
- preventing injury caused by electrolyte disturbances
- providing adequate calories
- preventing infection
- detecting and managing complications.

Evaluating the child's fluid volume status is critical. Monitor hemodynamic parameters, including right atrial pressure, pulmonary artery pressure (PAP), pulmonary wedge pressure, central venous pressure (CVP), vital signs, peripheral pulses, edema, and weight. Suspect worsening hypervolemia if right atrial pressure, PAP, CVP, blood pressure, heart rate, respiratory rate, edema, or weight increase. Strong, bounding peripheral pulses also indicate hypervolemia.

Maintain sodium and fluid restrictions, as prescribed. Divide the allowed fluid volume evenly over the day and evening hours; 100 ml may be reserved for nighttime hours. Offer fluids in small amounts spread out over the course of the day. Make sure the child has no access to fluids. Advise the child and parents that soups, ice cream, ice pops, and gelatin desserts are considered fluid intake. As prescribed, implement dialysis. Be sure to record fluid intake and output.

Electrolyte disturbances, especially hyperkalemia, may be life-threatening. Monitor the child's ECG and laboratory values and maintain prescribed sodium, chloride, and potassium restrictions. To correct electrolyte disturbances, administer Kayexalate or implement dialysis, as prescribed.

Nutritional support poses a challenge for the child with ARF. Dietary restrictions limit the types of foods allowed, and many children dislike low-sodium diets. To promote adequate dietary intake, encourage the child to assist in meal planning. Present meals in an attractive setting. Stay with the child at mealtimes, or encourage the parents to do so. Praise the child for eating. As prescribed, implement parenteral nutrition.

The child with ARF is at risk for infection because of poor nutritional status and decreased immune function. To guard against infection, implement infection prevention measures, such as protecting the child from known infection sources. Be sure to use aseptic technique during invasive procedures.

Closely monitor the child to detect changes that suggest complications. Document changes in neurologic status, monitor cardiopulmonary status, and evaluate laboratory values for indications of anemia and uremia.

Chronic renal failure

CRF is an irreversible disorder characterized by a slow, progressive loss of renal function. The progression rate varies with the cause of the disorder. Late-stage CRF (also called ESRD) occurs when the kidneys no longer can function effectively, even with medical intervention. Children with ESRD need dialysis to survive.

Etiology

Various diseases may lead to CRF. In children under age 5, CRF most commonly results from an anatomic abnormality, such as vesicoureteral reflux. In older children, CRF typically stems from a glomerular disorder, such as chronic glomerulonephritis or focal glomerulosclerosis (a form of nephrotic syndrome), or a hereditary disorder (such as hereditary nephritis or polycystic kidney).

Pathophysiology and clinical manifestations

In CRF, nephrons undergo progressive destruction. During the early stage, the child has a sufficient number of functioning nephrons and generally remains asymptomatic. However, renal reserve is diminished, reflecting reduced renal function.

During the middle stage of CRF, renal insufficiency develops. Although the child still has no symptoms, metabolic wastes start to accumulate in the blood. Laboratory findings include elevated BUN, serum creatinine, serum phosphate, and serum uric acid levels.

During the late stage of CRF, excessive amounts of urea and other nitrogenous waste products accumulate in the blood, thus causing uremia. The kidneys no longer can excrete metabolic wastes, and fluid and electrolyte regulation is impaired. The child now shows symptoms, and multiple pathophysiologic changes occur. (For details on these changes and related clinical manifestations, see *CRF and end-stage renal disease: Multisystemic effects,* page 336.)

Diagnosis

The physician suspects CRF from suggestive clinical findings and a history of renal disease. Because signs and symptoms arise slowly, diagnosis typically comes during the late stage of CRF, when laboratory analysis reveals elevations in BUN and serum creatinine along with hyperphosphatemia, hypocalcemia, hyperkalemia, and compensated metabolic acidosis.

CRF and end-stage renal disease: Multisystemic effects

Chronic renal failure (CRF) and end-stage renal disease can lead to multisystemic effects.

Azotemia and uremia
Inability of the kidneys to excrete metabolic wastes leads to uremia—accumulation of excessive nitrogenous waste products in the blood. Uremia may impair the child's platelet function, causing easy bruising, bloody stools, and bleeding gums. The child typically complains of "itchy" skin, caused by deposition of uremic crystals in the skin. Other signs and symptoms of uremia include anorexia, nausea, vomiting, diarrhea, headache, lethargy, fatigue, seizures, and coma.

Water and sodium retention
Inadequate renal excretion of excess water causes fluid to remain in the vascular system, leading to vascular congestion. This, in turn, causes signs and symptoms of water and sodium retention, such as edema, tachycardia, and hypertension. Congestive heart failure may follow.

Hyperkalemia
Potassium and other electrolytes accumulate as the kidneys fail to excrete excess electrolytes. Hyperkalemia (an elevated serum potassium level) can lead to life-threatening cardiac arrhythmias.

Hyperphosphatemia and hypocalcemia
Hyperphosphatemia (an above normal serum phosphorus level) results from inadequate renal phosphorus excretion. As the serum phosphorus level rises, the serum calcium level falls. This, in turn, causes the parathyroid gland to secrete parathyroid hormone (PTH). PTH secretion induces calcium resorption from the bones, leading to bone demineralization.

Inability of the kidneys to synthesize vitamin D (which is necessary for calcium absorption from the gastrointestinal tract) contributes to hypocalcemia. These disturbances cause growth failure, bone pain, and bone abnormalities (renal osteodystrophy).

Phosphorus and calcium disturbances contribute to growth failure in children with CRF. Poor nutrition also impairs growth. Sexual maturation may be delayed. Disturbances in sex hormone production impair spermatogenesis in males and cause amenorrhea in females.

Acidosis
Chronic metabolic acidosis occurs in CRF because the kidneys cannot excrete excess hydrogen ions or retain bicarbonate ions. However, the body typically compensates for this condition through buffering mechanisms.

Anemia
Several factors contribute to anemia in the child with CRF:
- insufficient erythropoietin production by the kidneys, which reduces red blood cell (RBC) production
- poor nutrition, which also decreases RBC production
- uremia, which promotes RBC destruction
- bleeding tendencies.

In the anemic child, pallor and fatigue reflect decreased oxygen-carrying capacity of the blood, secondary to reduced hemoglobin levels. The child needs frequent rest periods during the day and sleeps longer at night.

Increased susceptibility to infection
For unknown reasons, children with CRF are more prone to infections—especially those of the respiratory and urinary tracts.

Medical management
Medical goals are to promote the patient's remaining renal function, maintain fluid and electrolyte balance, detect and treat complications, and replace kidney function once ESRD develops.

To promote renal function, the physician orders dietary modifications and other measures to reduce the kidney's excretory demands. Dietary modifications also help to maintain fluid and electrolyte balance and limit the effects of CRF-related bone abnormalities (renal osteodystrophy). Dietary management also aims to provide sufficient calories for growth while reducing renal excretory demands. (For details on dietary modifications, see *Dietary management of the child with CRF.*)

Dietary management of the child with CRF

The child with chronic renal failure (CRF) requires a high-carbohydrate, moderate-fat, low-protein diet. Carbohydrates and fats should provide most of the child's calories. Protein is restricted because protein metabolism produces urea and other nitrogenous wastes. Any proteins that the child consumes should be high in essential amino acids to promote growth.

Intake of milk—the primary source of dietary phosphorus—is restricted to counter hyperphosphatemia and thus prevent hypocalcemia and calcium loss from bone. Unless the child has edema or hypertension, fluid and sodium intake are unrestricted. Potassium intake is not restricted unless creatinine clearance is below 35 ml/minute or the serum potassium level is abnormal (below 3.5 mEq/liter or above 5.0 mEq/liter).

The physician prescribes vitamins and drugs to limit the effects of phosphorus and calcium disturbances. Vitamin D supplementation, for example, makes more vitamin D available for calcium absorption from the GI tract. Vitamin D analogs, such as calcitriol, increase calcium absorption from the GI tract. Aluminum-phosphate binders (such as aluminum hydroxide [Amphojel]) prevent GI absorption of phosphorus. However, these drugs may cause aluminum toxicity, so their use is restricted to short-term therapy for hyperphosphatemia. Calcium carbonate, which acts as a phosphate binder when administered before meals, is a safer alternative. Calcium supplements, such as calcium carbonate and calcium gluconate, are used to prevent or treat renal osteodystrophy. When used to treat hypocalcemia, they must be given 1 to 2 hours after meals.

A child with hypertension requires a low-sodium diet, fluid restrictions, antihypertensive drugs, and diuretics (such as chlorothiazide [Diuril] or furosemide). Captopril (Capoten) is used to treat mild to moderate hypertension; propranolol and hydralazine, to treat severe hypertension.

The acidotic child receives drug therapy, such as sodium bicarbonate or sodium and potassium citrate, and must restrict protein and milk intake to reduce metabolic acid formation. The physician also may prescribe sodium bicarbonate or sodium and potassium citrate to treat acidosis. Because correcting acidosis too quickly may induce severe hypocalcemia, acidosis is treated only after the child regains a near-normal serum calcium level.

The anemic child receives iron and folic acid supplements, vitamin C supplements to increase iron absorption from the GI tract, and epoetin alfa (erythropoietin) to stimulate the bone marrow to produce RBCs. A child with severe anemia requires packed RBC transfusions.

Infections call for prompt antibiotic therapy. However, the physician uses caution when prescribing antibiotics that are excreted by the kidneys. The patient's decreased renal function may warrant lower antibiotic dosages; serum blood levels are monitored to prevent toxic drug accumulation.

The physician may prescribe growth hormone for a child with growth failure. Recent research shows that administering growth hormone to children with CRF achieves significant gains in physical growth. (Koch et. al., 1989)

Dialysis

The child with ESRD requires dialysis. This technique removes excess water, electrolytes, and waste products from circulating blood by means of osmosis, diffusion, and ultrafiltration. Hemodialysis and peritoneal dialysis are the most common methods of dialysis used to treat children with CRF.

Hemodialysis. This method is preferred for children with renal failure secondary to drug poisoning and for those with life-threatening hyperkalemia. It also is used in children who are poor risks for peritoneal dialysis—for instance, because of noncompliance with therapy or recurrent peritoneal infections.

Hemodialysis requires vascular access via a surgically created arteriovenous fistula or temporary access for short-term use. Once venous access is established, blood flows from the child to the hemodialyzer (dialyzing machine), where excess water, electrolytes, and waste products are removed. The blood returns to the child via the access site.

The child undergoes hemodialysis 3 times weekly, for 5 to 6 hours each session—commonly, as an outpatient at the hospital. However, home dialysis is possible for certain families that have adequate training.

Complications of hemodialysis, which stem from rapid changes in blood volume and blood chemistry, may include nausea, vomiting, abdominal and muscle cramps, headache, and dizziness. A few children have seizures resulting from cerebral edema secondary to sudden shifts in blood osmolarity. Clotting, bleeding, and infection may occur at the vascular access site.

Peritoneal dialysis. This method, preferred for most children with CRF, requires surgical implantation of a peritoneal catheter. The peritoneal lining acts as a semipermeable membrane through which water, electrolytes, and waste products may pass. Osmosis and diffusion remove excessive amounts of these substances.

Two types of peritoneal dialysis exist: continuous ambulatory peritoneal dialysis (CAPD) and continuing cycling peritoneal dialysis (CCPD). In CAPD, which is conducted four or five times daily, dialysate (dialyzing solution) is infused by gravity into the peritoneal cavity via the peritoneal catheter. Then, the catheter is clamped and the dialyzing bag is rolled up and placed in the child's pocket or secured to the body. After 4 hours, the clamp is released and the fluid is allowed to flow out of the body into the dialyzing bag. The procedure is repeated, using a fresh bag of dialysate.

Instillation and removal both take 15 to 20 minutes in CAPD. The volume of dialysate is measured (based on weight of the bag) before instillation and after the fluid flows out of the body. Fluid volume should be greater after outflow is completed, reflecting removal of excess water.

CCPD requires a dialysis cycling machine. It is performed during the night when the child sleeps, with six to ten dialysis cycles completed over 10 hours.

Peritoneal dialysis can take place in the home, eliminating time-consuming travel to a dialysis outpatient center. Because it is performed daily, it necessitates fewer dietary restrictions. Peritoneal dialysis also interferes less with daily activities; once the dialysate is infused, the child can participate in most activities. More frequent dialysis also makes normal serum electrolyte and BUN levels easier to maintain, thus minimizing fatigue and allowing the child to participate more fully in school- and peer-related activities.

Complications of peritoneal dialysis include sensations of abdominal fullness, peritonitis, and infection at the catheter insertion site. Mild respiratory compromise (resulting from pressure on the diaphragm) occurs occasionally—usually when the child is lying down.

Renal transplantation

Renal (kidney) transplantation is considered for children with ESRD who require dialysis. The procedure offers the child a chance to live a relatively normal life, unencumbered by day-to-day management of CRF. Transplants from cadavers are less successful than those from compatible living relatives.

Nursing management

Nursing goals for the child with CRF are similar to those for the child with ARF. The nurse aims to:
• detect changes in fluid volume status
• implement measures to reduce the kidney's excretory load
• provide adequate caloric intake
• minimize the effects of phosphorus and calcium disturbances
• detect and manage complications of CRF
• detect and manage complications of dialysis therapy
• help the child and family adapt to living with a chronic disease. (For details, see Chapter 15, Illness concepts.)

To detect changes in fluid volume status, stay alert for signs of vascular congestion, increased weight, and edema formation, all of which suggest deteriorating renal function. Periodically measure the child's blood pressure and weight. Observe for developing edema. If the child is monitored on an outpatient basis (as are most children with CRF), instruct the parents to keep track of the child's daily urine output. Evaluate laboratory results for values that suggest worsening renal function—chiefly, an increase in BUN or serum creatinine level. Teach parents about prescribed antihypertensive therapy.

To help reduce the kidney's excretory load, explain prescribed dietary restrictions to the child and family. Design appropriate meal plans in conjunction with a dietitian. Provide the child and parents with approved food lists. Explain that unrestricted amounts of carbohydrates and fats increase oral intake by making food more palatable and that including such foods as sugar, jam, and honey also boosts caloric intake. Stress that good nutrition helps promote the child's overall growth and reduces the severity of anemia.

Explain that vitamin therapy is important to the child's overall well-being and limits the effects of renal osteodystrophy. Depending on the purpose of supplemental calcium therapy, instruct the parents on correct timing of calcium administration. If the child has hyperphosphatemia, teach the parents to limit milk and dairy products, which have a high phosphorus content.

Closely monitor the child to detect changes that may indicate worsening renal status. Also teach the parents to watch for such changes—headache, pruritus (itchy skin), nausea and vomiting, increasing fatigue, and lethargy—all of which reflect uremia. Periodically evaluate laboratory test results for evidence of anemia and uremia.

To minimize neurologic complications of hemodialysis, slow the dialysis procedure or give phenobarbital to prevent seizures, as prescribed. Protect the venous access site from injury. Do not take blood pressure and perform venipuncture in the affected arm. Report signs or symptoms of infection to the physician. Control any bleeding at the access site by applying direct pressure.

For the child on home peritoneal dialysis, teach the family about the dialysis routine, peritoneal catheter care, signs of infection at the catheter site (redness, swelling, tenderness, and warmth), and signs of peritonitis (abdominal pain, abdominal tenderness, nausea and vomiting, fever, and cloudy dialysate return). Instruct parents to call the physician if signs of infection appear. Advise them to change the child's position if breathing becomes difficult during dialysis. Instruct them to slow the dialysate infusion rate if the child complains of abdominal fullness.

STUDY ACTIVITIES

Short answer

1. List at least three signs or symptoms of APSGN.

_____

2. Explain how edema develops in children with nephrotic syndrome.

_____

_____

_____

3. How does metabolic acidosis develop in children with CRF?

_____

_____

4. Martha, age 7, has MCNS. To detect changes in her fluid status and help prevent fluid retention, the nurse formulates the following nursing diagnosis: _Fluid volume excess related to hypoproteinemia._ The expected outcomes are that Martha exhibit diminishing edema and reduced proteinuria; maintain a urine output above 2 ml/kg/hour and a urine specific gravity of 1.012 to 1.020; and verbalize relief of abdominal distention. Identify three nursing interventions that would help achieve these outcomes.

_____

_____

_____

Multiple choice

5. Which of the following is most important for the nurse to include when formulating a teaching plan for a child with APSGN?
  A. Nutritional planning
  B. Infection control
  C. Blood pressure monitoring
  D. Prevention of streptococcal pharyngitis

6. In a child with APSGN, which assessment finding provides the first clue that the child's status is improving?
  A. Increased urine output
  B. Increased appetite
  C. Increased energy level
  D. Decreased diarrhea

7. In a child with nephrotic syndrome, What is the primary goal of corticosteroid therapy in a child with nephrotic syndrome?
  A. To reduce inflammation.
  B. To increase blood pressure.
  C. To prevent infection.
  D. To decrease proteinuria.

8. When caring for a child with suspected ARF, the nurse should stay alert for which early sign?
  A. Hypertension
  B. Decreased urine output
  C. Anemia
  D. Hematuria

9. Which sign suggests hypervolemia in a child with ARF?
A. Increased CVP
B. Decreased blood pressure
C. Increased urine output
D. Fever

10. The nurse should observe for which finding when caring for a child at risk for uremia?
A. Increasing fatigue
B. Cardiac arrhythmias
C. Bone deformities
D. Increased urine specific gravity

11. To detect peritonitis as early as possible in a child on peritoneal dialysis, the nurse should be alert for:
A. Redness at the catheter site
B. Abdominal tenderness
C. Abdominal fullness
D. Headache

12. Michael, age 6, has hyperphosphatemia secondary to CRF. His parents should eliminate which foods from his diet?
A. Meats
B. Carbohydrates
C. Fats
D. Dairy products

13. What is the primary purpose of administering epoetin alfa to a child with CRF?
A. To decrease the kidney's excretory load.
B. To prevent anemia.
C. To lower the serum phosphorus level.
D. To prevent renal osteodystrophy.

ANSWERS **Short answer**

1. Signs and symptoms of APSGN include general malaise, anorexia, fatigue, weight gain, hypertension, headache, periorbital and peripheral edema, urinary changes, and increased urine specific gravity.

2. In nephrotic syndrome, urinary excretion of proteins causes hypoproteinemia. This condition, in turn, causes plasma oncotic pressure to fall, which allows intravascular water to shift to the extravascular spaces. Thus, blood volume decreases and profound edema occurs.

3. In CRF, the kidneys cannot excrete excess hydrogen ions or retain bicarbonate ions. Hydrogen (an acid) then accumulates in the blood, causing metabolic acidosis.

4. Record Martha's intake and output. Record her urine specific gravity and monitor urine protein values. Weigh Martha daily. Measure her abdominal girth daily. Monitor heart rate, quality of pulses, and blood pressure every 4 hours. Maintain fluid and dietary sodium restrictions, as prescribed. Administer corticosteroids, albumin, and diuretics, as prescribed.

Multiple choice

5. C. Severe, life-threatening hypertension may occur in APSGN. Therefore, teaching the child's parents how to monitor blood pressure is the most important choice among those given.

6. A. Increased urine output typically is the first sign that APSGN is resolving. The other choices are not specific to APSGN.

7. D. The main goal of corticosteroid therapy in nephrotic syndrome is to decrease proteinuria (urinary excretion of proteins). Corticosteroids have no effect on blood pressure. Although they help reduce inflammation, this is not the purpose for their use in nephrotic syndrome. Corticosteroid use may predispose someone to infection rather than prevent it.

8. B. Decreased urine output (oliguria) is an early sign of ARF. Hypertension and anemia arise later. Hematuria is rare.

9. A. A rise in CVP may indicate hypervolemia. Blood pressure and weight increase, not decrease, in hypervolemia. Fever is not associated with hypervolemia.

10. A. Increasing fatigue is an early sign of uremia. Arrhythmias, bone deformities, and increased urine specific gravity do not indicate uremia.

11. B. Abdominal tenderness is a sign of peritonitis. Redness at the catheter site indicates a skin infection. Abdominal fullness is expected during dialysate infusion. Headache is not associated with peritonitis.

12. D. Dairy products contain large amounts of phosphorus, which must be restricted in patients with hyperphosphatemia.

13. B. The primary purpose of giving epoetin alfa to this child is to stimulate the bone marrow production of RBCs, thus preventing anemia.

CHAPTER 25

Musculoskeletal disorders

OBJECTIVES

After studying this chapter, the reader should be able to:

1. Describe the causes, pathophysiology, and clinical manifestations of muscular dystrophy.

2. Discuss medical and nursing management of children with muscular dystrophy.

3. Describe the causes, pathophysiology, and clinical manifestations of Legg-Calvé-Perthes disease, Osgood-Schlatter disease, and scoliosis.

4. Discuss medical and nursing management of children with Legg-Calvé-Perthes disease, Osgood-Schlatter disease, and scoliosis.

5. Describe the causes, pathophysiology, and clinical manifestations of osteomyelitis and septic arthritis.

6. Discuss medical and nursing management of children with osteomyelitis and septic arthritis.

OVERVIEW OF CONCEPTS

Musculoskeletal disorders in children have various causes, including genetic factors and infection. This chapter explores muscular dystrophy, an inherited disorder; osteomyelitis and septic arthritis, which occur secondary to infection; and Legg-Calvé-Perthes (LCP) disease, Osgood-Schlatter disease, and scoliosis, which a child may acquire during the school-age years or the adolescent growth period. For each disorder, the chapter reviews the underlying pathophysiology, discusses clinical manifestations, and presents medical and nursing management. (For information about neonatal congenital skeletal deformities, see Chapter 11, The infant with disturbances in physical development.)

Muscular dystrophy

Muscular dystrophy is a collective term for a group of congenital disorders characterized by progressive symmetrical wasting of skeletal muscles without neural or sensory defects. All forms of the disease cause progressive loss of muscle function. The primary muscles affected and the degree of disability vary with the specific form.

Duchenne muscular dystrophy, also called pseudohypertrophic muscular dystrophy, is the most common and severe form; this section focuses on this disease. In approximately 50% of patients, Duchenne muscular dystrophy is inherited through an X-linked recessive inheritance pattern; spontaneous mutations probably account for the remaining cases. The life span of children with Duchenne muscular dystrophy is 15 to 25 years, with death commonly resulting from respiratory infection or failure. Other forms of muscular dystrophy include Becker muscular dystrophy, congenital muscular dystrophy, facioscapulohumeral muscular dystrophy, limb-girdle muscular dystrophy, ocular myopathy, and myotonic dystrophy.

Pathophysiology

Children with Duchenne muscular dystrophy lack dystrophin, a protein found in skeletal muscle. Fatty infiltration (pseudohypertrophy), which may result from the lack of dystrophin, causes enlargement of calf, thigh, and arm muscles that feel firm and rubbery. During the terminal stage of the disease, respiratory muscles are affected. For unknown reasons, most children with Duchenne muscular dystrophy experience gradual loss of mental capacity.

Clinical manifestations

Initial signs and symptoms of Duchenne muscular dystrophy, which reflect muscle weakness, arise during the preschool-age period. Parents may first notice that the child cannot perform previously mastered motor skills, such as bicycle riding, stair climbing, or running. Muscle weakness first affects the muscles of the hip, shoulder girdle, and abdomen.

To compensate for weakened hip muscles, the child walks with a wide base and waddling gait. Diminished muscle strength causes difficulty rising from a supine or sitting position. To rise from a supine to standing position, the child uses a maneuver called Gowers' sign. (See *Identifying Gowers' sign,* page 346.)

Eventually, all muscles—both voluntary and involuntary—become weak. Muscles atrophy rapidly unless the child exercises; bed rest and inactivity reduce muscle strength markedly within just a few days. Muscle atrophy may lead to skeletal contractures. Lordosis, an inward curvature of the lumbar vertebrae, also develops. Scoliosis, a lateral spinal curvature, may appear later.

Some children with Duchenne muscular dystrophy become obese because of limited mobility caused by muscle weakness. Boredom and overeating may contribute to obesity, which strains weakened muscles and typically causes loss of ambulation by age 12.

Diagnosis

The child's signs and symptoms may suggest Duchenne muscular dystrophy. The diagnosis is confirmed by:

- elevated level of serum creatine phosphokinase, an enzyme normally found in muscle tissue
- muscle biopsy showing replacement of muscle tissue by fibrous tissue and fat
- abnormal electromyogram (EMG) results.

Identifying Gowers' sign

To move from a supine to a standing position, the child with Duchenne muscular dystrophy uses a maneuver called Gowers' sign. With hands placed on the floor, the child uses arm muscles to push up to a jackknife position, then moves the hands (one after another) up the legs in a walking-like motion until the child is upright.

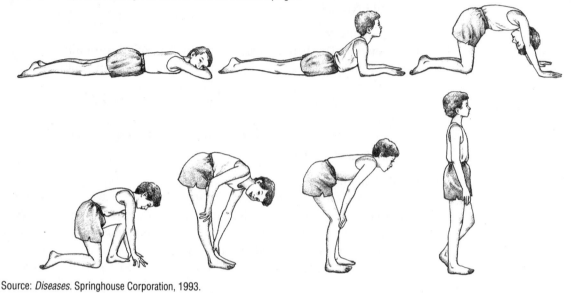

Source: *Diseases.* Springhouse Corporation, 1993.

Medical management

Because Duchenne muscular dystrophy is a terminal disorder, management is supportive and aims to maintain function in unaffected muscles. The child requires a multidisciplinary approach that includes the physician, the nurse, and physical, occupational, and nutritional therapists.

The therapeutic regimen includes at least 3 hours of physical activity daily (such as walking and swimming) and physical therapy to provide range-of-motion exercises. Bracing and surgery may help ease contracture deformities. The physician may order respiratory therapy to prevent complications of weakened respiratory muscles. An overweight child requires nutritional counseling. One who has trouble performing activities of daily living may require assistive devices, designed by the occupational therapist.

Nursing management

Nursing goals for the child with Duchenne muscular dystrophy are:
• promote physical mobility
• ensure respiratory function
• prevent or manage obesity
• promote independence
• encourage socialization

• provide emotional support.

Promoting physical mobility

Advise parents that exercise is crucial in maintaining the child's muscle function. Stress the importance of complying with the prescribed physical exercise program. However, explain that exercise will not halt disease progression. Advise parents to call the physician if the child is temporarily bedridden, such as during illness, because the exercise program should be modified at that time.

Ensuring respiratory function

If the child has had surgery, perform chest physiotherapy, as prescribed, to promote pulmonary drainage and lung expansion. Also implement exercise therapy to prevent atrophy from disuse. During the later stage of the disease, teach the parents how to perform postural drainage and chest physiotherapy to promote lung function and prevent pulmonary infection.

Preventing or managing obesity

In conjunction with a dietitian, review the child's nutritional requirements. If the child is overweight, instruct the parents to restrict the child's consumption of fats and concentrated sugar. Suggest fruit and pretzels as alternatives to fatty snacks, and frozen yogurt as a substitute for ice cream.

Promoting independence

Self-care skills give the child with Duchenne muscular dystrophy a sense of independence and self-worth. If the child is able, advise parents to let the child perform self-care tasks, such as grooming, dressing, and eating, unassisted. The child who has difficulty performing these tasks may need assistive devices.

Encouraging socialization

As the child's physical condition deteriorates, socialization opportunities may diminish. Encourage school attendance as one way for the child to socialize. Although few children with Duchenne muscular dystrophy can participate in sports, attending sporting events may provide an outlet for the child with an interest in sports.

Providing emotional support

Be sure to provide emotional support—especially during the early stage, when the family must confront the diagnosis of a progressive and fatal disease. Offer ongoing support as the disease progresses. As needed, coordinate multidisciplinary services. (For more information on the nurse's role in supporting the child and family with a chronic, life-threatening disease, see Chapter 15, Illness concepts.)

Legg-Calvé-Perthes disease

LCP disease is characterized by dysfunction of the femoral head caused by interruption of blood supply to the proximal femoral epiphysis. The cause of the interrupted blood supply is unknown.

LCP disease may involve the femur and hip on either side; in roughly 15% of cases, both hips are involved. LCP disease occurs in children ages 3 to 12, and affects more boys than girls.

LCP disease is self-limiting. Early diagnosis and full compliance with therapy improve the chance for full recovery of femur and hip function.

Pathophysiology

Interruption in blood supply to the proximal femoral epiphysis causes necrosis of the femoral head. Normal physical activity leads to minute fractures of the softened, necrotic bone tissue. Inflammation and synovitis may follow. Necrotic tissue is resorbed slowly, and fibrocartilaginous tissue fills in the areas of resorbed necrotic tissue. The femoral head then reossifies and reforms as new bone is produced—a process that may take 18 to 36 months.

Assessment

Signs and symptoms of LCP disease include intermittent or constant hip soreness or stiffness and a limp on the affected side. Some children also have pain near the knee. Range of motion (ROM) in the affected hip is limited. Pain worsens with physical exertion of the affected leg and subsides with rest.

The school nurse may be the first health care professional to identify the child with LCP disease. A common initial complaint is vaguely defined hip or knee pain after a physical education class. The child also may exhibit an intermittent limp.

Diagnosis

LCP disease is confirmed by X-rays showing characteristic bone changes.

Medical management

The goal of medical therapy is to prevent deformity of the femoral head by containing the necrotic femoral head beneath the acetabulum. Presumably, containment preserves the spherical shape of the femoral head as the bone reforms.

Most children with LCP disease are managed as outpatients and can attend school. During the early stage of the disease, the physician prescribes rest and restricts weight-bearing on the affected limb. Bracing (or occasionally casting) is used to contain the femoral head beneath the acetabulum. The child must continue to wear braces for 2 to 4 years until the disease process is complete.

A newer treatment option is surgical correction and containment, which allows the child to return to full physical activity within 6 months. In containment, the avascular femoral head must remain beneath the coverage of the acetabulum. This causes the new femoral head to be congruent with the acetabulum and results in a joint that glides smoothly through a range of motion.

Nursing management

Nursing goals include promoting normal femur and hip function and providing diversional activities.

To promote femur and hip function, explain the rationale for braces or serial casting therapy to the child and family. Teach self-management skills related to the prescribed therapeutic plan. Depending on the treatment approach, the child may be able to ambulate with or without crutches. However, some children are wheelchair-bound.

Stress the importance of complying with therapy to prevent femoral head deformity. Be aware that because braces can be removed, the child may not comply fully with this part of therapy.

A child accustomed to full activity may have a hard time adjusting to physical limitations. Suggest that the child take up a hobby that does not require ambulation, such as drawing, painting, building models, crafts, or stamp collecting. Also suggest age-appropriate board games, which many children enjoy.

Osgood-Schlatter disease

Osgood-Schlatter disease is an incomplete separation of the epiphysis of the tibial tubercle from the tibial shaft. A type of overuse injury caused by repeated traction or pull on the patellar tendon, it is most common in physically active boys ages 10 to 16. The disorder is self-limiting and resolves once the epiphyseal growth plates close.

Pathophysiology and clinical manifestations

Tendinitis of the patellar tendon and separation of the tibial tuberosity cause pain and tenderness over the anterior portion of the knee. The pain subsides with rest and worsens during activities that cause stress or pressure on the anterior knee or tibial tubercle.

Medical management

Treatment is supportive. The physician prescribes ibuprofen to relieve inflammation and discomfort, and advises the child to engage in physical activities when free of pain, to take short rest periods when pain occurs, and to avoid activities that cause pain.

Most children respond favorably to modifications in physical activity and frequent rest periods. Some need braces or casts to provide immobilization if pain persists.

Nursing management

The nursing goal is to help the child identify physical activities in which the child can participate comfortably. Such activities typically include swimming and bicycle riding.

Scoliosis

Scoliosis is a lateral curvature of the spine. The most common spinal deformity, it may occur in the thoracic, lumbar, or thoracolumbar spinal segment. It most commonly affects preadolescent girls.

Comparing the types of scoliosis

Scoliosis may be functional or structural. In *functional scoliosis,* a flexible spinal curvature is noticeable when the child stands. Functional scoliosis does not cause pain or vertebral changes. When the child bends forward at the hips, spinal curvature is normal.

Structural scoliosis is an inflexible spinal curvature that persists when the child bends forward. The spine and ribs are rotated toward the inward portion of the curvature. The thoracic cage is asymmetrical, and the sternum is displaced. When observed from behind, a prominent rib hump appears on the outward portion of the curvature when the child bends forward. The hip on the inward portion is elevated and the scapula on the outward portion is prominent.

Structural scoliosis may progress rapidly during the adolescent growth spurt. In severe cases, it compromises pulmonary function by causing displacement of internal organs. Unless significant structural changes have occurred, however, the disorder does not cause pain.

Classification

Scoliosis may be functional or structural. Functional scoliosis typically results from poor posture. Structural scoliosis is caused by changes in the vertebrae and supporting structures; it may be idiopathic (most common), congenital, or associated with another disorder. (For a comparison of functional and idiopathic structural scoliosis, see *Comparing the types of scoliosis.*)

Assessment

The nurse (particularly a school nurse) may identify the child with scoliosis through routine preadolescent screening. To screen for scoliosis, ask the child to remove all clothes except underpants. With the child standing upright and facing away from the nurse, observe for spinal deformity from behind. Note whether the child's head aligns with the gluteal fold. Then ask the child to bend forward at the hips, with the back at a right angle to the legs. Observing from behind, note the presence of a rib hump or flank asymmetry.

Diagnosis

Scoliosis is diagnosed from clinical findings and X-rays, which reveal the degree of the spinal curvature.

Medical management

Functional scoliosis is treated by correcting the underlying cause. Commonly, the physician prescribes exercises to strengthen abdominal and back muscles. Treatment of structural scoliosis may involve surgery. (For more information, see *Managing structural scoliosis.*)

Nursing management

Nursing goals for the child with idiopathic structural scoliosis include:
• protecting the surgical site from injury
• promoting postoperative comfort
• teaching the child and family about brace therapy

Managing structural scoliosis

The choice of therapy for a child with structural scoliosis depends on the severity of the spinal curvature. Treatment must begin early to stop the curvature from worsening as the child grows.

External bracing

A child with mild to moderate structural scoliosis requires external bracing. Although bracing does not correct the curvature, it does prevent it from worsening.

The Milwaukee brace, the most common choice, extends from the neck to the pelvis. Worn 23 hours a day, it is adjusted as the child grows. Although it appears cumbersome, it does not interfere with most activities. The child continues to wear the brace until spinal bones reach maturity (typically between ages 18 and 21), then wears only it at night for 1 to 2 years.

Electrical stimulation

For the child with mild to moderate structural scoliosis, the physician may prescribe electrical stimulation of muscles on the outward (convex) side of the curvature. Electrical stimulation causes these muscles to contract, helping to straighten the spine. It may be applied via electrodes on the skin or via surgically implanted devices. Conducted while the child sleeps, this therapy may not correct the curvature completely but does help halt its progression.

Surgery

Surgical correction of scoliosis typically is reserved for children with moderate to severe curvature, although it may be offered to certain children with milder scoliosis. Criteria for surgery include pain, diminished pulmonary function, and noncompliance with braces (usually because of self-image problems).

Preoperatively, the child with a severe curvature may require traction to provide partial correction. Generally, traction is applied with a halo device—a metal ring attached to the skull with pins, pulleys, and weights.

During surgery, the physician realigns the spine, inserts an internal fixation device (typically a Harrington rod), and fuses the realigned vertebrae. After surgery, the child is immobilized with a Stryker frame. After 8 to 12 days, a plaster cast is applied from the occiput to the pelvis. The cast is changed at 3 months, then maintained for a total of 6 months.

- promoting a positive body image.

Protecting the surgical site

If the child has undergone surgery, protect the surgical site from injury. Maintain the child on a Stryker frame and reposition the child, as prescribed. Be sure to maintain proper body alignment, with the spine kept straight. Caution the child to avoid twisting movements. Use log-rolling methods when turning the child from side to side. Maintain a dry, intact surgical dressing and observe the dressing for bleeding.

Promoting postoperative comfort

Surgery involving the spine is particularly painful. As prescribed, give narcotic analgesics to control pain. For many patients, the most efficient analgesic administration method is patient-controlled analgesia. (For a comprehensive discussion of pain management and nursing goals related to routine postoperative care, see Chapter 16, Management principles.)

Providing teaching

If the child must wear braces, reinforce teaching about brace application and removal (initially provided by the orthotist). Because compliance is critical to the success of brace therapy, be sure to stress the importance of wearing the brace for the prescribed time. Suggest ways to perform activities of daily living, such as dressing and getting out of bed.

Because the brace may rub against the skin and cause skin breakdown, instruct parents to inspect the child's skin daily for redness and other signs of breakdown. If redness persists, advise them to contact the orthotist, who will determine the need for brace adjustment. To protect the skin, advise the child to wear a thin cotton vest or T-shirt under the brace.

Promoting a positive body image

Developing a sense of identity and positive self-worth is a critical task during both the preadolescent period, when idiopathic scoliosis develops, and adolescence, when scoliosis treatment continues. The child with scoliosis may feel unattractive and different from peers because of braces, poorly fitting clothes (caused by pelvic and hip discrepancies or scapular prominence), and obvious deformities related to the spinal curvature.

To improve the child's body image, suggest oversized shirts to accommodate and camouflage the brace. Encourage the child to express feelings about wearing brace. Stress the positive outcome of complying with therapy.

Osteomyelitis

Osteomyelitis is a pyogenic infection of the bone, typically resulting from a combination of local trauma and an acute infection originating elsewhere in the body. Osteomyelitis commonly occurs in boys under age 16.

Staphylococcus aureus is the most common causative organism in older children; *Haemophilus influenzae* is more common in younger children. Although the infection typically remains localized, it may spread through the bone to the marrow, cortex, and periosteum.

Osteomyelitis may be acute or chronic. The acute form, which generally is blood-borne, affects rapidly growing children. Chronic osteomyelitis, characterized by multiple draining sinus tracts and metastatic lesions, lasts more than 4 weeks or does not respond to therapy.

Pathophysiology and clinical manifestations

Bacteria may enter the bone in one of two ways:
- by direct invasion, as from a puncture wound, an open fracture, or surgical contamination
- by indirect invasion of blood-borne pathogens originating from a primary infection source.

Indirect (hematogenous) invasion is more common. Primary sources of infection include boils, impetigo, otitis media, tonsillitis, infected burns, and tooth abscesses.

Bacterial invasion of the bone causes an inflammatory response. An abscess forms, and pus may seep into the metaphysis. Bony tissue within the abscessed area becomes necrotic. If the infection is not treated, pressure from accumulated pus may cause the periosteum to rupture, permitting bacteria to escape into the nearest joint spaces.

Hematogenous osteomyelitis typically involves a single bone. Signs and symptoms may arise suddenly and commonly include high fever, malaise, irritability, tachycardia, and tachypnea. Bone pain is severe enough to limit movement. The child refuses to bear weight on the involved bone; skin over the bone may be tender, warm, and swollen. In some children, systemic symptoms are absent, although bone pain always is present.

Diagnosis

Osteomyelitis is suspected from clinical findings. X-rays reveal soft-tissue swelling and movement of the periosteum away from the bone and its vascular supply. Bone aspiration and culture identifies the causative bacteria.

Medical management

Acute osteomyelitis calls for a 3- to 4-week course of high-dose antibiotic therapy. Initially, the child is hospitalized and receives intravenous (I.V.) antibiotics for 5 to 7 days to evaluate the therapeutic response. With a good initial response and available home care services, the child may be discharged with I.V. antibiotics. (Some physicians switch the child to oral antibiotics before discharge.) A child with chronic osteomyelitis requires additional therapy with an alternate antibiotic.

Some children require surgery to evacuate pus from the metaphyseal space and prevent rupture of the periosteum. After surgery, the wound is irrigated with antibiotics and a tube inserted for continuous drainage of pus and debris.

At home, the child is confined to bed until the infection is eradicated, which generally takes 3 to 4 weeks. The bone may be immobilized with a splint. Bed rest and immobilization help prevent the spread of infection to adjacent joints. Weight-bearing on the affected bone is prohibited because of the high risk of fracture.

Nursing management

The nurse's goals are to control infection, enhance bone healing, and promote comfort.

Controlling infection

Administer antibiotics, as prescribed. Evaluate the child's response to antibiotic therapy by measuring temperature, monitoring blood drug levels, and assessing for pain. Monitor closely for adverse effects of high-dose antibiotic therapy, such as renal toxicity and ototoxicity. Before discharge, stress the importance of compliance with antibiotic therapy.

Enhancing bone healing

Encourage the child to consume a diet high in calories, protein, and calcium. Stress the need to maintain bed rest and the prescribed immobilization device. Inform the child and parents that these therapies are necessary to protect the bone from injury. Teach the child to avoid weight-bearing on the affected limb.

Promoting comfort

Assess the child's pain and administer analgesics, as prescribed. Consider immobilizing and elevating the affected bone, which also may relieve pain. Supply or suggest diversional activities to distract the child and thus reduce the perception of pain.

Septic arthritis

Septic arthritis is a medical emergency in which bacteria invade a joint, thereby causing inflammation of the synovial lining. This disorder typically involves a single joint—most commonly, the hip, knee, or ankle. The incidence of septic arthritis is highest in children under age 2 and in adolescents. It affects more males than females.

Pathophysiology

Typically, septic arthritis arises from hematogenous spread of bacteria that originates from an infection elsewhere in the body. Less commonly, it develops from direct bacterial invasion of the joint secondary to a penetrating injury or surgery, from the spread of the infection to surrounding soft tissue, or from the spread of osteomyelitis into the joint space. *S. aureus* and *H. influenzae* are the most common causative bacteria.

The infection leads to joint inflammation and effusion. If left untreated, irreversible cartilage damage may occur.

Assessment

Signs and symptoms of septic arthritis include fever, joint swelling, erythema, tenderness, and limited ROM. Hip, knee, or ankle involvement may cause the child to limp.

Diagnosis

The physician diagnoses septic arthritis from clinical findings, such as a history of recent joint injury. Arthrocentesis confirms the diagnosis and identifies the causative bacteria. Laboratory findings reveal leukocytosis and an increased erythrocyte sedimentation rate.

Medical management

The physician may drain the infected joint surgically and prescribe I.V. antibiotics. A patient who responds well to I.V. antibiotics is switched to oral antibiotics. Antibiotic therapy continues for 3 weeks. The physician prescribes bed rest and joint immobilization and prohibits weight-bearing until healing is complete.

Nursing management

Nursing measures for the child with septic arthritis resemble those for the child with osteomyelitis. Goals include cleansing and decompressing the joint, eliminating the infection, and preventing secondary infection.

STUDY ACTIVITIES **Short answer**

1. Describe Gowers' sign in a child.

_____

_____

_____

2. Identify at least two diagnostic criteria for Duchenne muscular dystrophy.

_____

_____

_____

3. Describe the dysfunction that occurs in LCP disease.

_____

_____

_____

4. Summarize the pathophysiology of Osgood-Schlatter disease.

_____

_____

_____

5. What is the most common cause of functional scoliosis?

_____

6. Alan, age 5, has muscular dystrophy. To promote physical mobility, the nurse formulates the following nursing diagnosis: _Impaired physical mobility related to muscle weakness secondary to muscular dystrophy._ The expected outcome is that Alan will maintain strength in unaffected muscles and the ability to ambulate. Identify three nursing interventions that would help achieve these outcomes.

_____

_____

_____

7. Barbie, age 8, has osteomyelitis. To promote comfort, the nurse formulates the following nursing diagnosis: *Pain related to bone infection.* The expected outcomes are that Barbie will verbalize a decrease in pain and will remain free from physiologic indicators of pain, such as increased heart rate and blood pressure, diaphoresis, and facial tension. Identify three nursing interventions that would help achieve these outcomes.

_____

_____

Multiple choice

8. The nurse would expect which assessment finding in a child with muscular dystrophy?
- **A.** A waddling gait
- **B.** Pain
- **C.** Limited ROM
- **D.** Joint swelling

9. The nurse should arrange for a dietary consultation for Billy, who has muscular dystrophy, because children with this disease dystrophy are at risk for:
- **A.** Malabsorption
- **B.** Obesity
- **C.** Diarrhea
- **D.** Food allergies

10. Osgood-Schlatter disease typically results from:
- **A.** An infection of the bone
- **B.** An overuse injury
- **C.** Arthritis
- **D.** Disturbed blood flow to the bone

11. Cindy, age 13, was diagnosed with scoliosis recently. Her mother asks for how long she will need to wear a brace. What would be the nurse's best response?
- **A.** "About 6 to 8 weeks."
- **B.** "About 6 months."
- **C.** "About 2 to 4 years."
- **D.** "About 5 to 8 years."

12. Which assessment finding would alert the nurse to possible scoliosis?
- **A.** A discrepancy in leg lengths
- **B.** A limp observed after exercise
- **C.** A rib hump
- **D.** Pain near the hip

ANSWERS **Short answer**

1. The child places the hands on the floor and uses the arm muscles to push up to a jackknife position. Then, using the hands, the child "walks up" the legs until upright.

2. Diagnostic criteria for Duchenne muscular dystrophy include an elevated serum creatine phosphokinase level, replacement of muscle tissue by fibrous tissue and fat, as shown by muscle biopsy, and abnormal EMG results.

3. In LCP disease, interruption of blood supply to the proximal femoral epiphysis causes dysfunction of the femoral head.

4. In Osgood-Schlatter disease, repeated traction or pull on the patellar tendon (from overuse injury) causes an incomplete separation of the epiphyses of the tibial tubercle from the tibial shaft. This leads to pain and tenderness over the anterior portion of the knee.

5. Poor posture is the most common cause of functional scoliosis.

6. Make sure Alan's parents understand the importance of compliance with the prescribed physical exercise program. Stress the importance of exercise in maintaining muscle function. Encourage Alan to get at least 3 hours of physical activity daily. Advise Alan's parents to call the physician if he becomes temporarily bedridden.

7. Monitor Barbie's pain level. Administer analgesics, as prescribed. Supply or suggest diversional activities. Immobilize and elevate the affected bone.

Multiple choice

8. A. A wide-based, waddling gait is characteristic of muscular dystrophy. Pain, limited ROM, and joint swelling are rare.

9. B. Children with muscular dystrophy are at risk for obesity from inactivity associated with muscle weakness. Generally, children with muscular dystrophy do not have malabsorption problems, food allergies, or diarrhea unless there is another problem involved.

10. B. Osgood-Schlatter disease most commonly results from overuse injury.

11. D. Most children with scoliosis must wear a brace until the spine matures, which typically occurs between ages 18 and 21. This means that Cindy, age 13, may need to wear the brace for 5 to 8 years.

12. C. In a child with scoliosis, a rib hump can be observed when the child bends forward at the hips.

CHAPTER 26

Cancer

OBJECTIVES
After studying this chapter, the reader should be able to:
1. Identify the causes of common childhood cancers.
2. Describe signs and symptoms of cancer in children.
3. Identify common treatments for childhood cancer.
4. Discuss acute and long-term effects of childhood cancer treatments.
5. Describe the causes, pathophysiology, and clinical manifestations of leukemia in children.
6. Discuss medical and nursing management of leukemia.

OVERVIEW OF CONCEPTS
Childhood cancer is becoming increasingly common in the United States. Each year, approximately 7,600 children under age 15 are diagnosed with cancer. (Cancer Facts and Figures, 1990) A chronic disease, cancer can impede physical and psychosocial development as well as threaten the child's health — effects that the nurse must consider when planning care.

This chapter explores common childhood cancers. It summarizes the causes and compares the incidence rates of various childhood cancers. Then it describes assessment methods and discusses common treatments and their adverse effects. It concludes with a comprehensive discussion of childhood leukemia management. (For details on the psychosocial impact of chronic illness on children and their families, see Chapter 15, Illness concepts.)

Causes of common childhood cancers
The precise causes of most childhood cancers remain unknown. However, most experts believe cancer develops when a genetic alteration causes abnormal cells to proliferate.

Experts also have identified risk factors for certain types of cancer. For instance, ionizing radiation has been linked to thyroid cancer and leukemia; maternal history of diethylstilbestrol use, to adenosarcoma of the vagina; genetically based hereditary factors, to retinoblastoma, Wilms' tumor, and neuroblastoma. Chromosomal abnormalities, such as Down syndrome, have been associated with leukemia; immunodeficiencies, such as acquired immunodeficiency syndrome or those associ-

Common childhood cancers

Cancers that occur in children include leukemia, brain tumors, lymphoma, neuroblastoma, Wilms' tumor, rhabdomyosarcoma, osteogenic sarcoma, Ewing's sarcoma, and retinoblastoma.

Leukemia

A malignancy of the hematopoietic tissue, leukemia is characterized by replacement of normal bone marrow elements by abnormal, immature white blood cells. Leukemia accounts for roughly 30% of childhood cancer cases. Most common in Caucasian males, it peaks in incidence between ages 3 and 5.

Brain tumor

A neoplasm within the brain, a brain tumor may affect any brain tissue, including the blood vessels, cranial nerves, neurons, neuroglia, hypophysis, neuroepithelium, or the pineal gland.

Most brain tumors are infratentorial — located below the tentorium cerebelli in the posterior one-third of the brain, primarily the cerebellum or brain stem. Some are supratentorial — located above the tentorium cerebelli in the anterior two-thirds of the brain, primarily in the cerebrum.

Brain tumors account for about 20% of all cancer cases. Their incidence peaks between ages 5 and 10.

Lymphoma

Lymphoma includes Hodgkin's disease, a malignancy of the lymphoid tissue, and malignant lymphoma (also called lymphosarcoma), a solid tumor of the hematopoietic system. Hodgkin's disease accounts for 4 in every 1 million cancers; malignant lymphoma, for 8 in every 1 million cancers.

Both Hodgkin's disease and malignant lymphoma are more common in males than females. Hodgkin's disease peaks in incidence between ages 15 and 34; malignant lymphoma, between ages 7 and 11.

Neuroblastoma

A tumor of the sympathetic nervous system, neuroblastoma typically involves the adrenal medulla or the sympathetic ganglia of the abdomen and pelvis. It accounts for roughly 8% of childhood cancer cases. More common in males, neuroblastoma peaks in incidence from birth to age 2.

Wilms' tumor

This tumor of the renal parenchyma may have a genetic basis. Approximately 30% of cases seem to result from an autosomal dominant transmission pattern with variable penetrance. Wilms' tumor accounts for about 6% of childhood cancer cases (7 in every 1 million cancers). Its incidence peaks at age 3.

Rhabdomyosarcoma

This soft-tissue sarcoma derives from primitive striated muscle cells, most commonly affecting muscles of the head and neck. It accounts for about 6% of childhood cancer cases. More common in males and Caucasians, it peaks in incidence in children under age 5 and in older adolescents.

Osteogenic sarcoma and Ewing's sarcoma

Osteogenic sarcoma (also called osteosarcoma) is a tumor of the osteoid tissue — most commonly the metaphyses of long bones. Ewing's sarcoma is a tumor within the bone marrow spaces — typically within the shaft of long and trunk bones.

These forms of sarcoma account for approximately 4% of childhood cancer cases. They are more common in males and Caucasians, and peak in incidence between ages 15 and 19.

Retinoblastoma

A tumor of the retina, retinoblastoma commonly is inherited by autosomal dominant transmission when it occurs bilaterally; unilateral retinoblastoma is not inherited. The disease accounts for about 3% of childhood cancer cases. Peak incidence occurs from birth to age 2.

---

ated with organ transplantation, with various cancers. (For descriptions of cancers that occur in children, see *Common childhood cancers*.)

Assessment   Prompt recognition of cancer warning signs allows early detection and treatment. Although clinical manifestations vary with the specific type of cancer, the nurse should stay alert for the following signs and symptoms during a routine assessment of a healthy child:
- sudden tendency to bruise

- sudden eye or vision changes, including strabismus or a white reflection rather than the normal red pupil reflex
- prolonged, unexplained fever or illness
- excessive and rapid weight loss
- frequent headaches accompanied by vomiting
- an unusual mass or swelling
- unexplained pallor and energy loss
- persistent, localized pain
- limping.

Also note any changes in the child's personality or gait, which may indicate a brain tumor (Cancer Facts and Figures, 1990).

General medical management

Treatment of a child with cancer may involve chemotherapy, radiation therapy, surgery, bone marrow transplantation, or supportive measures. Typically, the physician chooses a combination of these treatments.

Chemotherapy

The goal of chemotherapy — administration of antineoplastic drugs — is to interfere with cellular reproduction. Chemotherapy may be the primary cancer treatment or used in conjunction with other treatments.

The child typically receives a combination of antineoplastic drugs (called combination, or multiple, drug therapy). This approach promotes optimal cancer cell destruction, decreases drug resistance by cancer cells, and minimizes toxic effects. (For information about commonly used chemotherapeutic drugs, see *Antineoplastic agents*, pages 361 to 363.)

Most children undergoing chemotherapy require multiple administrations. To avoid complications of multiple venipunctures, the physician may insert a venous access device, such as a Hickman catheter or Infusaport. Such devices also decrease the risk of soft-tissue injury resulting from accidental administration through an infiltrated or leaking intravenous (I.V.) line. For a child who requires multiple doses of intrathecal chemotherapy, an Ommaya reservoir may be implanted into the space surrounding the spinal cord to eliminate the need for repeated lumbar punctures.

Unfortunately, antineoplastic drugs do not affect only malignant cells. They also damage normal, healthy cells that proliferate rapidly, such as those of the bone marrow, hair, skin, and epithelial lining of the gastrointestinal tract. Destruction of normal cells accounts for many of the adverse effects of chemotherapy. (For details on the timing of adverse effects, see *When adverse effects of chemotherapy may occur,* page 364.)

Radiation therapy

Commonly used in conjunction with chemotherapy or surgery, radiation therapy interferes with cellular reproduction, damaging or destroy-

Antineoplastic agents

Antineoplastic agents destroy cancer cells by interfering with their growth and division. However, these agents also have toxic effects on normal cells. They typically are given in combination to improve the response rate and minimize toxicity.

Some antineoplastic agents cause ototoxicity (manifested by hearing loss and ringing in the ears) and neurotoxicity (manifested by numbness, ataxia, and weakness). Some antineoplastic agents are vesicants, which cause blistering and severe tissue damage if allowed to infiltrate surrounding tissue. Vesicants must be administered through an intact I.V. line (preferably a central line) by a nurse who is experienced in antineoplastic drug administration.

This chart describes the adverse effects and nursing considerations for drugs commonly used to treat cancer in children.

DRUG	ACTION	ADVERSE EFFECTS
asparaginase [L-asparaginase] (Elspar)	• Allergic reactions, including urticaria and anaphylaxis (manifested by stridor, facial edema, hypotension, and wheezing) • Fever • Mild nausea and vomiting • Anorexia • Weight loss • Arthralgia • Toxicity, as indicated by liver dysfunction, renal failure, hyperglycemia, and pancreatitis	• Before administering, have emergency drugs used to treat anaphylaxis available at bedside. • Administer I.M. or I.V., as prescribed. • Monitor patient's heart rate, respiratory rate, and blood pressure every 15 minutes for 1 hour after administration. Report allergic reactions immediately. • Monitor patient's weight. • Monitor urine for glucose.
cisplatin [cis-platinum] (Platinol)	• Severe nausea and vomiting, resulting in electrolyte disturbances (including hypomagnesemia, hypocalcemia, hypokalemia, and hypophosphatemia) • Allergic reactions, including urticaria and anaphylaxis • Ototoxicity, neurotoxicity, and renal failure • Mild bone marrow depression (2 to 3 weeks after administration)	• Have emergency drugs used to treat anaphylaxis available at bedside. • Premedicate with antiemetics before infusion, according to institutional protocol. • Administer I.V. with mannitol, as prescribed, to promote diuresis and prevent renal and bladder toxicity (hemorrhagic cystitis). • Assess patient's renal function before giving drug; monitor renal function after administration. • Give fluids to hydrate patient before and after administration. • Monitor for signs and symptoms of ototoxicity and neurotoxicity; report such signs immediately. • Monitor patient's heart rate, respiratory rate, and blood pressure every 15 minutes for 1 hour after administration. • Monitor serum electrolyte levels.
corticosteroids, such as prednisone (Deltasone)	• Moon face • Fluid retention • Weight gain • Increased appetite • Gastric irritation • Hypertension • Mood swings	• Administer orally with an antacid to minimize gastrointestinal irritation, as prescribed. • To mask bitter taste, have patient swallow tablets whole or use commercially available oral solution. • Monitor patient's weight and blood pressure. • Taper dosage, as prescribed, before discontinuing drug. • Prepare patient for changes in body image.

(continued)

Antineoplastic agents *(continued)*

DRUG	ACTION	ADVERSE EFFECTS
cyclophosphamide (Cytoxan)	• Nausea and vomiting (within 3 to 4 hours of administration); may be severe with high doses • Hemorrhagic cystitis • Bone marrow depression (10 to 14 days after administration) • Alopecia (10 to 14 days after administration) • Infertility	• Administer P.O. or I.V., as prescribed. • Premedicate with antiemetics. • Force fluids before administering and for 2 days afterward to prevent chemical cystitis. Some protocols use mesna (Mesnex) as a uroprotectant. • Encourage frequent voiding.
cytarabine [ARA-C, cytosine arabinoside] (Cytosar-U)	• Mild nausea and vomiting • Stomatitis • Immunosuppression • Diarrhea • Skin rash • Bone marrow depression (7 to 14 days after administration)	• Administer I.V. or intrathecally, as prescribed. • Monitor patient's liver function studies. • Drug crosses blood-brain barrier and may be useful to treat central nervous system leukemia.
daunorubicin (Cerubidine); doxorubicin (Adriamycin)	• Moderate nausea and vomiting • Stomatitis • Fever, chills • Alopecia (10 to 14 days after administration) • Bone marrow depression (7 to 14 days after administration) • Cardiac toxicity, as indicated by ECG changes, cardiomyopathy, and heart failure (up to years after administration because cardiac toxicity is a function of total cumulative lifetime dose); lower total dosages are required for patients who receive chest radiation	• Administer I.V., as prescribed. • Know that these drugs are vesicants. • Inform child and parents that drug may turn urine red for up to 12 days after administration; reassure them that this is not a cause for concern.
etoposide [VP-16] (VePesid)	• Mild to moderate nausea and vomiting • Hypotension (with rapid infusion) • Allergic reactions, including urticaria and anaphylaxis • Bone marrow depression (7 to 14 days after administration) • Alopecia (10 to 14 days after administration)	• Before administering, have emergency drugs used to treat anaphylaxis at bedside. • As prescribed, give by slow I.V. infusion, over 30 to 60 minutes. • Monitor patient's heart rate, respiratory rate, and blood pressure every 15 minutes for 1 hour after administration. Report allergic reactions immediately.
mercaptopurine [6-MP, 6-mercaptopurine] (Purinethol)	• Mild nausea and vomiting • Diarrhea • Stomatitis • Anorexia • Immunosuppression • Skin rash • Bone marrow depression (4 to 6 weeks after administration)	• Administer P.O., as prescribed. • Keep in mind that allopurinol may be prescribed if uric acid levels increase. Administer allopurinol cautiously because it impairs the metabolism of mercaptopurine, resulting in elevated serum levels and increased risk of toxicity. Lower dosages of mercaptopurine may be required. Monitor child closely for bone marrow depression.

Antineoplastic agents *(continued)*

DRUG	ACTION	ADVERSE EFFECTS
methotrexate (Mexate)	• Nausea and vomiting (severe with high doses) • Diarrhea • Stomatitis • Immunosuppression • Skin rash • Photosensitivity • Bone marrow depression (about 10 days after administration)	• Administer P.O., I.V., or intrathecally, as prescribed. • Monitor renal function in patients receiving high doses of this drug. Avoid concomitant administration with salicylates or sulfonamides because of increased risk of toxicity.
vincristine (Oncovin)	• Fever • Constipation • Neurotoxicity • Mild nausea and vomiting • Mild bone marrow depression (7 to 14 days after administration) • Alopecia (10 to 14 days after administration)	• Administer I.V., as prescribed. • Know that this drug is a vesicant. • Monitor patient's bowel function, checking for bowel sounds and constipation. As needed and prescribed, administer stool softeners. • Promptly report signs of neurotoxicity, which may require drug discontinuation.

ing cells. It may be prescribed to achieve a cure or to provide palliation (such as by shrinking a tumor and thus relieving symptoms.

Like chemotherapy, radiation also damages normal, healthy cells, causing adverse effects. Such effects may occur within weeks (acute effects) or may be delayed until years after radiation therapy ends. Acute effects vary with the area irradiated. (For specific adverse effects of radiation therapy, see *Radiation therapy: Acute and late effects,* page 365.)

Surgery
Most children who have solid tumors require surgery. The goal of surgery is to remove all traces of the tumor. A localized or encapsulated tumor generally is removed completely. The child may need preoperative radiation or chemotherapy to shrink the tumor; after surgery, radiation or chemotherapy may be repeated to help prevent metastasis. Palliative surgery may be performed if the tumor is large and cannot be removed completely without damaging adjacent tissues or organs.

Bone marrow transplantation
Bone marrow transplantation involves administration of near-lethal doses of chemotherapy and total-body irradiation therapy to kill all cancer cells, followed by I.V. administration of donor bone marrow (or the child's own previously obtained marrow) to restore the child's immune system and marrow. Transplanted bone marrow starts to produce normal blood cells within 21 days.

Bone marrow transplantation provides hope for a cure and is being used more commonly to manage childhood cancers. However, because

When adverse effects of chemotherapy may occur

Adverse effects of chemotherapy may arise within hours after drug administration (immediate effects), within 1 to 3 weeks (intermediate effects), or years later (late effects). This chart delineates immediate, intermediate, and late effects.

IMMEDIATE EFFECTS	INTERMEDIATE EFFECTS	LATE EFFECTS
• Allergic reactions (within 1 hour)	• Alopecia (hair loss)	• Adrenal dysfunction
• Nausea and vomiting (within 8 hours)	• Anorexia	• Cardiac toxicity
• Photosensitivity	• Bone marrow depression	• Chromosomal abnormalities
	• Cystitis	• Chronic cystitis
	• Neuropathy	• Cognitive deficits
	• Oral ulcers	• Infertility
	• Ototoxicity	• Cirrhosis
	• Pancreatitis	• Secondary malignancy
	• Renal toxicity	

of its inherent risks, it is reserved for children whose cancers cannot be cured by other means.

Potential complications include life-threatening infection (until the transplanted marrow produces sufficient granulocytes) as well as anorexia, oral ulcers, severe nausea and vomiting, and severe diarrhea (caused by high-dose chemotherapy and radiation therapy). Graft-versus-host disease (GVHD) also may occur. In GVHD, antigens in the donor marrow that do not match the child's antigens attack the child's cells, causing tissue and organ damage. To prevent or minimize the effects of GVHD, the child receives immunosuppressant drugs.

Supportive therapy

Supportive measures for the child with cancer include nutritional therapy and administration of various drugs and blood products.

Nutritional therapy

Because cancer cell reproduction and proliferation causes considerable energy expenditure, the physician prescribes a diet high in calories, carbohydrates, and proteins. Good nutrition also boosts immune system function, improves tolerance of chemotherapy, and provides nutrient reserves for use during periods of nausea, vomiting, diarrhea, and anorexia.

Allopurinol therapy

In a child who has undergone chemotherapy, cellular death may trigger release of uric acid. Administering allopurinol prevents uric acid accumulation in the renal tubules, which may cause tubular obstruction. In conjunction with allopurinol, the physician typically prescribes urinary alkalinizing agents. Sodium bicarbonate, which increases urinary pH, is used to minimize risk of uric acid crystal formation. I.V. flu-

Radiation therapy: Acute and late effects

Like chemotherapy, radiation therapy may cause adverse effects relatively soon after drug administration or up to years later.

Adverse effects that occur within weeks after radiation therapy begins include:

- alopecia
- anorexia
- bone marrow depression
- diarrhea
- fatigue
- nausea and vomiting
- skin erythema and desquamation
- tissue edema and inflammation.

Years after radiation therapy, a patient may suffer the following late effects:

- cataracts
- cognitive deficits
- dental problems
- endocrine dysfunction
- infertility
- delayed growth and short stature
- secondary malignancy
- soft-tissue fibrosis
- pulmonary fibrosis.

id therapy may be prescribed to ensure adequate hydration and sufficient urine output. Hydration therapy prevents deposition of uric acid crystals in the kidneys.

Antibiotic therapy

The physician may prescribe oral prophylactic antibiotics if the child is at risk for infection, I.V. antibiotics if the child has septicemia, and bacteriostatic or antifungal mouthwashes to prevent oral infections in a child who has oral ulcers.

Analgesic therapy

The physician may prescribe narcotic analgesics for a child with severe pain and topical anesthetics for a child who has oral ulcers.

Blood product replacement therapy

Bone marrow depression (resulting from chemotherapy or radiation therapy) impairs production of red blood cells (RBCs), white blood cells (WBCs), and platelets. Depending on the child's condition, the physician also may prescribe packed RBC transfusions to treat anemia, granulocyte transfusions to treat granulocytopenia, and platelet transfusions to treat thrombocytopenia.

Leukemia

Leukemia — cancer of the hematopoietic tissue — is the most common form of cancer in children. Its precise cause is unknown.

Classification

Leukemia is classified by cell type. Two predominant forms of leukemia are acute lymphocytic (lymphoblastic) leukemia (ALL) and acute nonlymphocytic (nonlymphoblastic) leukemia (ANLL). Alternate terms for ALL include acute lymphatic leukemia, acute lymphoid leukemia, and acute lymphoblastoid leukemia. Alternate terms for ANLL include acute myelogenous or myeloblastic leukemia, acute granulocytic leukemia, acute myelocytic leukemia, acute monocytic leukemia, acute monoblastic leukemia, and acute nonlymphoid leukemia. Each form of of ALL and ANLL has several subtypes.

Acute lymphoblastic leukemia

ALL accounts for about 80% of childhood leukemia cases. The most common form of childhood cancer, it represents roughly 30% of all new cancer cases in children. (Fernbach and Vietti, 1991).

Subtypes of ALL classified by morphology and cytochemical activity include L_1, L_2, and L_3. L_1 is the most common subtype. ALL also may be subtyped according to immunologic markers (cell-surface antigens): T cell, B cell, and null cell.

Acute nonlymphoblastic leukemia

ANLL accounts for roughly 20% of childhood leukemia cases. ANLL has four major subtypes classified by morphology and cytochemical activity: acute myelocytic, acute myelomonocytic, acute monocytic, and erythromycytic.

Prognosis

Among children with ALL, Caucasian girls between ages 2 and 10 with the null-cell, L_1 subtype have the best prognosis. ANLL carries a less favorable prognosis than ALL.

Pathophysiology and clinical manifestations

In leukemia, abnormal, immature WBCs replace normal bone marrow elements (RBCs, WBCs, and platelets). The pathophysiology and clinical manifestations of leukemia reflect WBC proliferation and subsequent "crowding out" of normal cells.

Bone marrow dysfunction

Leukemic cells depress normal bone marrow function by competing with mature blood cells for space and essential nutrients. Consequently, the marrow cannot produce sufficient amounts of mature WBCs, RBCs, and platelets. Clinical manifestations of bone marrow dysfunction include:
• infection caused by neutropenia (a decreased WBC count)
• anemia caused by a decreased RBC count
• bleeding tendencies, including petechiae and bruising, caused by thrombocytopenia (a decreased platelet count).

The child also may have fever, pallor, fatigue, persistent upper respiratory infection or pharyngitis, petechiae, bruising, and epistaxis. Marrow infiltration with immature WBCs may cause bone pain.

Liver, spleen, and lymph node disturbances

Infiltration of the liver, spleen, and lymph nodes by leukemic cells causes enlargement and eventual fibrosis of these organs. Hepatomegaly (liver enlargement) is the most common leukemia-related finding.

Central nervous system involvement

Infiltration of the meninges by leukemic cells leads to increased intracranial pressure (ICP), which in turn causes headache (commonly accompanied by vomiting), confusion, papilledema, lethargy, and irritability. However, not all children develop central nervous system (CNS) involvement.

Hypermetabolism

Leukemic cells require a tremendous store of nutrients and energy for reproduction. Eventually, they deprive normal cells of nutrients. This causes such changes as weight loss, muscle wasting, lethargy, and fatigue.

Diagnosis

Clinical and laboratory findings may suggest leukemia. Laboratory studies typically reveal anemia, neutropenia, and immature WBCs (as seen in a peripheral blood smear).

Definitive diagnosis and leukemia classification are based on the findings of bone marrow aspiration, which typically reveals hypercellular marrow with a predominance of blast cells (immature WBCs). Lumbar puncture is performed to detect CNS involvement.

Medical management

Regardless of the type of leukemia, treatment occurs in three phases: an induction phase, prophylactic CNS therapy, and a maintenance phase. The child who suffers a relapse (return of leukemic cells within the marrow) also goes through a reinduction phase.

Induction phase

The goal of the induction phase is to achieve a complete remission — disappearance of leukemic cells from the marrow. Children with ALL commonly receive vincristine, prednisone, and asparaginase — a regimen that achieves remission in approximately 95% of cases.

For children with ANLL, induction therapy involves cytosine arabinoside, prednisone, and doxorubicin or daunorubicin. Most children with ANLL achieve initial remission; however, they are more likely to suffer relapses than children with ALL.

The induction phase lasts 4 to 6 weeks. Initially, the child is hospitalized for placement of a venous access device and evaluation of the therapeutic response. The child who tolerates induction therapy is discharged and continues therapy as an outpatient, with close monitoring for adverse and toxic effects of therapy. Bone marrow depression is common during the induction phase.

Prophylactic CNS therapy

This therapy, which starts within 6 to 8 weeks of diagnosis, aims to prevent leukemic cells from infiltrating the CNS. (Most antineoplastic drugs do not cross the blood-brain barrier, making them ineffective against CNS infiltration.) The child may undergo cranial irradiation and receive methotrexate intrathecally. Alternatively, some children receive a combination of methotrexate, hydrocortisone, and cytosine arabinoside intrathecally without cranial irradiation. Because cranial irradiation may cause late adverse effects, such as cataracts and cognitive deficits, it commonly is reserved for children with CNS infiltration.

Maintenance phase

The goal of this treatment phase, which follows CNS prophylactic therapy, is to maintain remission and kill residual leukemic cells. For a child with ALL, maintenance typically includes daily oral doses of 6-mercaptopurine and weekly oral doses of methotrexate. The child also may receive I.V. vincristine and oral prednisone periodically.

The maintenance phase continues for 18 months in girls and 24 to 36 months in boys (who have a greater relapse rate). After it ends, boys undergo testicular biopsy to detect any testicular involvement; such involvement warrants testicular irradiation therapy and systemic chemotherapy.

During and after the maintenance phase, the child requires regular monitoring (including laboratory studies and bone marrow studies) to evaluate the therapeutic response, check for bone marrow depression, and detect a possible relapse. Therapy may be halted temporarily if the child's neutrophil count drops below $1,000/\text{mm}^3$ or if toxic effects occur.

Reinduction phase

The child who has a relapse undergoes a reinduction phase. Most relapses occur within 12 months after cessation of therapy. For the child with ALL, reinduction therapy involves oral prednisone, I.V. vincristine, and other drugs not used during the induction phase. CNS prophylaxis and maintenance therapy continue if remission occurs. Most children achieve a second remission, although the prognosis is less favorable with each relapse.

Bone marrow transplantation offers an additional treatment option. It may be recommended for children with ANLL who have achieved their first remission. Because ALL generally carries a more favorable prognosis, bone marrow transplantation is not recommended for children in their first remission. However, it may be an option for those with ALL in their second remission.

Nursing management

Nursing goals for the child with leukemia include:
- supporting the child and family
- implementing measures to eliminate leukemic cells
- preventing complications of bone marrow depression
- managing adverse effects of chemotherapy and radiation therapy
- preventing constipation
- ensuring adequate nutrition
- promoting a positive body image.

Supporting the child and family

The diagnosis of cancer can have devastating effects on both the child and family. Fear of cancer treatment and the possibility of the child's death may cause intense distress.

To help the family cope with the crisis, provide emotional support. Offer information about leukemia, its treatment, and home management. (For details on nursing care of the child with a life-threatening disease, see Chapter 15, Illness concepts.)

Implementing measures to eliminate leukemic cells

Administer the prescribed chemotherapy protocol and monitor for adverse effects. Assist the physician in giving intrathecal medications, as prescribed. Teach the family about outpatient chemotherapy administration, if prescribed.

Preventing complications of bone marrow depression

Bone marrow depression may cause anemia, thrombocytopenia, and neutropenia. As prescribed, administer blood transfusions. Encourage the child with anemia to rest. To help conserve the child's energy, assist with self-care tasks.

Thrombocytopenia places the child at risk for bleeding and spontaneous hemorrhage. To decrease the risk of bleeding, implement the following thrombocytopenic precautions:
- Administer platelets, as prescribed.
- Apply local pressure to bleeding sites.
- Use a soft-sponge toothbrush for mouth care.
- Avoid needle sticks.
- Avoid giving aspirin products, which promote bleeding.
- Restrict strenuous play, which could cause bleeding.

The child with neutropenia is at risk for infection. Administer antibiotics, as prescribed, and institute the following neutropenic precautions:
- Place the child in a private room.
- Prohibit visits by persons with infections.
- Do not take rectal temperatures (because this may introduce bacteria into the bloodstream through minute anal fissures or ulcers).
- Use aseptic technique for all invasive procedures.

Managing adverse effects of chemotherapy and radiation therapy

Chemotherapy and radiation therapy may cause a wide range of adverse effects, including nausea, vomiting, and oral and rectal ulcers.

Nausea and vomiting predispose the child to fluid and electrolyte imbalances. To prevent these problems, use measures to prevent or control nausea and vomiting. For example, give the child an antiemetic, as prescribed, before administering chemotherapy; continue antiemetic administration if nausea or vomiting occurs. Limit food intake during chemotherapy administration. Encourage the child to consume clear fluids in small to moderate amounts. As appropriate, use relaxation techniques to help reduce nausea.

Oral ulcers are painful and are likely to become infected; some ulcers may interfere with food intake. To prevent or minimize ulcer development, implement oral hygiene measures. Clean the child's teeth, gums, and tongue with a soft-sponge toothbrush at least three times a day. After every meal and before bedtime, rinse the child's mouth with clear water, 0.9% sodium chloride (normal saline) solution, an over-the-counter mouthwash, or a prescription mouthwash (depending on the physician's preference). If oral ulcers develop, apply topical anesthetics and administer topical antibiotics as prescribed, provide a bland diet, and avoid giving the child citrus products.

Rectal ulcers also are painful and place the child at risk for sepsis. To prevent rectal ulcers, keep the child's perianal area meticulously clean. Clean the perianal area after each bowel movement, and dry gently after cleaning; also, teach the child and parents to do this. To increase the child's comfort, use sitz baths and a protective skin barrier, as appropriate. To promote healing, leave ulcerated skin exposed to the air.

Preventing constipation

If the child is receiving vincristine, take measures to prevent constipation. For example, give stool softeners, as prescribed; ensure an adequate fluid intake; encourage exercise; and provide a high-fiber diet. The child may need suppositories or enemas to empty the bowel completely. However, these treatments are prohibited in the neutropenic child because they may introduce infectious organisms.

Ensuring adequate nutrition

Nutritional support is an important component of cancer treatment. Chemotherapy may cause nausea and changes in taste; some children develop an aversion to foods they previously liked. Along with hypermetabolism, these responses contribute to nutritional and caloric deficits.

During periods of nausea, limit the child's oral intake. Offer dry crackers, toast, and clear fluids. If the child has a poor appetite, allow any food the child desires — calories from any source are preferable to none. Reassure parents that the child will eat more when the appetite improves.

Once the child's appetite returns, include the child in meal planning. Provide high-carbohydrate, high-protein foods in an attractive setting. To boost caloric intake, encourage the family to provide nutritional supplements, such as breakfast shakes. Stay with the child during mealtimes, or encourage the parents to do so.

Promoting a positive body image

Alopecia (a potential adverse effect of chemotherapy or radiation therapy) places the child at risk for a disturbed body image. Reassure the patient that hair loss is temporary and that hair will grow back once the treatment ends. Suggest ways to minimize the effects of hair loss before it occurs. For example, suggest that the child obtain a baseball cap, bandanna, or wig before hair loss begins. Encourage good grooming and advise the child to wear attractive clothing to promote a positive self-image.

Because thinning hair or baldness places the child at risk for injury from sun exposure or cold, teach the child to apply sunscreen and cover the head before exposure to the sun and to cover the head before exposure to wind or cold.

STUDY ACTIVITIES

Short answer

1. Identify at least three risk factors associated with cancer in children.

_____

_____

2. What precautions should the nurse take before administering asparaginase? Why are these precautions necessary?

_____

_____

3. Define the term *vesicant,* and identify at least two antineoplastic agents classified as vesicants.

_____

_____

4. Identify at least three factors that may lead to nutritional deficiencies in children with cancer.

_____

_____

5. Josie, age 3, has leukemia. To conserve her energy and improve her activity tolerance, the nurse formulates the following nursing diagnosis: *Activity intolerance related to decreased RBC count secondary to bone marrow depression.* The expected outcomes are that Josie will participate in activities of daily living, as tolerated, and regain a normal RBC count. Identify three nursing interventions that would help achieve these outcomes.

_____

_____

_____

Matching related elements
Match the form of cancer on the left with the affected body system or tissue on the right.

6. ___ Rhabdomyo-   **A.** Renal system
     sarcoma

7. ___ Leukemia   **B.** Hematopoietic tissue

8. ___ Hodgkin's   **C.** Striated muscle
     disease

9. ___ Neuroblastoma   **D.** Bone

10. ___ Osteosarcoma   **E.** Sympathetic nervous system

11. ___ Wilms' tumor   **F.** Lymphoid tissue

Multiple choice
12. Brian, age 3, has just been diagnosed with leukemia. He seems tired and sleeps most of the day. Based on the known pathophysiologic effects of leukemia, the nurse suspects Brian's fatigue results from:
    A. Nutritional deficiencies
    B. Sleep disturbances related to hospitalization
    C. A decreased RBC count
    D. Leukemic CNS infiltration

13. Brian is receiving methotrexate. When is he most likely to suffer associated bone marrow depression?
    A. Within hours after receiving the drug
    B. 2 weeks after receiving the drug
    C. 1 month after receiving the drug
    D. After completing induction therapy

14. Which of the following is a common relapse site in boys who have completed treatment for leukemia?
    A. Bone
    B. Testes
    C. Lung
    D. Liver

15. Susie, age 8, loses her appetite during chemotherapy. What should the nurse tell Susie's parents when teaching them how to care for her?
  A. "Offer dry crackers or toast."
  B. "Withhold all food and fluids."
  C. "Ignore her lack of food intake."
  D. "Let her eat any food she wants."

ANSWERS **Short answer**

1. Ionizing radiation has been linked to thyroid cancer and leukemia; maternal history of diethylstilbestrol use, to adenosarcoma of the vagina; genetically based hereditary factors, to retinoblastoma, Wilms' tumor, and neuroblastoma; chromosomal abnormalities, to leukemia; and immunodeficiencies, to various cancers.

2. The nurse should have emergency drugs at bedside before administering asparaginase because the drug may cause anaphylaxis.

3. A vesicant is a substance that can cause severe tissue damage if allowed to infiltrate the tissue surrounding an I.V. site. Daunorubicin, doxorubicin, and vincristine are vesicants.

4. Nausea, changes in taste, aversion to foods the child previously liked, and hypermetabolism may lead to nutritional deficiencies.

5. Administer blood transfusions, as prescribed. Encourage Josie to rest. Assist Josie with self-care tasks.

Matching related elements

6. C
7. B
8. F
9. E
10. D
11. A

Multiple choice

12. C. A child with leukemia may develop anemia from bone marrow depression (such as from chemotherapy or replacement of normal marrow elements by immature WBCs). Anemia results in fatigue, lack of energy, and activity intolerance.

13. B. Bone marrow depression is most likely to occur 10 days after methotrexate administration.

14. B. The testes are a common relapse site in boys who have completed treatment for leukemia.

15. D. The nurse should instruct the parents to let Susie eat any food she wants, because any caloric intake is better than none. Dry crackers should be offered to children experiencing nausea. The other options are inappropriate.

CHAPTER 27

Fractures

OBJECTIVES

After studying this chapter, the reader should be able to:

1. Describe the causes, pathophysiology, and clinical manifestations of fractures in children.

2. Discuss the pathophysiologic effects of the prolonged immobilization necessary for bone healing.

3. Describe the various traction systems used to treat fractures.

4. Discuss medical and nursing management of children with fractures.

OVERVIEW OF CONCEPTS

A fracture is a traumatic injury in which the continuity of the bone tissue is broken. Because of skeletal immaturity, children suffer more fractures than adults. However, fractures heal more quickly in children and are less likely to cause extensive tissue damage.

Most fractures in children result from accidental injury, such as falls, motor vehicle accidents, and pedestrian-automobile and bicycle-automobile accidents. Because these accidents are relatively uncommon in infants, fracture of a rib or a long bone in an infant may indicate child abuse.

This chapter explores fractures in children. It reviews fracture classifications and discusses the stages of bone healing. Then it explores the pathophysiologic effects of the prolonged period of immobility required for bone healing. After discussing assessment of fractures, the chapter covers medical and nursing management, focusing on casting and traction.

Classification of fractures

Fractures typically are described as open or closed, depending on how they communicate with the outside environment. The direction of the fracture line or the position of the bony fragments also may be used to describe fractures. Fractures fall into the following categories:

- In a *closed,* or *simple,* fracture, skin over the fractured bone is intact.
- In an *open,* or *compound,* fracture, the fractured bone breaks through the skin, creating an open wound.
- In a *complicated fracture*, fragments from the fractured bone damage surrounding tissue or organs.

Stages of bone healing

Stage 1: Hematoma formation
This stage starts at the time of the fracture and continues for 24 hours afterward. Immediately after a fracture, muscles near the fractured bone contract to support the injured area. A hematoma forms as blood seeps from torn vessels in the bone and surrounding tissue into the fragments of the fractured bone. The hematoma serves as the base for new tissue growth. Granulation tissue develops and osteoblastic (bone-forming) activity is stimulated.

If the initial injury causes contusion of soft tissues, blood seeps into the damaged tissue. In some cases, severe hemorrhage may occur.

Stage 2: Cellular proliferation
During this stage, which occurs 24 to 72 hours after the fracture, blood supply to the fracture site increases, drawing calcium, phosphate, and fibroblasts to the area. Fibroblasts convert to osteoblasts (bone-forming cells). The ends of the bony fragments become necrotic, and then are reabsorbed.

Stage 3: Callus formation
This stage occurs 1 to 3 weeks after the fracture. Osteoblasts multiply and form a soft callus around the fracture site. The callus holds the bone together but is not strong enough to support the child's body weight.

Stage 4: Ossification
Starting the third week after the fracture, mature bone tissue replaces the callus. Ossification continues through the tenth week.

Stage 5: Consolidation and remodeling
Roughly 9 months after the fracture, the callus is resorbed fully and the bone marrow cavity is restored.

- In a *comminuted fracture*, bone fragments become embedded in surrounding tissue.
- In a *longitudinal fracture*, the fracture runs parallel to the long axis of the bone (the shaft).
- In a *transverse fracture*, the fracture occurs across the shaft, at right angles to the long axis of the bone.
- In an *oblique fracture*, the fracture breaks the bone at an angle (relative to the bone's axis).
- In a *spiral fracture*, the fracture line runs through the bone in a coiling direction.
- In a *greenstick fracture*, the bone is partially broken and bent.

Pathophysiology   After a fracture, a bone heals in predictable stages, starting with hematoma formation and ending with consolidation and remodeling. (For details about these stages, see *Stages of bone healing*.)

The type of fracture and the child's age, nutritional status, and health status influence the speed of bone healing. Gaps between the fractured bone ends and fragments delay healing. The younger the child and the better the nutritional status and overall health, the faster the bone heals.

Children with severe fractures requiring traction and those confined to bed during bone healing are at risk for complications of immobility. These include muscle atrophy, edema, contractures, bone demineralization (leading to osteoporosis and hypercalcemia), retention of pulmonary secretions (leading to atelectasis and pneumonia), abdominal distention, constipation, urine retention, difficulty voiding, renal calculi, orthostatic hypertension, skin breakdown, venous stasis, and thrombi formation.

Assessment The most common signs of a fracture are swelling over the injury site, pain with movement, and decreased function of the injured bone. Some patients also have bruising, muscle rigidity, crepitus (a grating sensation at the fracture site), and obvious deformity.

Nerve injury, vessel damage, or tissue injury and swelling may occur secondary to the trauma. Displaced bone fragments may cause internal injury. Tissue damage and swelling or direct injury to vessels or nerves may lead to neurovascular compromise, as indicated by pain, pallor of the affected extremity, absence of pulses distal to the injury site, paresthesia (decreased sensation in the affected extremity), and inability to move the affected extremity voluntarily.

Diagnosis
X-rays confirm a fracture and may help classify it. However, the bones of infants and young children contain radiolucent growth cartilage, making radiographic examination difficult. To detect changes indicating fracture in these children, the physician must compare X-rays of the affected extremity with those of the unaffected extremity.

Medical management Treatment of a fracture involves three steps: realigning bony fragments, retaining alignment until the bone heals, and restoring function to the injured bone.

Realigning bony fragments
Depending on the type of fracture, realignment is accomplished through reduction or traction.

Reduction
Reduction may be closed or open. In *closed reduction,* the physician externally manipulates bone fragments into place, then applies a cast.

Open (surgical) reduction is reserved for patients with fractures that cannot be realigned through closed reduction or those who have soft-tissue, vascular, or nerve injury. The physician surgically manipulates bone fragments into place, then inserts rods, plates, or screws to maintain bone alignment. After surgery, a plaster splint may be applied. Although the splint is removed after a few weeks, the child cannot use the injured extremity until full ossification occurs.

Traction

Traction allows realignment of bony fragments by tiring the involved muscles and reducing muscle spasm. Traction systems maintain the bone in alignment by applying forward force (traction), a counterforce (countertraction), and frictional force between the child's body and the bed. Typically, traction is used to treat fractures of the humerus, femur, or vertebrae, which are hard to realign through closed methods.

For countertraction, a pulling force is applied in the direction opposite that of traction. Oppositional forces, generated by the forward pull of traction and the backward pull of countertraction, keep the bone in alignment. Countertraction, which generally can be achieved by the child's own weight, may be increased by raising the foot of the bed.

Traction may be applied either to the skin or directly to the bone. *Skin traction* is used if the child has minimal bone displacement and muscle spasticity; tissue damage contraindicates this type of traction. Because skin traction provides only a small pull, it can realign only simple, uncomplicated fractures.

Skin traction is applied directly to the skin surface and indirectly to the bone. Traction straps are applied to the child's skin, and the weight and pulley system is applied over the straps and held in place with adhesive material or elastic wrap. Depending on the physician's preference, skin traction may be applied continuously or intermittently.

Skeletal traction is used when a strong pull is needed to achieve realignment and immobilization. The physician inserts a pin or wire directly into the bone, then attaches the traction system to the skeletal pins to apply traction directly to the bone. (For more information on traction, see *Comparing traction systems,* page 378.)

Retaining alignment

After closed reduction, the physician may apply a cast to immobilize the bone and thus maintain alignment. The cast remains in place until ossification is complete.

If a fractured bone has been realigned through traction, the child remains in traction to maintain realignment and promote bone healing. Once sufficient healing takes place, a cast is applied until full healing occurs.

Restoring function

Once the fractured bone heals, the immobilization device (cast or traction system) is removed. Normally, the child's preinjury activity patterns are sufficient to restore normal function to the affected extremity. Some children, however, require physical therapy.

Comparing traction systems

To realign bony fragments of a fracture, the physician may order one of the traction systems described below.

Bryant's traction
This traction system is used to treat femur fractures or congenital hip dislocation in children under age 2 who weigh less than 30 lb. Skin traction is applied bilaterally to the lower extremities, which are suspended above the bed. The child's hips are flexed at a right angle and the buttocks are elevated slightly. A restraining jacket prevents rotation of the pelvis and hips.

Buck's extension
This system applies skin traction to the child's lower extremity, which is maintained in an extended position. It is used for short-term immobilization or to correct bone deformities or contractures.

Russell's traction
Used to treat hip and femur fractures and knee injuries, this system applies skin traction to the child's lower extremity. The extremity is suspended above the bed, with a sling placed under the knee. The hip is flexed at the prescribed angle, with the knee flexed to maintain the lower leg parallel to the bed.

90-90 traction
This system, used to treat femur fractures in children over age 2, applies skeletal traction to the lower extremity. A cast is applied to the child's lower leg, and skeletal pins are placed through the distal femur. Traction is applied to the skeletal pin and to pins embedded in the cast. The child's hip and knee are flexed at a 90° angle.

Overhead suspension
Used to treat humerus fractures, overhead suspension applies skin or skeletal traction to the upper extremity. Two systems are used—one applied to the child's upper arm and the other to the lower arm. The arm is bent at the elbow and suspended vertically by skin or skeletal traction.

Balanced suspension with Thomas splint and Pearson attachment
Used to suspend the leg in flexion to relax the hip and hamstring muscles, this traction system may be used with or without skin or skeletal traction. The child's leg is suspended in a flexed position. A Thomas splint extends from the groin to midair, above the foot. A Pearson attachment supports the child's lower leg.

Nursing management Nursing goals for the child with a fracture depend on the medical treatment plan.

General nursing goals
Nursing goals common to all children with a fracture include:
- maintaining correct alignment (as prescribed)
- promoting comfort and relieving pain
- detecting complications of neurovascular compromise
- reducing fear and anxiety
- maintaining function in unaffected extremities.

Promoting comfort and relieving pain

To reduce pain and discomfort, administer pain medications, as prescribed, and use nonpharmacologic strategies, such as distraction or ice application. Support the affected extremity and limit its movement, using pillows and rolls as appropriate. Be aware that positioning the fractured part above heart level promotes venous return and decreases edema; this may promote comfort by diminishing pressure on nerve endings.

Detecting complications of neurovascular compromise

Monitor the child for the following signs and symptoms, which indicate neurovascular compromise:

- increasing pain, decreased sensation, pallor, or slow capillary refill of the affected extremity
- weak or absent pulses distal to the fracture site
- inability to move the affected extremity or digits distal to the fracture site.

Report any of these signs to the physician immediately. If the child is discharged from the hospital with a cast, teach the parents to recognize these signs.

Reducing fear and anxiety

Trauma, pain, a strange environment, and medical treatment contribute to the child's fear and anxiety. To put the child and parents at ease, explain the treatment plan. Prepare them for the prescribed procedures. Encourage a family member to stay with the child to provide comfort and security.

Maintaining function in unaffected extremities

Normally, children are active and need little encouragement to use their large and fine muscle groups. However, their high activity level puts them at risk for reinjuring the fractured bone. Collaborate with the physician to design an activity plan for the child that promotes use of unaffected muscles and joints while protecting the injured bone.

Cast care

Nursing goals include preparing the child for cast application, teaching the parents how to manage the cast at home, and preparing the child for cast removal. Recently developed casting materials, which use fiberglass and polyurethane resins, have made casts more lightweight and water-resistant. Although more expensive than plaster casts, they are easier to clean, resist soiling better, and are stronger than plaster casts. They dry and harden within minutes after application and cannot be dented. Such casts commonly are used for immobilizing arms and for hip spica casts.

Cast application

Before the cast is applied, explain the casting procedure to the child, such as by using a doll to demonstrate. Then, gently clean the skin where the cast will be applied, and remove any jewelry from the affected extremity. Perform a baseline neurovascular assessment. Provide comfort by staying with the child as the cast is applied.

After cast application, gently clean the skin around the cast edges to remove any debris. To reduce swelling and edema formation, elevate the casted extremity above heart level, using pillows. Reposition the child every 3 to 4 hours to promote cast drying and prevent skin breakdown. Depending on the size and thickness of the cast, plaster casts may take 24 to 72 hours to dry. Let the cast air dry; do not use heat lamps or blow dryers to hasten drying.

Perform neurovascular assessments every hour for the first 4 hours after cast application, then every 4 hours. Once the cast dries completely, the cast edges should be covered with soft moleskin to provide a smooth edge surface. If the child will be discharged immediately after cast application, teach the parents how to do this at home.

Before discharge, caution the child and parents never to put anything underneath the cast. If itching occurs, advise the child or parents to scratch the skin near the cast edge gently. Instruct parents to avoid using lotions or powders on the skin near or underneath the cast because this may predispose the child to skin irritation and breakdown.

Teach parents how to provide daily cast care. Instruct them to inspect the skin at the cast edges and beneath the cast twice daily, noting its condition and checking for drainage and odors. Advise them to report skin breakdown, drainage, or foul odor to the physician.

Cast removal

The physician removes the cast with a special saw, which can be especially frightening to the child. Explain the procedure in advance, and demonstrate use of the saw. Reassure the child that the saw will not cut through the skin. Stay with the child during cast removal. As necessary, use distraction to decrease anxiety.

After the cast is removed, inspect the child's skin. Use warm soapy water to remove any dead skin, then apply lotion to soften the skin.

Care during traction

Nursing goals for the child in traction include preventing injury caused by the traction system, preventing skin breakdown, providing diversional activities, and preventing complications of immobility.

Preventing injury

The nurse is responsible for maintaining the traction system. At the beginning of each shift, inspect the system to make sure it is working properly. Verify that the weights and pulleys are maintained in a free position — not resting against the end of the bed. Clean the skin around the skeletal pins twice daily according to institutional policies. As prescribed, apply topical antibiotic ointment. Position the child to maintain the prescribed joint angles.

Preventing skin breakdown

Skin traction places the child at risk for skin breakdown; friction from traction tape contributes to this risk. To help prevent skin breakdown, inspect the skin surrounding the traction system for such signs as redness. Because all body areas — especially the skin and tissue surrounding skin traction sites — are prone to breakdown during immobility — inspect the child's entire body for signs of pressure injury. To stimulate circulation and prevent injury, gently massage reddened areas.

Place the child on an low-air-loss mattress to help prevent pressure injury and skin breakdown. Change the child's position every 2 hours and remove sources of friction, such as sheet wrinkles, from the bed.

Providing diversional activities

To minimize monotony and boredom, provide access to diversional activities, such as television, board games, crafts, and reading. Encourage social interaction by wheeling the child's bed and traction system to the hallway or playroom, if space allows. Read to the child, as appropriate.

Preventing complications of immobility

Immobility during bone healing can lead to multisystemic problems. To help prevent respiratory complications of immobility, reposition the child every 2 hours. Teach the child to use an incentive spirometer, and encourage deep breathing and coughing.

To minimize cardiovascular complications, apply elastic stockings to unaffected lower extremities as prescribed. Reposition the child every 4 hours to prevent thrombus formation, and perform range-of-motion exercises in unaffected extremities to promote venous return.

To minimize muscle and joint complications, maintain the child in correct body alignment and encourage active range of motion to unaffected muscles.

To help prevent renal complications, provide adequate fluids, acidify the urine, and pour warm water over the child's suprapubic area to stimulate voiding.

To minimize bowel problems stemming from immobility, provide adequate fluids, add fiber to the child's diet, and administer stool softeners and laxatives as prescribed.

To minimize skin problems, reposition the child frequently, use a low air-loss mattress, gently massage reddened skin areas, and keep the bed free from friction sources.

STUDY ACTIVITIES

Short answer

1. Name three factors that influence bone healing in children.

_____

_____

2. Identify three pathophysiologic effects of immobility.

_____

3. Name at least three signs of fracture.

_____

4. Sherry, age 6, is in traction to treat a fracture of the femur. To promote skin integrity during immobilization, the nurse formulates the following nursing diagnosis: _High risk for impaired skin integrity related to immobility._ The expected outcome is that Sherry will maintain clear, intact skin. Identify two nursing interventions that would help achieve this outcome.

_____

_____

Matching related elements

Match the traction system on the left with its description on the right.

5. ___ Russell's traction   **A.** Skin traction applied bilaterally to the lower extremities

6. ___ Bryant's traction   **B.** Skin or skeletal traction applied to an upper extremity

7. ___ Overhead suspension   **C.** Skin traction applied to an extended lower extremity

8. ___ 90-90 traction   **D.** Skin traction applied to a lower extremity, with the extremity suspended above the bed and a sling placed under the knee

9. ___ Buck's extension   **E.** Skeletal traction applied to a lower extremity

Multiple choice

10. Eddie, age 7, fractured his left femur during a motor vehicle accident and has a full-length cast on his left foot. The nurse notices that the toes on his left foot are edematous. Which nursing action would be _most_ appropriate?

   A. Massage the toes.

   B. Apply ice to the foot.

   C. Elevate the foot of the bed.

   D. Place Eddie on his right side.

11. When teaching parents how to provide cast care for a child with a broken arm, the nurse should provide which instruction?

    A. Ask the child to wiggle the fingers at least twice daily.

    B. Have the child keep the casted arm close to the side to prevent injury.

    C. Insert a finger down the side of the cast to check for tightness.

    D. Use a blow dryer to hasten cast drying.

ANSWERS

Short answer

1. Factors that influence bone healing in children include fracture characteristics, the child's age, the child's nutritional status, and the child's health status.

2. Pathophysiologic effects of immobility include muscle atrophy, edema, contractures, bone demineralization, retention of pulmonary secretions, abdominal distention, altered bowel and bladder function, renal calculi, orthostatic hypertension, skin breakdown, venous stasis, and thrombi formation.

3. Signs of a fracture include pain with movement, limited function in the affected extremity, swelling over the injury site, bruising, muscle rigidity, crepitus, and obvious deformity.

4. Reposition Sherry frequently. Place Sherry on a low-air-loss mattress. Gently massage reddened skin areas. Keep Sherry's bed free from sheet wrinkles and other friction sources. Inspect Sherry's entire body — particularly the skin and tissue surrounding skin traction sites — for signs of pressure injury.

Matching related elements

5. D

6. A

7. B

8. E

9. C

Multiple choice

10. C. To relieve edema, the nurse should raise the affected extremity above heart level, such as by elevating the foot of the bed. The other choices would not help reduce the swelling.

11. A. The nurse should teach the parents to monitor for signs of neurovascular compromise, such as by asking the child to wiggle the fingers twice daily. A blow dryer should not be used because of the risk for burns.

CHAPTER 28

Burns

OBJECTIVES

After studying this chapter, the reader should be able to:

1. Identify the causes of burns in children.

2. Discuss local and systemic pathophysiologic responses to thermal injury.

3. Describe how to assess the extent, depth, and severity of a burn.

4. Discuss emergency care for the child with a burn.

5. Discuss medical and nursing management of children with minor burns, major burns, and critical burns.

OVERVIEW OF CONCEPTS

Burns are the second leading cause of accidental death in children. All burns damage the skin; severe burns may affect nearly every body system. Children with severe burns face extensive hospitalization followed by a prolonged period of rehabilitative therapy — sometimes lasting several years.

The nurse caring for a child with a burn must know how to assess burn extent, depth, and severity and must understand burn management principles. The nurse also must be familiar with special considerations for managing pain in burn victims and must be prepared to provide extensive psychosocial support to the child and family.

This chapter focuses on care of the child with burns who it hospitalized. It discusses causes of burns, pathophysiologic responses to a burn, and burn complications. The chapter tells how to assess a burn, reviews emergency burn care, and discusses medical and nursing management of children with burns. (For further information on correcting related fluid and electrolyte imbalances and managing pain in children, see Chapter 15, Illness concepts, and Chapter 16, Management principles.)

Causes of burns

Burns result from contact with thermal, chemical, electrical, or radioactive agents. Young children are curious about their environment; without adequate supervision, they are prone to burns and other accidental injuries. More boys than girls suffer burns.

Most burns occur in children under age 4 and result from thermal injury — typically from scalding liquids. Children under age 2 are at greatest risk for thermal injury. In children over age 4, contact with flames causes most burns.

Some parents and other caregivers inflict burns on children as a form of punishment; most common with children under age 4, this is considered a form of child abuse. Younger children and emotionally disturbed children may set fires deliberately and subsequently suffer a burn. Younger children also may suffer electrical burns after biting or gnawing on electrical wires.

Pathophysiologic responses to burns

Superficial burns hurt for 2 to 3 days. Damaged skin sloughs off within 7 to 10 days, and scarring is minimal.

Partial- and full-thickness burns cause edema, fluid loss, and changes in capillary circulation. Capillary damage resulting from thermal injury increases capillary permeability, causing intravascular fluids, electrolytes, and proteins to shift to the interstitial spaces. This produces significant edema, which peaks by the fourth day after the injury. Then, edema fluid mobilizes slowly, shifting back into the intravascular spaces. Loss of the protective skin barrier causes fluid loss at the injury site (via evaporation). Along with fluid shifts, such fluid loss may lead to hypovolemic shock.

In a partial-thickness burn, circulation to the burned area is impaired initially but returns to normal within 5 days. A thin layer of dried exudate forms over the burned skin as it heals, then sloughs off in 10 to 14 days. Once healed, the skin may appear pink and shiny; scarring is minimal. However, a deeper partial-thickness burn may take 4 to 6 weeks to heal fully and may result in scarring.

A full-thickness burn severely compromises capillary circulation. Capillary stasis and thrombi formation obstruct blood flow completely, with subsequent ischemia and necrosis. Within 3 days, necrotic tissue and exudate form a thick, leathery crust called *eschar*.

Systemic responses

The patient with a partial- or full-thickness burn may suffer systemic pathophysiologic responses.

Cardiovascular responses

Initially, severe fluid shifts and fluid loss cause a significant drop in cardiac output. Within 3 or 4 days after the injury, cardiac output returns to normal. In most children, the cardiovascular system can compensate for the decreased cardiac output. However, hypovolemic shock may develop with large thermal injuries. Clinical manifestations of hypovolemic shock include reduced capillary refill, decreased urine output, and decreased central venous pressure and blood pressure.

Hematologic responses

Anemia may result from red blood cell (RBC) destruction secondary to exposure to heat (which occurs initially) and infection (which occurs later), active wound bleeding, and bone marrow depression related to sepsis.

Renal responses

Hypovolemia impairs renal blood flow; this, in turn, decreases urine production. Oliguria occurs during the first 3 to 4 days after the burn injury.

A few days after the patient begins fluid therapy, urine output should increase because of mobilization of edema fluid and a subsequent increase in cardiac output. A child who does not respond to this therapy may suffer acute renal failure.

Blood urea nitrogen and serum creatinine levels rise as a result of tissue breakdown. Hematuria may result from RBC destruction.

Endocrine responses

In an attempt to restore equilibrium, the body increases secretion of epinephrine. Aldosterone and antidiuretic hormone secretion also increase.

Metabolic responses

The patient's metabolic rate rises significantly after a burn — probably from the energy needed to evaporate water from damaged skin surfaces. As a result, the child's energy requirements may be twice that of a normal, healthy child. With partial-thickness burns, evaporative fluid losses peak within the first 24 hours after the injury and persist until the burned tissue heals completely. With full-thickness burns, evaporative losses peak during the first 4 days after the injury and persist until the burned areas are covered completely by grafts.

Growth and developmental changes

Bone growth slows or stops altogether after a serious burn, and the child's weight drops as the burn heals. Once healing is complete, the child's bone growth and weight generally increase significantly.

Secondary sex characteristics may develop 2 to 3 years early in children who have experienced severe thermal burns. Experts believe the increased secretion of growth hormone that follows a thermal burn contributes to this phenomenon.

Prognosis

The prognosis for recovery from a thermal injury depends on the child's age and the extent of the burn. Children under age 2 have the highest mortality. In children over age 2 with burns involving less than 30% of body surface area, roughly 90% survive. Approximately half of children over age 2 with burns involving less than 60% of body surface area survive. Only 20% of children with burns involving more than 80% of body surface area survive.

Assessment

Accurate assessment of the child's burn is critical to burn management. The health care team assesses the extent, depth, and severity of the burn.

Burn extent

Burn extent is expressed as a percentage of the patient's body surface area. Because body proportions vary with age, standard burn charts that are used to assess burn extent in adults are inappropriate for children. For a more accurate estimation of the percentage of body surface area burned in children, use body charts and tables specific to the child's age-group.

Burn depth

A burn may be superficial (first-degree), partial-thickness (second-degree), or full-thickness (third-degree).

A *superficial burn* causes minimal tissue injury. Expect the skin to appear red with no blisters; pain is the most common complaint. Superficial burns rarely cause systemic effects or infection. The burned skin heals quickly, typically without scarring.

A *partial-thickness burn* damages only part of the skin — the epithelium and part of the dermis. The remaining unaffected dermis is capable of regenerating new tissue. The patient's skin appears moist, red, and blistered, and blanches with pressure. Severe pain is common. A partial-thickness burn heals over time and does not require grafting. Scarring is minimal.

A *full-thickness burn* destroys all skin layers and may injure subcutaneous tissue, muscles, and bones. The burned area does not blanch with pressure, and appears dry and leathery; it may be brown, deep red, white, or black. Because the nerve endings have been destroyed, the child feels little pain in the burned area itself. However, adjacent skin surfaces that are less severely burned are painful. A full-thickness burn typically causes scarring. It does not heal spontaneously and requires a graft.

Burn severity

A burn may be minor, major, or critical in severity. This type of classification delineates the injuries and complications expected and helps the nurse anticipate the treatment the child will need. For descriptions of these classifications, see *Classifying burn severity,* page 388.

Emergency care The goals of emergency care for the child with a burn injury are to:
• stop the burning process
• stabilize the child
• transport the child for further medical evaluation and care, as needed.
Measures used to stop the burning process vary with the type of burn. Small areas burned by scalding water, flames, or hot objects may be immersed in cool water. However, because of the risk of hypothermia, a child with extensive burns should not be immersed in water.

If the child's clothing is on fire, help the child to a supine position and roll the child in a blanket or towel; to prevent inhalation of toxic fumes, leave the child's head exposed. If towels or blankets are unavail-

Classifying burn severity

To estimate the severity of a burn, the health care team correlates burn depth and burn extent.

Minor burns include partial-thickness burns involving less than 10% of total body surface area (BSA) in patients over age 2, and full-thickness burns involving less than 2% of BSA in patients over age 2. The child with minor burns may be treated as an outpatient.

Moderate burns include partial-thickness burns involving 10% to 25% of BSA in patients over age 2, and full-thickness burns involving less than 10% of BSA in patients over age 2. The child with major burns may be treated in a general pediatric inpatient unit.

Critical burns include:
- partial-thickness burns involving more than 25% of BSA in patients over age 2
- partial-thickness burns involving less than 25% of BSA in patients under age 2
- full-thickness burns involving more than 10% of BSA in patients over age 2
- full-thickness burns involving less than 10% of BSA in patients under age 2
- penetrating electrical burns
- partial- or full-thickness burns of the feet, hands, face, or perineum
- burns complicated by other injuries, such as soft- tissue injury, fractures, or respiratory tract damage
- burns in patients with a history of chronic illness.

The child with critical burns must be treated in a special burn unit.

---

able, help the child to a supine position and roll slowly from side to side. If the child has been burned by a caustic liquid, rinse the skin thoroughly with clear water.

Once the burning stops, the health care team carefully assesses the child for further injury. After initial assessment of airway patency, breathing pattern, and cardiovascular status, the health care team monitors these factors continually. They cover the burn wound with a dry, clean cloth or bandage. If the child has extensive burns, they place a warm blanket over the child to prevent hypothermia. Ointments and salves are avoided.

For the child with a major or critical burn, emergency medical technicians institute fluid and oxygen therapy at the injury scene, then transport the child to the nearest burn center facility for further evaluation and care. A child with minor burns may be transported by car to an ambulatory care facility for further care.

Medical and nursing management

Specific measures depend on burn severity and other factors. For example, elasticized (Jobst) garments help reduce scar hypertrophy.

Managing minor burns

Most children with minor burns can be treated in an ambulatory care setting. The health care team cleans the wound with a mild soap solution and removes all dead skin. Blisters may or may not be left intact. Some physicians prefer to remove blistered skin to prevent infection;

others believe the intact blistered skin acts as a natural biologic dressing.

Next, the wound is rinsed with 0.9% sodium chloride (normal saline) solution. Depending on physician preference, the wound is covered with a dry, sterile dressing or a dressing containing antimicrobial cream. Then, the wound is wrapped in a dry gauze dressing.

After treatment, instruct the parents to remove the child's dressing once or twice daily. To reduce discomfort, advise them to soak the dressing in clean water or 0.9% sodium chloride (normal saline) solution before removing it. Instruct them to inspect for and report any edematous or reddened wound margins or purulent drainage before redressing the wound. (If the physician suspects the parents may be unable to provide wound care at home, the child must return to the health care facility for daily wound care.) If necessary, provide a home health care referral.

Managing moderate and critical burns
The goals of medical and nursing care for children with moderate or critical burns include:
• maintaining an adequate airway
• providing fluids
• performing wound care
• providing adequate nutrition for healing
• controlling pain
• managing complications
• supporting the child and family.

Maintaining an adequate airway
Respiratory problems associated with a burn commonly result from airway edema. Monitor the child closely for respiratory distress; suspect respiratory compromise if the child exhibits air hunger, anxiety, or wheezing. If necessary, assist the physician with insertion of an endotracheal tube to maintain an open airway.

To relieve bronchospasms caused by inhalation injury, place the child in high-Fowler's position and administer highly humidified oxygen, as prescribed. The child with circumferential chest wounds may have respiratory difficulty caused by inadequate chest and lung expansion. To permit full chest expansion with respiratory effort, assist the physician in cutting away constricting eschar, as prescribed.

Providing fluids
To prevent or correct hypovolemia and electrolyte disturbances, administer isotonic solutions (0.9% normal sodium chloride or lactated Ringer's solution), colloid solutions (albumin or Plasmanate), or hypertonic saline solutions (3% sodium chloride solution) for fluid replacement therapy, as prescribed. Routinely assess the child's fluid and electrolyte balance. To evaluate fluid status, carefully monitor level of consciousness, weight, intravenous intake, urine output, urine specific gravity,

capillary refill, arterial and central venous pressures, and laboratory test results.

With adequate fluid replacement, interstitial fluid gradually shifts back into the vascular spaces. Within 4 to 5 days after fluid therapy begins, urine output should rise markedly. During this time, the child who has received excessive fluids is at risk for congestive heart failure and pulmonary edema. To detect these conditions, monitor vital signs, weight, fluid intake and output, hemodynamic parameters, and breath sounds.

Performing wound care

To treat a full-thickness burn, the physician debrides (removes) dead tissue, orders measures to prevent infection, and closes the wound. Debridement may involve hydrotherapy (soaking in the Hubbard tank or hose therapy) or excision of loosened, dead tissue. Because debridement is extremely painful, administer narcotic analgesics, as prescribed, before the procedure.

After hydrotherapy, apply topical antimicrobial agents directly to the burn wound, as prescribed, to inhibit bacterial growth. (Capillary circulation is impaired after a burn, thus rendering systemic antibiotics ineffective against wound infection.) Commonly used agents include silver nitrate 0.5%, silver sulfadiazine 1%, and mafenide acetate 10%.

The physician covers a partial-thickness burn with a dry, sterile dressing; a deep partial- or full-thickness burn, with a temporary biologic dressing. These dressings protect the wound from infection and trauma, limit fluid loss, reduce pain, and speed epithelization (new tissue growth).

Split-thickness pigskin or cadaver grafts generally are used as temporary dressings for burn wounds in children. Autografts harvested from healthy skin areas (most commonly the thighs and buttocks) are used for permanent skin grafting. Some physicians prefer to cover a newly grafted burn wound with a dry dressing; others choose to leave it uncovered. If the wound is covered, remove the dressing, as prescribed.

To prevent accumulation of serum, fluids, or blood under the graft (which may prevent the graft from being vascularized), remove serum by rolling the wound carefully from the center to the edges. Apply gentle pressure to any bleeding sites. Cover donor graft sites with fine gauze. Leave the dressings in place until they fall off; changing them can damage the tender, newly regenerated epithelial tissue.

Providing adequate nutrition for healing

Because of hypermetabolism and protein breakdown, a child with moderate or critical burns needs additional calories and proteins. To obtain sufficient nutrients for healing and to prevent a negative nitrogen balance, the child may need two to three times the normal caloric and protein requirements. Additional calories should come from carbohydrates because fats do not prevent protein breakdown.

To maximize oral intake, help the child select foods high in calories, carbohydrates, and protein. Encourage the parents to bring favorite foods from home. Sit with the child during meal times, or encourage the parents to do so. Be sure to document nutritional intake.

To supplement oral intake and provide additional calories and protein, administer nasogastric feedings or parenteral nutrition, as prescribed. Also administer vitamin and iron supplements, as prescribed.

Controlling pain

During the immediate recovery period, the child experiences pain — not only from the burn wound itself but also from wound care. Because the pain is so severe and persists until the wound heals completely, the child may feel helpless from lack of control over the pain. This may lead to irritability, anger, hostility, or depression.

To help relieve pain during the early stages of burn healing, provide narcotic analgesics, as prescribed. For optimal analgesic effectiveness, be sure to give adequate doses and use an appropriate dosing schedule.

To help relieve pain during debridement, consider using nonpharmacologic strategies, such as distraction, relaxation techniques, and imagery. (For details on pain management, see Chapter 16, Management principles.)

Managing complications

Burns can cause complications in many body systems.

Infection. To help prevent wound infection, use aseptic technique and apply topical antimicrobial agents when performing wound care, as prescribed. Obtain wound cultures, as prescribed. If the child has bacteremia, administer systemic antibiotics, as prescribed, and maintain isolation precautions. Monitor the child's temperature, white blood cell count, and white blood cell differential.

Stress ulcer. Give prophylactic antacids, as prescribed. Observe for gastric bleeding or discomfort. Monitor the child's abdominal status and note any changes.

Joint contractures. The physician may order splinting and physical therapy to treat contractures. Encourage physical mobility. Maintain the child in proper body alignment and perform range-of-motion exercises, as prescribed.

Wound contracture and scar tissue formation. The physician may revise scar tissue surgically. They physician also may prescribe physical therapy or use of elastic bandages or elasticized garments. As appropriate, instruct parents on proper use of elastic bandages or elasticized garments. If the child has extensive burns, inform them that the child's heat regulation may be impaired during hot weather or fever (because scar tissue lacks sweat glands).

Severe itching of newly healed wound and scar tissue. As prescribed, give oral diphenhydramine hydrochloride (Benadryl) or hydroxyzine

Anticipating complications in the burn patient

The child with a burn injury is at risk for complications in multiple body systems.

Cardiovascular complications

Massive fluid losses and fluid shifts may cause hypovolemic shock within 4 days after a burn. Signs and symptoms of hypovolemic shock include decreased blood pressure and central venous pressure, poor capillary filling, slow capillary refill, rapid and thready peripheral pulses, and mottled skin. Hypertension may occur once cardiac output returns to normal.

Respiratory complications

Respiratory complications are the most common cause of death immediately after a thermal injury. Inhalation of hot air may damage upper airway tissue. As this tissue becomes edematous, airway obstruction and asphyxiation may occur. Signs and symptoms of airway obstruction, which may arise at any time within the first 24 hours after injury, include wheezing, crackles, a prolonged expiratory phase, air hunger, blackened pulmonary secretions, and anxiety.

The patient may suffer carbon monoxide poisoning if the burn occurred in an enclosed space. Clinical manifestations, which arise immediately after the injury, include headache, nausea, confusion, and coma.

Inhalation of sooty particles can lead to chemical pneumonitis within a few days. Signs and symptoms of pneumonitis include tachypnea, crackles, and impaired gas exchange.

Bacterial pneumonia may result from contamination of the airway via intubation, spread of infection from the burn wound, or airborne infection. With circumferential chest burns, immobility and decreased chest expansion set the stage for pneumonia. Signs and symptoms of pneumonia resemble those of pneumonitis.

Pulmonary embolism, although rare, may occur when the child first starts to ambulate after being immobilized during a prolonged recovery. Ambulation may cause release of thrombi in the lower extremities, which then travel to the pulmonary vasculature, causing embolism.

Pulmonary edema may result from rapid administration of large volumes of fluid to correct hypovolemia—especially when fluid mobilizes from the interstitial spaces.

Sepsis

Wound infection is most common within 5 days of injury. Infections arising during this period typically result from autocontamination with *Staphylococcus* organisms. After a few days, the wound becomes colonized with *Pseudomonas* organisms. Decreased capillary blood supply, an impaired immune response, and factors that promote infection (such as heat, moistness, and necrotic tissue) contribute to the development of wound infection.

Septicemia may arise from wound infection or bacterial invasion of indwelling catheter sites. Potentially fatal, this complication typically occurs within 2 weeks of the burn. Assessment findings include confusion, fever, paralytic ileus, and an elevated white blood cell count. If septicemia is not treated, septic shock may occur.

Gastrointestinal complications

Paralytic ileus may develop within a few days after the injury. Signs and symptoms include nausea, decreased bowel sounds, and abdominal distention.

Stress ulcer is a common complication during the first 4 weeks after injury. Clinical manifestations include nausea, blood-tinged emesis, black or tarry stools, and abdominal distention and discomfort.

Neurologic complications

Personality changes—particularly irritability and depressed mood—are common in children recovering from burns. Hypoxemia and electrolyte disturbances may cause seizures.

Musculoskeletal complications

Wound contractures and scarring may lead to joint contractures and limited range of motion.

---

hydrochloride (Atarax) to relieve itching. Apply moisturizers, such as cocoa butter or Eucerin cream. Inform parents that itching will subside over time. Advise them to use cool compresses to relieve the child's itching.

For information on other complications to expect in a patient with burns, see *Anticipating complications in the burn patient*.

Supporting the child and family

Burns are among the most stressful and frightening injuries for both the child and family. Besides coping with the stress caused by severe pain, they must deal with the child's altered physical appearance and the prospect of unattractive scars after the burn heals.

To help relieve stress, maintain a positive attitude. Explain the stages of wound healing. Inform the family that physical activity and compliance with splinting and use of elastic bandages will decrease the wound contracture and scarring. To help the child feel more attractive, encourage good grooming. Encourage parents to provide attractive clothing to enhance the child's self-image.

Arrange for a hospital-based school tutor, and encourage the child to return to school and participate in normal social activities as soon as possible. Be aware, however, that a burn victim may be ashamed of the appearance and thus fear going back to school. Encourage the child to express feelings about returning to school. If possible, visit the child's school to describe the injury to the child's classmates and to explain the healing process and special splints or garments the child will require.

STUDY ACTIVITIES

Short answer

1. Compare and contrast the physical appearance of superficial, partial-thickness, and full-thickness burns.

_____

_____

_____

2. Explain why a thermal injury can lead to hypovolemia.

_____

_____

3. Why do children with extensive burns require a diet high in calories, carbohydrates, and proteins?

_____

_____

_____

4. List at least three signs of airway obstruction.

_____

_____

Multiple choice

5. Which of the following indicates a stress ulcer in a child with burns?

    A. Diarrhea

    B. Black stools

    C. Decreased urine output

    D. Weight loss

6. Which nursing diagnosis takes *highest* priority for a patient in the early stages of burn recovery?

    A. *High risk for infection*

    B. *Impaired physical mobility*

    C. *Body image disturbance*

    D. *Constipation*

7. Regan, age 10, has suffered full-thickness burns. She is scheduled for hydrotherapy to debride her burn wounds. What must the nurse do before beginning hydrotherapy?

    A. Provide nutritional supplements.

    B. Administer fluids.

    C. Implement pain control measures.

    D. Administer antibiotics.

8. What is the most important parameter when assessing a child with a circumferential chest burn?

    A. Breathing pattern

    B. Pulse rate

    C. Temperature

    D. Wound characteristics

ANSWERS Short answer

1. A superficial burn appears red but does not blister. A partial-thickness burn is moist, red, and blistered, and blanches with pressure. A full-thickness burn is dry and leathery and may appear brown, deep red, white, or black; the burned area does not blanch when pressure is applied.

2. A thermal injury may can to hypovolemia because it causes evaporative fluid loss and results in shifting of intravascular fluid to the interstitial spaces.

3. Children with extensive burns experience hypermetabolism and protein breakdown. To obtain sufficient nutrients for healing and to prevent a negative nitrogen balance, they may need two to three times the normal caloric and protein requirements. Carbohydrates help prevent protein breakdown.

4. Signs of airway obstruction include wheezing, crackles, a prolonged expiratory phase, air hunger, blackened pulmonary secretions, and anxiety.

Multiple choice

5. B. Stress ulcer is associated with black or tarry stools, which are evidence of gastric bleeding. The other choices are not associated with stress ulcers.

6. A. Infection is a serious risk for a patient in the early stages of burn recovery. The other diagnoses listed may take lower priority.

7. C. Hydrotherapy is painful, so the nurse must implement pain control measures before this treatment begins. Nutritional supplements and fluids can be administered at any time and are not associated with hydrotherapy. Antibiotics, if prescribed, would be administered according to a specified schedule without regard to hydrotherapy treatments.

8. A. Although all the choices are important, breathing pattern is the most important factor to assess because eschar impedes chest expansion in a child with a circumferential chest burn, thus causing difficulty breathing.

Selected References

Behrman, R. and Vaughn, V. *Nelson Textbook of Pediatrics* (14th ed.). Philadelphia: W.B. Saunders, 1992.

Boynton, R., Dunn, E., and Stephens, G. *Manual of Ambulatory Pediatrics.* Philadelphia: J.B. Lippincott, 1994.

Cancer Facts and Figures. New York: American Cancer Society, 1990.

Committee on Psychosocial Aspects of Child and Family Life. *Guidelines for health supervision, II.* Elk Grove Village, Ill.:American Academy of Pediatrics, 1987.

Craft, M. and Denehy, J. *Nursing Interventions for Infants and Children.* Philadelphia: W.B. Saunders, 1990.

Duvall, E. *Marriage and family development* (5th ed.). Philadelphia: J.B. Lippincott, 1977.

Engel, J. *Pocket Guide to Pediatric Assessment.* St. Louis: Mosby, Inc., 1989.

Fernbach, D., and Vietti, R. *Clinical Pediatric Oncology.* St. Louis: Mosby, Inc. 1991.

Foster, R., Hunsberger, M., and Anderson, J. *Family Centered Nursing Care of Children.* Philadelphia: W.B. Saunders, 1989.

Friedman, M. *Family Nursing: Theory and Practice.* Norwalk, Conn.: Appleton-Croft-Lange, 1992.

Garbarino, J. (1977). The human ecology of child maltreatment. *Journal of Marriage and the Family,* 39: 721-736, 1977.

Glick, I., Weiss, R., and Parkes, D. *The First Year of Bereavement.* New York: John Wiley, 1974.

Hazinksi, M. *Nursing Care of the Critically Ill Child.* St. Louis: Mosby, Inc., 1992.

Jackson, D., and Saunders, R. *Child Health Nursing.* Philadelphia: J.B. Lippincott, 1993.

Jackson, P., and Vessey, J. *Primary Care of the Child with a Chronic Condition.* St. Louis: Mosby, Inc., 1991.

Klaus, M.H., and Fanaroff, A.A. (eds.). *Care of the High-Risk Neonate.* Philadelphia: W.B. Saunders, 1993.

Koch, V., et. al. "Accelerated growth after recombinant human growth hormone treatment of children with chronic renal failure." *Journal of Pediatrics,* 115: 365-371, 1989.

Korones, S. *High Risk Newborn Infants: The Basis for Intensive Nursing Care.* St. Louis: Mosby, Inc., 1986.

Kübler-Ross, E. *On Death and Dying.* London: Weidenfeld and Nicolson, 1965.

Leavell, H., and Clark, A. *Preventive Medicine For Doctors in the Community.* New York: McGraw-Hill, 1965.

Lindemann, E. "Symptomatology and management of acute grief." *American Journal of Psychiatry,* 101: 141-148, 1944.

Murray, R. and Zentner, J. *Nursing Assessment and Health Promotion.* Norwalk, Conn: Appleton-Croft-Lange, 1993.

Robertson, J. *Young Children in Hospitals.* London: Tavistock Publications, 1970.

Smith, S. *Communication in Nursing.* St. Louis: Mosby, Inc. 1992.

Spitz, R. "Hospitalism: An inquiry into the genesis of psychiatric conditioning in early childhood." In P. Fenichel (ed.), *Psychoanalytic Studies of the Child,* 1: 53-74. New York: International University Press, 1945.

State Education Department. *The identification and reporting of child abuse and maltreatment.* Albany, N.Y.: The University of the State of New York, 1990.

Whaley, L. and Wong, D. *Nursing Care of Infants and Children.* St. Louis: Mosby, Inc., 1991.

Williams, R., and Miller, C. *Preventive health care of young children: Findings from a 10-country study and directions for United States policy.* Arlington, Va.: National Center for Clinical Infant Programs, 1991.

Index

i refers to an illustration; t refers to a table

i refers to an illustration; t refers to a table

i refers to an illustration; t refers to a table

i refers to an illustration; t refers to a table

i refers to an illustration; t refers to a table